Oligodendroglia

Advances in Neurochemistry

SERIES EDITORS

B. W. Agranoff, *University of Michigan, Ann Arbor*
M. H. Aprison, *Indiana University School of Medicine, Indianapolis*

ADVISORY EDITORS

J. Axelrod	F. Margolis	P. Morell	J. S. O'Brien
F. Fonnum	B. S. McEwen	W. T. Norton	E. Roberts

Volumes 1–4 Edited by B. W. Agranoff and M. H. Aprison

Volume 5 OLIGODENDROGLIA
Edited by William T. Norton

Volume 6 AXONAL TRANSPORT IN NEURONAL GROWTH
AND REGENERATION
Edited by John S. Elam and Paul Cancalon

A Continuation Order Plan is available for this series. A continuation order will bring delivery of each new volume immediately upon publication. Volumes are billed only upon actual shipment. For further information please contact the publisher.

Oligodendroglia

Edited by
William T. Norton
Albert Einstein College of Medicine
Bronx, New York

PLENUM PRESS • NEW YORK AND LONDON

Library of Congress Cataloging in Publication Data

Main entry under title:

Oligodendroglia.

   Includes bibliographical references and index.
   1. Oligodendroglia. 2. Neurochemistry. I. Norton, William T., 1929–
QP356.3.O45   1984   599′.01′88   84-4821
ISBN 0-306-41547-X

© 1984 Plenum Press, New York
A Division of Plenum Publishing Corporation
233 Spring Street, New York, N.Y. 10013

Printed in the United States of America

CONTRIBUTORS

JOYCE A. BENJAMINS • *Department of Neurology, Wayne State University School of Medicine, Detroit, Michigan 48201*

JOSEPH BRESSLER • *Surgical Neurology Branch, National Institutes of Health, Bethesda, Maryland 20205*

RICHARD P. BUNGE • *Department of Anatomy and Neurobiology, Washington University School of Medicine, St. Louis, Missouri 63110*

WENDY CAMMER • *The Saul R. Korey Department of Neurology, and the Department of Neuroscience, Albert Einstein College of Medicine, Bronx, New York 10461*

JEAN DE VELLIS • *Laboratory of Biomedical and Environmental Sciences, Mental Retardation Research Center, and Departments of Anatomy and Psychiatry, University of California, Los Angeles, School of Medicine, Los Angeles, California 90024*

SEUNG U. KIM • *Division of Neurology, University of British Columbia, Vancouver, B. C. V6T1W5, Canada*

SHALINI KUMAR • *Laboratory of Biomedical and Environmental Sciences, Mental Retardation Research Center, and Departments of Anatomy and Psychiatry, University of California, Los Angeles, School of Medicine, Los Angeles, California 90024*

PIERRE MORELL • *Department of Biochemistry and Nutrition and Biological Sciences Research Center, University of North Carolina at Chapel Hill, Chapel Hill, North Carolina 27514*

STEVEN E. PFEIFFER • *Department of Microbiology, University of Connecticut Health Center, Farmington, Connecticut 06032*

DAVID PLEASURE • *Children's Hospital of Philadelphia and Departments of Neurology and Pediatrics, University of Pennsylvania, Philadelphia, Pennsylvania 19104*

DONALD H. SILBERBERG • *Children's Hospital of Philadelphia and Department of Neurology, University of Pennsylvania, Philadelphia, Pennsylvania 19104*

NANCY H. STERNBERGER • *Center for Brain Research, University of Rochester Medical Center, Rochester, New York 14642*

ARREL D. TOEWS • *Department of Biochemistry and Nutrition and Biological Sciences Research Center, University of North Carolina at Chapel Hill, Chapel Hill, North Carolina 27514*

DANIEL P. WEINGARTEN • *Life Technologies Incorporated, Chagrin Falls, Ohio 44022*

PATRICK WOOD • *Department of Anatomy and Neurobiology, Washington University School of Medicine, St. Louis, Missouri 63110*

PREFACE

This series has addressed a constituency of scientists possessing biochemical background with the goal of providing them with specialized reviews of neurobiological interest. Since its initiation, neurochemistry and neuroscience have come of age, and the editors initiate with this volume the concept of a central theme. It is planned that each subsequent volume will also be topical. We note with sadness the passing of Dr. Henry Mahler who served as an advisory editor since the initiation of this series. He played a major role in building the bridge between biochemistry and neurochemistry and will be missed. We are pleased to welcome two new editors, Drs. William Norton and Bruce McEwen.

B. W. Agranoff
M. H. Aprison

FOREWORD

Oligodendroglia constitute one of the three principal cell types of the central nervous system. These cells, together with their elaborated membranes, account for at least 25 percent of the dry mass of an adult rat brain and an even greater percentage of the central nervous system of larger animals. Knowledge of the biochemistry of these cells has advanced rapidly in recent years. This progress has, in part, been made possible by the development of new tissue culture systems, by improvement in the methods for the isolation of intact cells, and by the use of immunocytochemistry for identifying specific cell types and detecting their differentiated products. The purpose of this book is to provide a comprehensive critical review of the biochemistry of oligodendroglia as determined from results of both the newer as well as the earlier experimental approaches. It should serve equally the experienced investigator or the newcomer seeking a foundation in this important area of neurochemistry.

The stimulus for this book came indirectly from Byron Waksman, Director of Research Programs of the National Multiple Sclerosis Society. In 1980 Dr. Waksman realized that progress in basic research on oligodendroglia had been so rapid that the society was justified in sponsoring a conference of interested scientists. Dr. Waksman and I organized an intensive international meeting, held at Airlie House, Virginia in early summer, 1981, which seemed to be received enthusiastically by all participants. At that time we decided not to publish a proceedings volume. In the interim, largely because of my involvement in that meeting, I had suggested to Bernard Agranoff and Morris Aprison, editors of *Advances in Neurochemistry,* and Kirk Jensen of Plenum Press that a thematic volume on the biochemistry of oligodendroglia would be timely and appropriate for their series, *Advances in Neurochemistry,* and this suggestion was adopted. The selection of authors for this book from the many excellent scientists who attended the Airlie House Conference was difficult. Those chosen, all of whom accepted the task, have been major contributors to the topics included.

The first chapter, by Patrick Wood and Richard Bunge, reviews and synthesizes information on the biology of oligodendroglia. The biological perspective is essential for proper design and interpretation of neurochemical experiments, but is sometimes poorly appreciated by neurochemists. In constructing a new formulation of oligodendroglial development, these authors have identified gaps in our knowledge and have posed crucial questions that may eventually be answered by neurochemical approaches.

In the next two chapters Pierre Morell, Arrel Toews, and Joyce Benjamins discuss the *in vivo* metabolism of oligodendroglial lipids and proteins. As these authors point out, the major known function of oligodendroglia is the synthesis and maintenance of myelin, thus we know a great deal about the metabolism of oligodendroglia through studies of myelin and myelin-specific components. Except in the early stages of the developing nervous system, myelin constitutes the bulk of the oligodendrocyte and can be isolated readily from whole tissue. Therefore studies of the metabolism of myelin reflect a major part of oligodendroglial metabolism. Such investigations have led to more information about oligodendroglial metabolism *in vivo* than is available, for example, for astrocytes. The biochemistry of many cell-specific molecules can be studied *in vivo,* but the ability to obtain a purified cell-specific membrane (myelin) also makes it possible to study the biochemistry of ubiquitious compounds, such as lipids, which are not cell specific, but whose cellular origin is known.

In Chapter 4 Nancy Sternberger has reviewed the developmental distribution of oligodendroglial antigens *in situ* and has shown how useful the immunocytochemistry of oligodendroglial antigens has been for studies of oligodendrocytes in culture. Throughout, she has cast a critical eye on the concept of cell-specific markers and on the nature of immunocytochemical evidence.

The results of advances in tissue culture are reviewed in Chapters 5 and 7. A major advantage of tissue culture is that the cellular environment may be modified at will. Chapter 5, by David Pleasure and colleagues, serves as the *in vitro* counterpart to Chapter 2. They have surveyed information on oligodendroglial lipid metabolism that has been derived from different types of culture systems, related these data to those obtained from *in vivo* experiments, and discussed their relevance to the central question of metabolic regulation. In Chapter 7, Steven Pfeiffer has taken on the extremely difficult task of synthesizing all available information on the development of myelinogenic properties in oligodendroglia studied in *in vitro* systems. In doing so he has encompassed nearly the entire range of oligodendroglial biochemistry and myelinogenesis.

Wendy Cammer, in Chapter 6, has examined the enzymes of oligodendroglia that are involved in specific functions of the cell, as well as those enzymes that appear to be relatively cell specific. Some of the new findings she discusses confirm long-standing speculations about pathways of glucose metabolism. The functional implications of some of the high enzyme activities found in these cells are not yet understood, but are subjects of active investigation. The final chapter by Weingarten and colleagues discusses the critical problem of how the differentiated functions of these cells are regulated by hormones during development. Much of the pioneering work in this relatively new field has been done in the laboratories of the authors.

I have not attempted to eliminate the inevitable areas of overlap in these chapters. In most cases repetitions occur in different contexts and from different viewpoints, and their elimination would interrupt the narrative and destroy the unity of each chapter. In some cases the careful reader will find that the authors disagree in their interpretations, a sign that this is a young field, still in flux. Finally I would like to thank the authors for their cooperation and their thoughtful and scholarly contributions. I hope the readers find this book as interesting and educational as I have and that many can use it to help plan their own investigations in the central problem of oligodendroglial biochemistry—the regulation of myelinogenesis.

William T. Norton

CONTENTS

CHAPTER 3

PROTEIN METABOLISM OF OLIGODENDROGLIAL CELLS IN VIVO

JOYCE A. BENJAMINS

CHAPTER 4

*PATTERNS OF OLIGODENDROCYTE FUNCTION SEEN BY
    IMMUNOCYTOCHEMISTRY*

NANCY H. STERNBERGER

CHAPTER 5

IN VITRO STUDIES OF OLIGODENDROGLIAL LIPID METABOLISM

DAVID PLEASURE, SEUNG U. KIM, AND DONALD H. SILBERBERG

CHAPTER 6

OLIGODENDROCYTE-ASSOCIATED ENZYMES

WENDY CAMMER

Chapter 7

OLIGODENDROCYTE DEVELOPMENT IN CULTURE SYSTEMS

Steven E. Pfeiffer

CHAPTER 8

*REGULATION OF DIFFERENTIATED PROPERTIES OF
   OLIGODENDROCYTES*

DANIEL P. WEINGARTEN, SHALINI KUMAR, JOSEPH BRESSLER, AND JEAN DE
   VELLIS

THE BIOLOGY OF THE OLIGODENDROCYTE

PATRICK WOOD and RICHARD P. BUNGE

1. INTRODUCTION

Certain problems in defining the oligodendrocyte cell type should be pointed out at the onset. The interfascicular oligodendrocyte is commonly defined as the cell responsible for the formation and maintenance of central myelin. Direct demonstration of the connections between oligodendrocyte somas and myelin sheaths is inherently very difficult, however, and it is possible that there are substantial numbers of cells in white matter, resident among the myelin-related oligodendrocytes, that do not directly husband myelin segments. This possibility must be seriously considered because it is now known from tissue-culture studies (detailed in Section 6) that oligodendrocytes may express myelin-specific components when not directly connected to myelin sheaths. Also, recent detailed studies of remyelination in adult white matter suggest that glial reserve or stem cells (resident, but as yet unrecognized, in white matter) are responsible for the production of new oligodendrocytes prior to remyelination.

A second problem concerns the source and nature of these stem or reserve cells. Are mature oligodendrocytes that have formed and retained connections

PATRICK WOOD and RICHARD P. BUNGE • Department of Anatomy and Neurobiology, Washington University School of Medicine, St. Louis, Missouri 63110 to myelin segments capable of renewed proliferation to expand their cell numbers and subsequently to participate in remyelination? Alternately, are there a small number of stem cells among the oligodendrocytes of white matter that proliferate to provide a new population of myelinating cells? Both mechanisms can be observed in body tissues. In the liver, which is capable of considerable repair, it is clear that functional parenchymal hepatocytes have the capability of proliferating and expanding the hepatic-cell population during the regenerative process (Harkness, 1957). On the other hand, skeletal-muscle regeneration occurs when a small number of inconspicuous satellite cells (adjacent to but separate from the functional multinucleate muscle cells) expand their numbers to supply myoblasts for new muscle-fiber formation (Bischoff, 1979). At the time of this writing, it is not clear whether one of these cellular mechanisms or both are operative during the process of remyelination of damaged adult white matter.

Whereas we cannot entirely resolve the two problems outlined above on the basis of present data, we will propose a possible resolution in a third area of uncertainty—the issue of oligodendrocyte origins. In this case, the problem is to define the stage at which the oligodendrocyte and astrocyte cell lines diverge during development. New evidence that the astrocyte line is established very early (prior, in fact, to the birth of many neurons) (Levitt *et al.,* 1981), as well as accumulated observations on the appearance of oligodendrocytes and their immediate precursors, lead us to suggest that a separation of these cell lineages may occur very early in development.

We begin this chapter with a historical review of the definition of the oligodendrocyte and a description of the cell type as recognized at present. Subsequent sections deal with oligodendrocyte origin and maturation, the process of remyelination in adult white matter, and factors known to influence oligodendrocyte development. We also briefly consider the contributions of tissue-culture studies to understanding oligodendrocyte biology.

2. HISTORICAL PERSPECTIVES

It is generally accepted that the first description of the oligodendrocyte was given by Robertson (1899). Experimenting with metal impregnation of CNS tissues, he noted that among other tissue elements blackened by his technique, there were small branching cells "of very characteristic aspect" found throughout the cortex and in the white matter. These were small cells with a rounded nucleus surrounded by a sparse cytoplasm extending into 3–6 delicate processes; these processes tended to branch a short distance from the cell, often in "a distinctly dichotomous fashion." The branching processes exhibited small varicose swellings and were not attached to blood vessels or clearly related to other cellular elements. He concluded that these cells were manifestly different from the neuroglial cell then well known—the astrocyte—in that the branching of the cellular processes was much less profuse. The similarity between the cells he depicts in Figure 9 of his 1899 paper and the type I oligodendrocyte (See Figure 3) described by del Rio Hortega (see below) is striking; there is little doubt that he was describing the oligodendrocyte.

The cell visualized by Robertson was to receive its name and its definitive description several decades later in the extensive reports of the Spanish histologist del Rio Hortega (1921, 1928) With del Rio Hortega's silver carbonate stain (Figures 1 and 2), the cell was again seen in profile, with little information regarding specific cytoplasmic components. It is not surprising, then, that the cell's name derived from the profile of the somal region and the attached processes. The cell was marked by its comparatively small somal size and smooth contour. In contrast to the dozens of processes emanating in many directions from the typical astrocyte soma, the number of oligodendrocyte processes was few (often between 2 and 10); thus, del Rio Hortega named it the "cell with few branches," the *oligodendrocyte.* These cells could be distinguished from another small but poorly branched cell type, the microglia, in that microglial nuclei were frequently substantially elongated and distorted in shape (as was the entire form of the cell) and microglial processes were seen to egress from the elongate soma of the cell to form a spine-covered secondary extension. In contrast, except for modest (though frequent) varicosities, oligodendrocyte processes were remarkably smooth.

Shortly after the definition of the oligodendrocyte, its cytoplasmic characteristics were surmised from observations with a variety of staining techniques. In his extensive review of neuroglial cytology, Penfield (1932) pointed out that whereas oligodendrocytes shared with astrocytes the presence of a centrosome, Golgi apparatus, lipofuscin, and mitochondria, they differed from astrocytes in lacking perivascular feet and cytoplasmic fibrils. Unlike astrocytes, the form of which varied substantially according to position, the general morphology of oligodendrocytes was similar in all parts of the nervous system where they occurred. Oligodendrocytes were observed only in those regions of the CNS that contained myelin. Regions that contained exclusively unmyelinated nerve fibers, such as retina (in many species) or the molecular layer of the cerebellum, did not contain oligodendrocytes. The contrast with PNS tissues, in which Schwann cells accompany and ensheath unmyelinated as well as myelinated nerve fibers, should be noted.

In his extensive description of oligodendrocytes, del Rio Hortega classified these cells first in regard to their position: (1) perineuronal (if the cell body was adjacent to a neuronal soma) and (2) interfascicular (for oligodendrocytes interposed between myelinated nerve fibers in white matter). A second classification derived from his analysis of the number and branching patterns of the

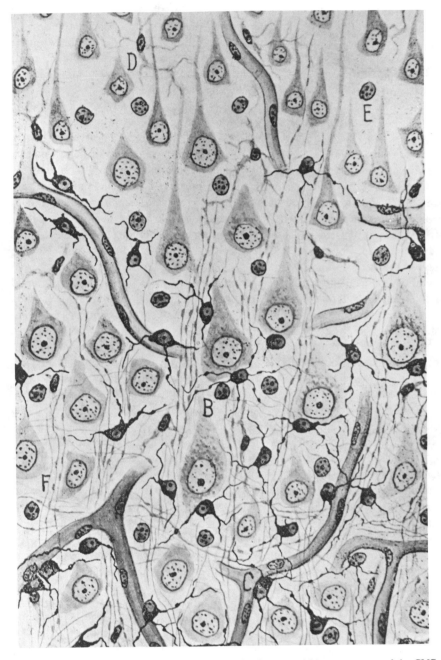

FIGURE 1. Depiction by del Rio Hortega of oligodendrocytes within gray matter of the CNS. The cytoplasm and processes of the oligodendrocytes are stained black by the silver carbonate method. Note that all cells depicted have several processes, most with substantial secondary branching. Although these cells are stationed near neuronal somas (shown in gray) and capillaries, the processes do not relate to these structures, but are often related to linear elements (presumably small myelinated fibers) traversing the field. From del Rio Hortega (1921).

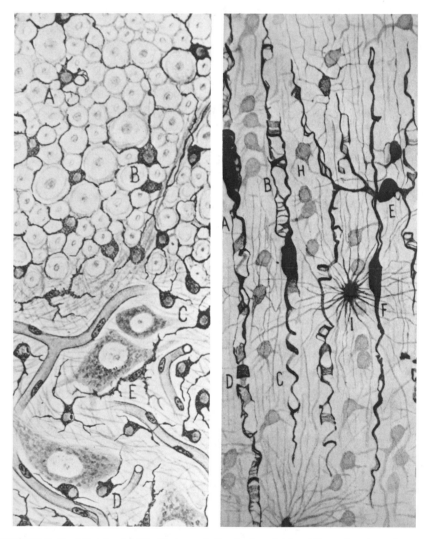

FIGURE 2. Depiction by del Rio Hortega of oligodendrocytes in white matter shown in cross section (*left*) and in longitudinal section (*right*). The sections are stained as in Figure 1. This type of preparation was probably prepared from a young animal in which oligodendrocyte processes retained some of the increased volume present during active myelin formation. *Left:* (E) Microglial cell. *Right* (A–D, B–C, F) Type IV oligodendrocytes; E type III oligodendrocyte; (H) type I oligodendrocyte (see Figure 3 for a description of types). (I) Astrocyte. From del Rio Hortega (1928).

processes. Del Rio Hortega (1928) found four patterns that he believed described the branching patterns of the processes of all oligodendrocytes, whether perineuronal or interfascicular (see Figures 1–3). The first two types of oligodendrocyte had branches scattering in many directions; the other two forms dispatched processes disposed parallel to adjacent myelin sheaths and therefore assumed a much more linear overall pattern.

Type I oligodendrocytes possess a small soma (10–20 μm, varying with species) with relatively frequent processes (5–10 but sometimes as many as 20) arising from the soma. These processes are long and very thin with periodic knotlike expansions of protoplasm and with branching frequently occurring at obtuse angles. Type I is the most abundant of all the oligodendrocyte types.

Type II oligodendrocytes are found frequently in the white matter, especially within fascicles of thinly myelinated axons, and also in gray matter closely related to the cell bodies of neurons (and thus termed perineuronal). Type II oligodendrocytes have larger cell somata than type I, but fewer primary processes (3–5). These processes are larger in diameter and divide at T or Y branches into smaller secondary processes that are long and thin as in type I cells. This form is found in white matter only and is intermediate in frequency between type I and types III and IV.

Types III and IV oligodendrocytes are more elongated than the other two types and have only one or two processes. Both are prominent in white matter in relation to the largest myelinated axons. They differ in that type III cells often have two processes, each reticulating over the surface of an adjacent myelinated fiber. Type IV cells, along with their processes, are flattened over the surface of a single large myelinated axon. Del Rio Hortega (1922, 1924) noted their similarity to the Schwann cells related to the large myelinated axons of the PNS.

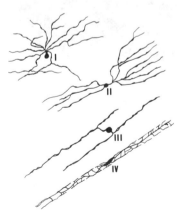

FIGURE 3. The four types of oligodendrocyte profile recognized by del Rio Hortega (1928) and confirmed by Stensaas and Stensaas (1968). Type I is presumably related to many small myelin segments traveling through the tissue (as in gray matter) at many different angles. Type II is similar but related to segments of myelin within a fascicle containing many axons coursing in the same direction. Type III is a cell related to two large segments of myelin; type IV, to one large segment. Del Rio Hortega was struck by the similarity of the relationship between the type IV oligodendrocyte and the Schwann cell to the underlying myelin segments, indicating that the oligodendrocyte was the central homolog of the cell of Schwann.

Del Rio Hortega's classification of oligodendrocytes has been confirmed and correlated with electron-microscopic (EM) observations in a study of neuroglia in the amphibian spinal cord by Stensaas and Stensaas (1968). They confirmed that four basic types of oligodendrocytes could be identified in this tissue and supplemented the analysis by three-dimensional reconstructions of several oligodendrocyte somata from serial-section electron micrographs of very high quality. They added the observation that the various profile classes of oligodendrocyte all shared common ultrastructural characteristics within their cytoplasm (see below). Thus, as we discuss in Section 4, while there are many steps in oligodendrocyte maturation, and whereas the general form of the oligodendrocyte differs substantially, there may be just one basic mature cellular type in terms of cytoplasmic density, content, and function.

The characterization of the oligodendrocyte as viewed in the EM was initially complicated by a period of confusion regarding the identification of astrocytes and oligodendrocytes [see discussion in R. P. Bunge (1968)]. In retrospect, it seems likely that this confusion resulted from the propensity of oligodendrocytes to undergo cytoplasmic swelling under certain anoxic conditions. When swollen, its normally compact cytoplasm resembles that of the normally "clear" cytoplasm of the astrocyte. This type of change, mentioned prominently in the review by Penfield (1932), could certainly have occurred during the less than optimal immersion fixation and embedding procedures used in the earliest years of EM study of central neural tissues.

When optimally fixed for EM the mature oligodendrocyte is a small cell (10–20 μm in diameter) with marked density of both nucleus and cytoplasm (Peters *et al.,* 1976). Within the round or oval nucleus, the substantial amounts of heterochromatin occupying the nuclear periphery contribute to its dense appearance. Generally, the largest mass of cytoplasm lies to one side of the nucleus, with the remainder of the nucleus being surrounded by a thin rim of cytoplasm. The density of the oligodendrocyte cytoplasm is thought to be contributed by densely staining material (of unknown nature) occupying the cytosol between the organelles (Peters *et al.,* 1976; Mori and Leblond, 1970). There are no unique organelles within the oligodendrocyte cytoplasm. The rough endoplasmic reticulum is well developed, and the cisternae tend to be flattened, arranged in stacks, and appear empty. Ribosomes are present on the surface of the rough endoplasmic reticulum, the outer aspect of the nuclear envelope, and within the cytoplasm, where they are often grouped into polysomes. The Golgi apparatus of the oligodendrocyte contains cisternae that are electron-lucent and often appear distended. The mitochondria are relatively inconspicuous within the dense cytoplasm and show no unusual features. They tend to be short with their cristae arranged transversely. Some mature oligodendrocytes contain distinct lamellar bodies (of unknown function) that appear to increase with age (Mori and Leblond, 1970; D. Vaughn and Peters, 1974).

Mature oligodendrocytes have also been found to contain numerous microperoxisomes that often appear as clusters within the cytoplasm of the perikaryon (McKenna *et al.*, 1976). The authors postulate that peroxisomes may have some as yet undemonstrated role in lipid metabolism related to myelin synthesis or maintenance.

The oligodendrocyte is distinguished from the astrocyte by the general density of its cytoplasm and the lack of cytoplasmic fibrils, glycogen granules, and frequent dense bodies (Skoff *et al.*, 1976a). Oligodendrocytes and astrocytes do share, however, a substantial cytoplasmic content of microtubules; these tend to be more conspicuous in the oligodendrocyte. Like the microtubules in neurons, these are 25 nm in diameter and are randomly arranged throughout the perikaryal cytoplasm. They are extended into the processes of the oligodendrocyte, where they tend to be arranged parallel to one another. Because there are substantial numbers of microtubules in oligodendrocytes, axons, and dendrites, these processes may have a very similar appearance. Dendrites can be differentiated, however, in that they frequently receive synapses, have less cytoplasmic density, and are frequently seen to give rise to spines. Axons can usually be distinguished from oligodendrocyte processes in that axons often contain filaments, while oligodendrocyte processes do not.

In their study of neuroglial cells in the spinal cord of the frog, Stensaas and Stensaas (1968) have emphasized that oligodendrocytes appear to have a firm or turgid cell body that is never seen to be indented by adjacent cellular components.This aspect distinguishes oligodendrocytes from the phagocytic microglia to which they have some resemblance. Microglia frequently have elongated nuclei, and both the nucleus and the cytoplasm are seen to be distorted and altered in configuration by adjacent cell processes. Another distinguishing characteristic of microglia is the frequent presence of residual bodies indicative of their phagocytic activity.

In what appears to be the earliest light-microscopic (LM) description of the cells (later termed oligodendrocytes) during myelination, Hardesty (1904, 1905) puzzled over the fact that there seemed to be cells very directly related to the forming myelin sheaths. These cells, in fact, formed "signet-ring" configurations around the forming myelin sheaths and seemed to be directly involved in the formation of the underlying myelin. The observation that the cytoplasm of these cells appeared to disappear after the active period of myelination left Hardesty uncertain regarding the relationship of these neuroglia to the mature myelin sheath. The resolution of the LM was simply inadequate to illustrate the direct connections present between mature oligodendrocytes and fully formed myelin sheaths.

It should be noted that these connections are difficult to demonstrate even in the modern era of the EM. When examining mature white matter in the

EM, it is possible to demonstrate that associated with the internal and external aspect of the compact myelin, there are regions of cytoplasm that have the density and microtubule content that characterize oligodendrocyte processes. It is also possible to section through the cell bodies of oligodendrocytes and follow by serial reconstruction the course of the processes that leave the cell body and approach the surrounding myelin sheaths (Stensaas and Stensaas, 1968). It is extremely difficult, however to demonstrate the continuity between the cytoplasm of these oligodendrocyte processes and that associated with the mature sheath. This continuity has been easier to demonstrate in developing white matter.

In his pictures of the white matter from young animals, del Rio Hortega (1928) frequently demonstrated extensions from the oligodendrocyte somal region that provide a spirally disposed process in relation to a forming myelin sheath. There seems little doubt that these processes were in fact the cytoplasm directly related to the myelin sheath in either the external or the internal aspect. Similarly, it has been possible, by studying developing white matter during the period of active myelination, to directly visualize continuity between processes extending from oligodendrocytes to the external aspect of the forming myelin sheath (Bunge et al., 1962; Peters, 1964). It has also been possible to demonstrate directly that oligodendrocytes are frequently involved in the formation of more than one segment of myelin on adjacent axons. A determination of the actual number of myelin segments that a single oligodendrocyte can maintain has been done, not by serial-section reconstruction, but by calculation of the number of myelin segments present in a specific portion of a well-defined central nerve tract and an evaluation of the number of oligodendrocytes present to provide these segments. This type of calculation was done for the optic nerve of the rat by Peters and Vaughn (1970), with the conclusion that oligodendrocytes must frequently support in the range of 40 segments of myelin.

More recently, the use of antibodies to specific myelin components has allowed the direct demonstration of the continuity between oligodendrocyte cell body and forming myelin sheaths as discussed by Sternberger in Chapter 4. Sternberger et al. (1978a) have been able, by serial reconstruction of LM preparations stained for myelin basic protein (MBP), to demonstrate direct continuity between a single oligodendrocyte and ten adjacent myelin segments. Moreover, they were able to show that these myelin segments may not be localized to a specific central tract, but could belong to nerve-fiber bundles coursing in different directions within the neuropil.

The fact that MBP is not present in substantial amounts in mature oligodendrocyte cytoplasm precludes utilizing this immunocytochemical method for direct analysis of connectivity between oligodendrocyte and myelin sheath in the adult. The concordance between the early pictures obtained with metal impregnation of oligodendrocytes and the immunocytochemically demonstrated relationship between oligodendrocytes and forming myelin segments, as well as the EM demonstration that there is cytoplasm very similar to that found in oligodendrocytes associated with myelin sheaths in mature animals, leaves little doubt that a continuity between oligodendrocytes and myelin segments is retained in the adult animal.

Because the direct demonstration of the connection between the oligodendrocyte and myelin segments can only rarely be achieved, it does not seem possible to rule out that some interfascicular oligodendrocytes are adjacent to, but not in direct continuity with, myelin segments. Thus, it is possible that among the population of interfascicular oligodendrocytes, there are mature oligodendrocytes not connected to myelin sheaths, as well as a small number of "stem cells" or oligodendroblasts capable of proliferation and the production of a new oligodendrocyte population (see Section 3).

Is the perineuronal oligodendrocyte not an example of a non-myelin-related oligodendrocyte? Perineuronal oligodendrocytes have now been shown to be involved in myelin formation during remyelination (Ludwin, 1979b) (also see Chapter 4). Because neuronal-cell bodies are often in close relation to adjacent myelinated axons and because perineuronal oligodendrocytes are not numerous (expecially when compared to the satellite cells of peripheral ganglia), it seems reasonable to suggest they may be myelin-related cells, the cell soma of which happens to reside near a neuronal-cell body. In their comprehensive study of frog neuroglia, Stensaas and Stensaas (1968) state that they did not observe oligodendrocytes as neuronal satellites in this species. This view that perineuronal oligodendrocytes are involved in myelination is supported by the observations by Penfield (1932) that "satellite cells, wherever found, have roughly the same morphology" and "they do not surround the (anterior) horn cells closely" and "the satellite expansions (processes) pass around the nerve cell and off toward other structures."

3.　OLIGODENDROCYTE ORIGINS

The family of cells defined morphologically as oligodendrocytes first appears (rather suddenly) just prior to the beginning of myelination and increase rapidly in number as myelination progresses (J. E. Vaughn, 1969; Skoff *et al.,* 1976b). There is evidence (discussed below), however, that most myelinating oligodendrocytes no longer display mitotic activity; thus, the beginning of myelination may not correspond to the true "origin" of this cell type, but rather to the final transformation of precursors into the myelinating cells. How these oligodendrocyte precursors are generated is still a major unresolved question.

Early precursors of the oligodendrocytes are thought to be among the proliferating cells of the primitive neural tube and are morphologically identical to the precursors of neurons and astrocytes (Sauer, 1935; S. Fugita, 1963; Hinds and Ruffett, 1971). In the early LM studies, cells that could be recognized as distinct from neurons were detected in the developing neural tissue only after the major period of neuronal production had ceased (Smart and Leblond, 1961; H. Fugita and S. Fugita, 1964). When compared to neurons, these cells were smaller and contained small and more densely staining nuclei. These small cells were called glioblasts (from Gr. *glia,* "glue") in accordance with the belief that they would mature into either oligodendrocytes or astrocytes as development proceeded (H. Fugita and S. Fugita, 1964). This view was given some support by the finding that these small cells were strongly labeled immediately after an injection of tritiated thymidine ([^{3}H]-TdR), while mature oligodendrocytes and astrocytes contained little label (Smart and Leblond, 1961; S. Fugita, 1964). After longer periods of survival, the labeling index declined in the glioblast population, but increased in the astrocyte and oligodendrocyte groups. These early autoradiographic experiments thus provided the first evidence that mature glia might be mitotically inactive and the observed labeling sequence was consistent with the idea of the transformation of a multipotential "glioblast" into the mature glial cells.

More recent observations of Skoff *et al.* (1976*a,b*) and Imamoto *et al.* (1978) have clearly shown that the more advanced blast forms of astrocytes and oligodendrocytes that occur during postnatal development in rodents are morphologically distinct cell types, but the multipotential glioblast is still thought to exist during the embryonic period of development. However, because conclusive observations confirming its supposed properties have not been reported, the existence of this hypothetical cell, even during the embryonic period, must still be open to question. The possibility that the astrocyte and oligodendrocyte lineages may arise separately from primitive ventricular or subventricular cells has been raised (Skoff, 1980), but does not seem to have been considered very seriously. After reviewing carefully the limited number of studies dealing with oligodendrocyte origin, we believe that the reported observations contain evidence for two extremely immature but still distinct cell types, and these cell types may be the early representatives of distinct astrocyte and oligodendrocyte cell lines.

The first systematic study of the origin of mature glial cells with the EM was reported by Caley and Maxwell (1968). They examined the cerebrum in young postnatal rats at successive stages of maturation and described a "continuum" of cell types ranging from "indifferent cells" to the more easily recognized immature astrocytes and oligodendrocytes. These latter cells were referred to as astroblasts and oligodendroblasts, although these authors presented no evidence for their division. All the nonneuronal cells, including the "indifferent" cells seen in this study, were characterized by a clumping of nuclear chromatin near the nuclear envelope. The "indifferent" cells had a thin rim of cytoplasm with no processes and few organelles. A second form of immature glial cell, the "spongioblast," had processes but could not be classified as either astrocyte or oligodendrocyte. The cytoplasm of the spongioblast contained numerous mitochondria, many free ribosomes, and a prominent Golgi complex, but little rough endoplasmic reticulum. While the authors did not report quantitative data on the number of these cells they stated that at birth, nearly all the nonneuronal cells were of the "indifferent" type, but after 10 days, these cells were found only rarely, and instead many spongioblasts were evident. The spongioblast was thought to be able to generate either astroblasts or oligodendroblasts.

Although the cytoplasm of immature glial cells was not as distinctive as that of mature glia, the astroblast and oligodendroblast could be distinguished from one another by criteria based on the morphology of mature forms. In addition, it was noted that the morphology of the processes and the relationship of these processes to axons was different for the two cell types. The thin oligodendroblast processes appeared to contact and begin to enclose axons, whereas the broad astrocyte processes appeared to grow by the axons and to form perivascular and subpial end-feet. Cytoplasmic filaments not present in immature oligodendrocytes could often be found in the immature astrocytes, thus aiding in their identification.

A more quantitative EM study of gliogenesis in the optic nerve of the rat was reported by J. E. Vaughn (1969, 1971), in which both embryonic and postnatal tissues were examined. As Vaughn pointed out, the optic nerve is an ideal location for the study of gliogenesis because neuronal cell bodies are absent and because the nerve is relatively small, a feature that should facilitate the tracing of cells and their processes as the nerve develops. In addition, the glial cells in this nerve are all believed to arise from cells that make up the optic stalk (Skoff, 1980), with very little migration of glial precursors from areas outside the stalk. Vaughn described a range of cells that were similar to those that Caley and Maxwell (1968) had found in the cerebral cortex just after birth. Again, the maturity of these cells was measured by the degree of organization of the cytoplasm and by the formation of processes. In general, maturation was signified by a relative decrease in the free ribosome content and a relative increase in the length and number of cisternae of rough endoplasmic reticulum and in the prominence of the Golgi complex. Vaughn named three distinct types of immature glial cells: the small glioblast, the large glioblast, and the large glial precursor.

An important role in gliogenesis was assigned by Vaughn to the cell he calls the small glioblast. This cell was characterized by increased numbers of mitochondria and slightly more abundant rough endoplasmic reticulum than the more primitive intermitotic cells. Most important, it also had processes that extended into the neighboring neuropil. These processes, however, were not well characterized. J. E. Vaughn (1971) reported that at 15½ days of gestation, some cells very similar to the small glioblast were found in the optic stalk, where some of them contributed to the glial limitans (suggestive of an early astroglial function for these cells). Vaughn believed that becoming a small glioblast was the first step in differentiation made by the primitive mitotically active derivatives of the neuroectodermal cells. These small glioblasts could then either differentiate further or continue to divide. Vaughn thought that prior to becoming more specialized, the small glioblast would grow to become the cell that he designated a large glial precursor. As seen in the electron micrographs, this process-bearing cell could either exhibit no cytoplasmic specialization or show an organelle content indicative of differentiation along either astrocyte or oligodendrocyte lines.

J. E. Vaughn (1969) found in addition to the small glioblast a larger cell that he called the large glioblast. The large glioblast appeared to be less specialized than the small glioblast, with relatively less cytoplasm and no processes, regardless of the plane of section. The cytoplasm contained numerous ribosomal clusters and very little rough endoplasmic reticulum. Chromatin patterns suggestive of early stages of mitosis were seen in many of these cells. Vaughn therefore assigned to this cell a position in the cell cycle of the small glioblast and felt that the collection of cells that included the small and large glioblasts and the large glial precursors would probably correspond to the "spongioblast" group described by Caley and Maxwell (1968). We will propose that an alternative interpretation of these data is that the process-bearing small glioblast may be an astrocyte precursor and that the large glioblast may be a precursor of the oligodendrocyte. A relationship of the astrocyte to the small glioblast is clearly suggested by similarities between these cells.

In an EM analysis of gliogenesis in the more slowly developing spinal cord of the pilot monkey, Philips (1973) found that nearly all the cells that could be classified as glioblasts in the marginal zone of the 49 to 70 day fetus became astroglia, with many transitional forms observed between these two types. On the other hand, the formation of oligodendrocytes seemed to depend on the migration from the mantle zone of cells that he called "oligoblasts." Few transitional forms could be found between the cells classified as glioblasts and oligoblasts in the marginal zone. Philips postulated that any transformation from glioblast to oligoblast would have to occur in the mantle zone before migration of the oligoblast. As shown in Philips's electron micrographs, the migrating "oligoblast" was similar to the large glioblast of J. E. Vaughn (1969) in that it exhibited primitive, sparse cytoplasm and lack of processes.

While the use of the EM to study gliogenesis brought a greater degree of certainty in identifying the different classes of glial cells in immature tissue, there is an inherent limitation in the number of cells that can be examined. More recently, the combination of the resolution of EM with the analytical power of LM autoradiography has been used in efforts to extend our conception of the early events of gliogenesis. [^{3}H]-TdR has been used in these studies both to assess the mitotic activity of the cells and to trace the relationship between mitotic cells and their descendants.

The use of this methodology in the study of gliogenesis was first reported in 1973 by Leblond and co-workers in a series of papers (Ling *et al.*, 1973; Ling and Leblond, 1973; Paterson *et al.*, 1973) about glial maturation in the cerebral cortex and corpus callosum of the young rat. This group had previously (Mori and Leblond, 1969, 1970) gone to great length to identify each of the glial-cell classes in electron micrographs of metal-impregnated tissue, thus firmly establishing the equation of images in electron micrographs with the profiles described by classic histologists. They (Ling *et al.*, 1973) then showed that images of glial nuclei in toluidine-blue-stained semithin sections corresponded reproducibly to images of specific glia in electron micrographs. Thus, a method of identifying nuclei in autoradiograms of semithin sections was obtained in which large numbers of cells could be surveyed. The identity of cells could be checked in electron micrographs of adjacent thin sections.

The stage of development studied was later than those discussed above in that 1-month-old rats were used. Myelination was well under way in both cortex and corpus callosum, and the period of peak astrocyte proliferation had passed. Most of the new glia being formed were oligodencrocytes. Most of the immature glia seen in corpus callosum in this study were called "free subependymal cells," denoting their probable migration into the corpus callosum from the subependymal zone. These cells had been described in detail earlier by Privat and Leblond (1972). The scanty cytoplasm of the free subependymal cells resembled that of the large glioblast described by J. E. Vaughn (1969), but the cells appeared to be much smaller. They were shown as elongated cells without processes and with evenly dispersed chromatin. In general, they were quite unlike the small glioblast of J. E. Vaughn (1969). The "free subependymal cells" retained a high level of mitotic activity even at this relatively late stage of development. After a pulse of [^{3}H]-TdR, about 85% of them were labeled. The kinetics of the rise and decay of the labeling index of these cells relative to that of the oligodendrocytes suggested that the free subependymal cells were precursors of the oligodendrocytes. In contrast, however, no clear relationship could be demonstrated between the "free subependymal cell" and the astrocyte in this study.

A combined quantitative LM and EM analysis of gliogenesis in mouse corpus callosum from birth to adulthood was reported by Sturrock (1976). He described three coexisting classes of immature glia including the "early" glioblast, a "small" glioblast, and a "large" glioblast. The properties of the small and large glioblasts are remarkably close to those described by J. E. Vaughn (1969) for cells given the same names. The "early" glioblast was similar to the "large" glioblast, but a little bigger, and had a very homogeneous, lightly staining nucleoplasm. The early glioblasts had disappeared by 11 days after birth. On the basis of differential cell counts and shared morphological properties, Sturrock proposed that the large glioblasts were primitive oligodendrocytes and that the small glioblasts were the primitive astrocytes. The early glioblasts were proposed by Sturrock to be multipotential cells that could transform into the other two classes.

A comparison of the pictures and descriptions contained in the reports just mentioned indicated that there are two very different immature glial-cell types in developing tissue. One of these cell types has no processes, very little cytoplasm, and a relatively large, essentially euchromatic nucleus of about 5–6 μm in size; the other cell type has processes, relatively more cytoplasm, and a small, largely heterochromatic nucleus of about 3–4 μm in size. While these two forms have sometimes been interpreted as different forms of a single cell type, this concept does not appear to be justified by the evidence presented in the studies mentioned and was to receive even less support in subsequent studies.

Skoff et al. (1976a,b) used the combined techniques of EM analysis and LM and EM autoradiography in a careful study of gliogenesis in the optic nerve of fetal and young rats. They conclusively demonstrated that immature cells resembling oligodendrocytes (which appeared in the rat optic nerve at 5 days after birth) were mitotically active (see Figure 4). Many of these cells had incorporated [^{3}H]-TdR by 1 hr after an injection, so they could properly be called oligodendroblasts; as such, they probably correspond to the cells called young oligodendrocytes or possibly to some of the large glial precursors described by J. E. Vaughn (1969). More mature oligodendrocytes did not incorporate thymidine. The oligodendroblast at 5 days postnatally (at the beginning of myelination) was very similar to the oligodendroblast found at later stages of myelination. This was in marked contrast to the labeling pattern among the astroglia, in which astrocytes showing a wide range of cytoplasmic differentiation became labeled by 1 hr after the injection.

Skoff et al. (1976b) pointed out that whereas oligodendroblasts could be found at 5 days of age in the optic nerve, at 2 days of age they could not. At 2 days, nearly all (85–95%) of the cells could be identified as astroglia by mor-

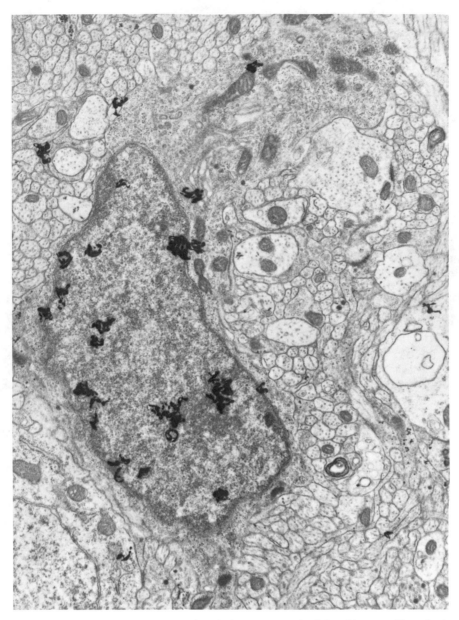

FIGURE 4. EM autoradiogram from the spinal gray matter of a 7-day-old mouse. The animal was sacrificed 1 hr after an injection of [³H]-TdR. The labeled cell is an oligodendroblast and is characterized by the eccentric position of the nucleus, low contrast between chromatin and nucleoplasm, Golgi apparatus adjacent to the nucleus, numerous mitochondria, ribosomal rosettes, and scattered microtubules. The immature oligodendrocyte has fewer cisternae of endoplasmic reticulum than the mature form. ×20,000. Micrograph kindly provided by Dr. R. P. Skoff.

phological criteria (e.g., filaments). The remaining cells could not be classified. They were relatively small mitotic cells, with very scanty cytoplasm, and evenly dispersed chromatin. According to this description, they resemble the "indifferent" cells described earlier by Caley and Maxwell (1968) in the neonatal rat cerebral cortex, the large glioblasts described by J. E. Vaughn (1969), "immature subependymal cells" as described by Privat and Leblond (1972), and the "early" or "large" glioblast described in corpus callosum by Sturrock (1976). They were distinctly different from the small glioblast described by J. E. Vaughn (1969) in lacking processes and in their paucity of cytoplasm. They make up 10% of the mitotic cells in the 2-day-postnatal optic nerve.

In agreement with the findings of J. E. Vaughn (1969), Skoff and co-workers showed that some glial cells could be identified as astroglia as early as the 15th day of gestation in the embryonic optic nerve. This result suggests quite strongly that astroglia might arise directly from ventricular cells in the optic stalk. Alternatively, the astroglia might exist as a subpopulation among the less differentiated ventricular cells. The morpholgy of these embryonic astroglia in the optic nerve is very similar to the morphology of the radial glia found in other areas of the CNS (Del Cerro and Schwarz, 1976; Henrikson and Vaughn, 1974).

Although the radial glia are greatly elongated bipolar cells that for the most part do not contain bundles of 90 Å filaments, as do astrocytes, forms intermediate between between radial glia and astrocytes have been described (Schmechel and Rakic, 1979) in tissue impregnated by the Golgi method. These intermediate forms may exhibit both a single elongated, radially oriented process and many stellate processes characteristic of the astrocyte. Furthermore, it has recently been demonstrated that radial glia contain glial fibrillary acidic protein, a component of the 90 Å filaments common in astrocytes (Levitt et al., 1981). It has thus been possible to trace a line of cells with astrocyte characteristics to very early stages of neural-tube development, at a time when neuronal proliferation is still ongoing.

Gliogenesis in corpus callosum at the onset of myelination has recently been reexamined by Imamoto et al. (1978). Their object was to determine whether or not mature glia incorporated thymidine. All the immature oligodendrocytes, astrocytes, and unclassifiable cells were grouped together and referred to as "immature" glia. The mature glia included light, medium, and dark oligodendrocytes (the characteristics of which are described in Section 4) and astrocytes. Only the immature cells incorporated thymidine, and (as was reported earlier) (Paterson et al., 1973) a clear relationship was demonstrated between the immature cells and the oligodendrocytes by the sequential appearance of label first in the immature cells and later in the mature oligodendrocytes. It should be noted that whereas the astroblast and the oligodendroblasts shown in this study had relatively advanced and distinctive morphologies, the cytoplasm of other cells included in the "immature" cell category was extremely primitive.

The work of Skoff *et al.* (1976*a,b*) and Imamoto *et al.* (1978) has clearly shown that the immediate precursors of astrocytes and oligodendrocytes are differentiated enough to be quite distinct from each other and yet are capable of proliferation. Skoff (1980) has thus formally proposed that after birth, the cell lineages for astrocytes and oligodendrocytes may be entirely separate, with multipotential glioblasts possibly existing only during the embryonic period in the rodent. The astroglial lineage can be definitely traced into the embryonic period (a few astrocytes in the rat optic nerve become postmitotic by as early as the 15th day of gestation), whereas the oligodendroglial lineage can be clearly traced only back to the 2nd postnatal day.

In reviewing some of this literature, we noted that two assumptions have been made consistently in interpreting the static images of the electron micrographs. These are that an increasing complexity of the cytoplasm within the immature cell and the formation of cellular processes are the first reliable indicators of commitment to a specific cell line. These trends would appear to be valid for cells in the astrocyte lineage, but both cytoplasmic differentiation and process formation may be relatively late events for cells in the oligodendrocyte lineage, heralding the approach of the final round of division. The properties of the earliest oligodendrocytes might be similar to those that have been generally attributed to the uncommitted or unclassifiable cells. Thus, they would lack extensive processes, which might make migration a simpler task. During embryonic development, they would proliferate slowly to form a small resident nonmyelinating population within the neuropil. Just before myelination, they would proliferate rapidly, produce cellular processes, and transform into readily recognized oligodendrocytes. In the studies we have reviewed, these juvenile oligodendrocytes might have been classified as "indifferent" cells (Caley and Maxwell, 1968)), "large glioblasts" (J. E. Vaughn, 1969), "oligoblast" (Philips, 1973), "free subependymal cells" (Paterson *et al.*, 1973), "early" glioblast (Sturrock, 1976), "unclassifiable" cell (Skoff *et al.*, 1976*a,b*), and "immature cell" (Imamoto *et al.*, 1978). The astrocyte lineage characterized by the possession of cellular processes from its earliest stages of development could arise as radial glia or in the form of the "small" glioblast (J. E. Vaughn, 1971; Sturrock, 1976).

This scheme of gliogenesis is summarized diagrammatically in Figure 5. It is essentially the same as that proposed by Skoff *et al.* (1976*b*) except that the oligodendrocyte and astrocyte lineages would be viewed as entirely separate, from their earliest origins in the ependymal zone; no multipotential glioblast is included.

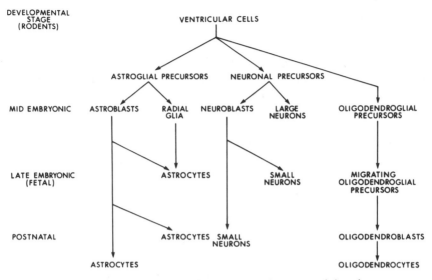

FIGURE 5. Proposed scheme of gliogenesis and neurogenesis in rodents.

4. OLIGODENDROCYTE MATURATION

The general description of the oligodendrocyte given earlier was for the mature form. In fact, the oligodendrocyte class exhibits a considerable diversity in both cell size and overall cytoplasmic composition, even in adult animals (Kruger and Maxwell, 1966). This diversity is now partly understood to represent different states of maturation of the myelinating oligodendrocyte, rather than different cell types or functions within the family of oligodendrocytes. Although the coexistence of different stages of maturation throughout the period of myelination has made a precise correlation between morphological profiles and biochemical activity difficult, the general features of oligodendrocyte maturation can now be described with reasonable confidence.

J. E. Vaughn (1969), in his study of gliogenesis in rat optic nerve, commented on the dramatic contrast in electron micrographs between the mature oligodendrocyte and those found during early stages of myelination. These later cells were called "active" oligodendrocytes and were bigger and displayed more processes than those found later. When compared to the more mature oligodendrocyte, the "active" cells had much "more obvious" cisternae of Golgi complexes and rough endoplasmic reticulum. The nucleus of the active oligodendrocyte was large and filled with evenly dispersed chromatin and contained prominent nucleoli, whereas that of the mature oligodendrocyte had aggregates of chromatin around its rim. All these features in "active" oligodendrocytes were considered appropriate to a cell engaged in very active biosynthesis of processes and membranes.

Mori and Leblond (1970) recognized that the diverse forms of oligodendrocytes seen in electron micrographs of adolescent rat corpus callosum could be arranged in a continuous spectrum. All the cells that could not be classified as either astrocytes or or microglia by metal-impregnation methods were included in this spectrum. They were arranged according to size and electron opacity (as these features varied in parallel). Large cells containing electron-pale cytoplasm and many processes were at one end of the spectrum and small cells with electron-dense cytoplasm and few processes at the other. Three classes were described in detail and were called "light," "medium," and "dark" oligodendrocytes, and cells intermediate between these classes were seen as well.

The distinguishing features of these cells were as follows: The light oligodendrocyte was characterized by a large euchromatic nucleus with very few chromatin masses. This cell had abundant cytoplasm that was filled with organelles, and many free ribosomes or polysomes or both. It contained very little rough endoplasmic reticulum and a rather variable Golgi apparatus. It had many fine processes. The medium oligodendrocyte was smaller and was more electron-dense than the light one and its nucleus was also smaller with more clumps of chromatin beneath the nuclear envelope. The cytoplasm was decreased in volume, with fewer free ribosomes, but it contained a more prominent Golgi apparatus and longer and more regularly stacked cisternae of rough endoplasmic reticulum. The resemblance between the photographs of these medium oligodendrocytes and the "active" oligodendrocytes described by J. E. Vaughn (1969) is striking, and they probably correspond to the same cell. The medium oligodencrocyte had fewer processes than the light variety. The dark oligodendrocyte was smaller still, with a small electron-dense nucleus and electron-dense cytoplasm. It contained stacks of relatively elongated lucent cisternae of rough endoplasmic reticulum and a somewhat smaller Golgi apparatus, also with lucent cisternae. The relative percentages of the light, medium, and dark oligodendrocytes found by Mori and Leblond (1970) in their study in young rats were 6, 25, and 40% of the total glial population. Some of the light and a few of the medium oligodendrocytes were labeled as soon as 1 hr after an injection of [^{3}H]-TdR, but dark oligodendrocytes became labeled only several days after the injection.

Mori and Leblond (1970) proposed that the continuum of cellular profiles they observed represented different maturational stages of oligodendrocytes during differentiation. The light oligodendrocyte was considered to be the myelinating cell and the dark oligodendrocyte a mature cell engaged in myelin maintenance. This proposal was supported by the changes observed in rat cerebral cortex and corpus callosum in the relative percentages of these three classes of oligodendrocytes from adolescence to adulthood (Ling and Leblond, 1973). At early ages, the light and medium variety together made up from 30 to 60% of the total oligodendrocyte population, but the numbers of cells in these two categories decreased in the mature adult, so that the dark variety came to make up more than 90% of the total oligodendrocytes. These workers believed that the light oligodendrocyte was capable of further division while maintaining its processes and that the light-oligodendrocyte stock was partly replenished by this division.

The relationship among light, medium, and dark oligodendrocytes was further investigated by autoradiographic techniques in two much more detailed studies of rat corpus callosum reported by Paterson *et al.* (1973) and Imamoto *et al.* (1978). The numbers of each of these cells that were labeled after an injection of [^{3}H]-TdR were recorded successively for up to 5 weeks after the injection. The label appeared sequentially in the light, medium, and dark oligodendrocytes, with kinetics that clearly supported the interpretation that the light oligodendrocytes were transforming into the medium and then into the dark form. The average duration of the different stages could be calculated from the numerical data. It was found that the light stage lasted 4–5 days, the medium stage 12–14 days, and the dark stage more or less indefinitely. The duration of each stage was to some extent dependent on the age of the animal. It is interesting that the duration of the medium stage ($\approx$12–14 days) was about the time estimated by Skoff *et al.* (1976*b*) to be required for the postmitotic oligodendrocyte to differentiate morphologically. However, Skoff presented electron micrographs of oligodendrocytes at 2 and at 4 weeks after the cells shown had presumably undergone a terminal division and remained permanently labeled. The 2-week-postmitotic cells [compare Figure 13 in Skoff *et al.* (1976*b*) with Figure 7 in Mori and Leblond (1970)] still looked more like light oligodendrocytes, while the 4-week-postmitotic cell resembled the medium oligodendrocytes [compare Figure 14 in Skoff *et al.* (1976*b*) with Figure 10 in Mori and Leblond (1970)]. Thus, the length of the light, medium, and dark phases may vary.

The beginning of myelination coincides very closely in time with the termination of cell division for some oligodendrocytes, but there is very little evidence that oligodendroblasts begin synthesizing myelin components prior to their final cell division. In their study of gliogenesis in postnatal rat optic nerve, Skoff *et al.* (1976*b*) found that most of the oligodendrocytes could be permanently heavily labeled by [^{3}H]-TdR injected before the 14th postnatal day. At this time, only about a third of the axons had been myelinated. Furthermore, the earliest point at which oligodendrocytes could be permanently heavily labeled was at 5 days postnatally, which was a day or two before a few myelin segments were also present. In direct biochemical analysis of developing rat optic nerves (Tennekoon *et al.*, 1980), the kinetics of the appearance of myelin-specific proteins and lipids corresponded quite closely to the time–course of permanent heavy labeling of oligodendrocyte nuclei by [^{3}H]-TdR injections (Skoff *et al.,* 1976*b*). Lipid synthesis appears to begin slightly earlier than protein synthesis in these studies. However, in immunocytochemical studies, which are probably more sensitive than direct biochemical analyses, oligodendrocytes that contained myelin basic protein (MBP) or myelin-associated glycoprotein could be demonstrated a few days before the myelin sheaths themselves were present (Sternberger *et al.,* 1978). The mitotic activity of these cells was not determined.

As mentioned earlier, it was noted by Skoff *et al.* (1976*a*) that the appearance in EM autoradiograms of oligodendroblasts at 5 days of age was the same as the appearance of oligodendroblasts at 14 days of age. They contained many small mitochondria, some stacks of Golgi cisternae, and free ribosomes. The cytoplasm was similar to that observed in "young" oligodendrocytes (J. E. Vaughn, 1969), but was more electron-opaque and perhaps smaller than that of the light oligodendrocyte (Mori and Leblond 1970). Skoff *et al.* (1976*a*) did not find label in cells that showed greater maturity. Furthermore, they felt that postmitotic cells were larger, with a rounder nucleus that contained more evenly dispersed chromatin. Thus, the postmitotic oligodendrocytes they describe might correspond to the light oligodendrocyte described by Mori and Leblond (1970). However, the labeling that Mori and Leblond (1970) observed of light and even of a few medium oligodendrocytes suggested to them that substantial numbers of this class were blasts. Their observations seemed to be confirmed by Paterson *et al.* (1973) in a later, more detailed study. Finally, however, Imamoto *et al.* (1978) found that light oligodendrocytes were not labeled initially and were for the most part postmitotic. Of 600 light cells examined, only 1 was labeled. The many discrepancies noted here could be explained by the slightly different criteria used for classifying the immature forms of the oligodendrocyte or by differences in preparative procedures.

The organelle content of either the light or the medium oligodendrocyte could be said to be consistent with myelinating activity. The profiles of these oligodendrocytes during the peak period of myelination show an abundant cytoplasm containing numerous free ribosomes or polysomes, several moderate lengths of rough endoplasmic reticulum that are occasionally arranged in stacks, and several prominent Golgi complexes. The subcellular pathways of myelin synthesis and the possible involvement of specific organelles with the various aspects of myelin synthesis are discussed in detail in Chapter 3. Here we might briefly mention that some recent evidence suggests that proteolipid protein, the major integral membrane protein of myelin, may be synthesized and inserted into the membrane in the rough endoplasmic reticulum in the oligodendrocyte perikaryon and transported with some delay (via the Golgi apparatus) into the forming myelin sheath, whereas MBP may be synthesized on free polysomes in the myelinating oligodendrocyte processes (Colman *et al.,* 1982). The Golgi apparatus may also play some role in the sulfation of lipids and possibly proteins (Tennekoon *et al.,* 1977).

After myelination is completed, the morphology and the numbers of mature or dark oligodendrocytes change very little; in rats, no significant changes were observed between 3 and 27 months of age (D. Vaughn and Peters, 1974; Imamoto *et al.,* 1978). This remarkable stability is consistent with the major function of these cells, which is to maintain the many myelin sheaths to which each of them is connected. In several studies, they could not be directly labeled by [^{3}H]-TdR injection, even in young animals in which myelination was proceeding (H. Fugita and S. Figita, 1964; Skoff *et al.,* 1976*b*; Imamoto *et al.,* 1978). Thus, fully mature oligodendrocytes appear not to divide. In Section 5, in which we discuss the process of remyelination of adult tissue, we will suggest that oligodendrocyte precursors, rather than mature oligodendrocytes, are involved in this process.

The reaction of mature oligodendrocytes during Wallerian degeneration in the optic nerve of young adult rats has been studied with the EM (Skoff, 1975) and by autoradiographic techniques (Skoff and Vaughn, 1971). Other than a slight hypertrophy and an increase in the content of lysosomes, the number and appearance of these cells showed very little change during the course of Wallerian degeneration, in contrast to the behavior of both astrocytes and microglial cells. This is also in marked contrast to the reaction of myelinating Schwann cells during Wallerian degeneration. Schwann cells have been shown to autophagocytose myelin membranes and debris and to divide vigorously during myelin breakdown in peripheral nerves (Abercrombie and Johnson, 1946; Asbury, 1975; Hall and Gregson, 1975; Salzer and Bunge, 1980). At advanced stages of Wallerian degeneration, oligodendrocytes appear to produce membranes that surround their own surfaces or ensheath astrocytic processes (J. E. Vaughn and Pease, 1970). The production of membranes by axon-deprived mature oligodendrocytes has also been noted in cultures of bulk-isolated cells (Poduslo *et al.,* 1982). One may conclude from these observations that the mature oligodendrocyte, if not itself damaged, may be relatively indifferent to drastic changes in its environment.

5. CENTRAL NERVOUS SYSTEM REMYELINATION

It is now firmly established that remyelination of central axons that have undergone demyelination may occur in a variety of experimental conditions (for reviews see R. P. Bunge, 1968; Ludwin, 1981; Sears, 1982). Because CNS axons generally do not regenerate, preservation of axon continuity is required for remyelination to occur. Remyelination frequently, though not invariably, is accompanied by varying degrees of astrocytic scarring. It is not our purpose here to review the various agents that may cause central demyelination; this has been done recently in admirable detail by Ludwin (1981). He points out that demyelination may result from direct damage to the myelin sheath or by damage to oligodendrocytes, with subsequent damage to the myelin sheath. Examples of the latter situation include viral infections of the oligodendrocyte by JHM mouse hepatitis virus and papovavirus (causing progressive multifocal leukoencephalopathy). Under the heading of conditions that primarily affect the myelin sheath, Ludwin (1981) lists hexachlorophene toxicity, lysolecithin-induced demyelination, cyanide toxicity, and the immune-mediated diseases experimental allergic encephalomyelitis (and neuritis), as well as immune-mediated viral diseases such as canine distemper virus demyelination. Demyelination can also be caused by physical damage, as in mechanical compression and CSF barbotage. The human neurological disease multiple sclerosis (MS) is thought to involve both viral and immune mechanisms. In each of these diseases, some degree of remyelination occurs; the relative paucity of remyelination following the extensive demyelination in MS remains an enigma.

The mechanisms by which new myelin sheaths are constructed in remyelination appears to be similar to that seen in initial myelin formation (R. P. Bunge, 1968) and will not be detailed here. Instead, we will review those cases in which substantial study of the cellular events leading up to remyelination is available. It should be noted that central remyelination can also be accomplished by Schwann cells in certain instances (see, for example, Blakemore, 1976; Dal Canto and Lipton, 1980).

Remyelination was first studied in detail in demyelination of the spinal cord caused by CSF barbotage (M. B. Bunge *et al.,* 1961). This manipulation causes, by mechanisms that are not understood, an acute loss of myelin and oligodendrocytes in superficial portions of the spinal cord white matter. Within 2 weeks , the demyelinated area is invaded by reacting glial cells, and both astroglial scarring and remyelination occur during the next several months. The invading cells were manifestly hypertrophic as they undertook this dual activity; later, definitive astrocytes and oligodendrocytes were identified in the lesion. The authors comment on the similarity of cells seen early in the lesion to reactive astrocytes. In light of the foregoing discussion of glial precursor cells, and the early date of this study, it now seems reasonable to suggest that more than one type of reacting glial cell may have been present in the early lesion. A separate autoradiographic study of the barbotage lesion (Koenig *et al.,* 1962) presented evidence that proliferation of a small glial cell (considered to be an oligodendrocyte) was occurring along the borders of the lesion early in the demyelinating period.

A second study presenting evidence on the source of cells responsible for remyelination involved the use of JHM mouse hepatitis virus (Herndon *et al.,*

1977). The response varies somewhat from that described above in that little astrocytic scarring occurs in this lesion and a remarkably complete remyelination is observed. This brief report presented evidence that the remyelinating oligodendrocytes contained [^{3}H]-TdR from an injection made several days previously. This observation indicated that these cells had undergone prior cell division, but did not establish whether the cells labeled at the time of thymidine injection were derived from mature oligodendrocytes or from undifferentiated precursors.

The most complete studies of remyelination have been carried out following the administration of the toxic agent Cuprizone (Ludwin, 1978). The advantages of the Cuprizone model of demyelination and remyelination in the mouse are that the demyelination occurs consistently in a predictable region— the superior cerebellar peduncle—and that remyelination occurs along axons in a predictable temporal pattern. Oligodendrocyte degeneration is seen 2 weeks after the onset of treatment, followed by myelin breakdown; after 6–8 weeks, all the axons of the superior cerebellar peduncle are demyelinated, and after several additional weeks, a substantial astrocytosis occurs. Within 1 week after the animals are returned to normal diet, remyelination commences. The axons are invested by the cytoplasmic processes of oligodendrocytes that insinuate themselves between the bare axons and the copious astrocyte processes. These processes wrap around the axons in a spiral fashion, forming inner and outer cytoplasmic tongues as the myelin sheath begins to form. Ludwin points out that an interesting feature of this remyelination is the presence of clusters of remyelinated axons, suggesting that all the axons in the neighborhood of a single oligodendrocyte and its processes may be myelinated at the same time. After 6 or 7 weeks on a normal diet, remyelination has progressed substantially throughout the peduncle.

In a detailed LM and EM autoradiographic study of cellular proliferation in the various phases of this lesion, Ludwin (1979a) observed labeled cells (immediately after thymidine injection) from about the 3rd week of demyelination; these remained numerous until demyelination was almost complete. In the 1st week of remyelination, labeled cells were seen infrequently and thereafter very rarely. In animals injected during the 5th and 6th weeks of demyelination and killed at later times, labeled cells were seen up to the 3rd week of remyelination.

EM autoradiography allowed identification of the labeled cells. The first labeled cells (those labeled between the 2nd and 3rd weeks of demyelination) were macrophages. During the 3rd through 6th weeks of demyelination, many astrocytes were labeled. From the 5th week of demyelination, labeled cells described as immature or reactive glial cells (Ludwin, 1979a) became apparent and could be found up to the 1st week of remyelination. Many of these cells had large nuclei with clumped heterochromatin with cytoplasm containing abundant ribosomes, microtubules, and endoplasmic reticulum. Some resembled light or medium oligodendrocytes; mature oligodendrocytes did not take up the label at any stage during the experiment (if the animals were injected just prior to sacrifice). In animals injected with thymidine in the demyelinating phase and killed after 3 weeks or remyelination, labeled nuclei were seen in dark oligodendrocytes involved in remyelination. No evidence of mitotic activity was observed in the nearby subependymal zone of the 4th ventricle.

Of particular interest were the proliferating immature glial cells that appeared during the 4th and 5th weeks of the lesion. In commenting on these cells, Ludwin (1981) states:

> It is often difficult at this stage to determine whether these cells are of oligodendrocytic or astrocytic origin. The cells, which continue to undergo mitosis up to about the 6th or 7th week, then show features of maturation along oligodendroglial lines. There is a progressive darkening of their cytoplasm, with a increase in the number of microtubules. Their nuclei become rounder and darker and more clumping of the chromatin occurs. The maturation of these cells copies that seen in normal development of oligodendrocytes.

Ludwin concludes that

> the majority of the proliferating oligodendrocytes were derived from . . . immature glia . . . probably derived from undifferentiated reserve cells in the rodent brain.

By repeatedly administering Cuprizone to mice, E. S. Johnson and Ludwin (1981) have also been able to study recurrent demyelination in the CNS. In contrast to the first demyelination caused by Cuprizone, the recurrent demyelination was markedly protracted and resulted in a reduced inflammatory and glial reaction. The second remyelination occurred at a slower rate, varied in completeness, and appeared to be associated with a diminished regeneration of oligodendrocytes. The authors interpreted autoradiographic observations after thymidine injection as indicating that the cellular response resulting in oligodendrocyte regeneration was markedy diminished during the second bout of demyelination. Both this study and studies of very long-term demyelination with Cuprizone (Ludwin, 1980) suggest that a limiting factor in remyelination is the availability of cells capable of generating a new population of oligodendrocytes during the cellular reaciton to demyelination.

It is worth noting that in each of these three cases, substantial proliferation of glial cells at the borders of the lesion was documented, and thus one is led to the conclusion that proliferative activity may be a prerequisite for CNS remyelination. The precise nature of the reserve cells in adult remyelination is an unresolved question, as is the precise nature of the precursors of oligodendrocytes during embryonic development (see above). Is the reserve cell in adult white matter a nonmyelinating precursor cell capable only of differentiation as an oligodendrocyte? Or is the reserve cell a multipotential glioblast capable of generating both oligodendrocytes and astrocytes? Alternatively, it is possible that fully differentiated oligodendrocytes may detach from their myelin segments and undergo a proliferative phase prior to undertaking the process of remyelination? This latter possibility appears unlikely, but it should be noted that there is evidence that Schwann cells committed to myelin formation may (subsequent to myelin breakdown) undergo a proliferative phase prior to remyelination (for a review, see Salzer and Bunge, 1980).

Nonetheless, the most reasonable explanation for the capacity of adult white matter to remyelinate would appear to be that there exists undetected among the cells called interfascicular oligodendrocytes a reserve glial population not related to myelin segments. As Ludwin (1981) has recently pointed out, the understanding of the signal that engenders proliferation in this cell type would seem important in understanding why the process of remyelination is sometimes minimal (as in MS and in diptheria toxin demyelination) and in other cases is remarkably complete (as in the JHM mouse hepatitis virus lesion).

6. TISSUE-CULTURE STUDIES OF OLIGODENDROCYTE DEVELOPMENT

Nearly all of what we now know about oligodendrocytes has been learned from studies of this cell *in situ*. However, whereas the general timetable and some descriptive aspects of oligodendrocyte development and function have been reasonably well sketched out, as discussed in the previous sections, relatively little information has appeared about what factors influence oligodendrocyte differentiation. Both intrinsic facts (e.g., genetic controls or internal "clocks") and extrinsic factors (e.g., the cellular and humoral environment) are undoubtedly important. In recent years, several investigators have begun using cell- and tissue-culture methods in the hope of gaining new insights into how oligodendrocytes and other cells in the nervous system function. Within the past two years, at least four new methods for the bulk isolation of oligodendrocytes have been reported, all of which yield viable cells capable of being maintained for long periods in culture, in high purity (Gebicke-Harter *et al.*, 1981; McCarthy and de Vellis, 1980; Szuchet *et al.*, 1980; Lisak *et al.*, 1981). Such preparations have been used mainly to determine the biochemical properties of these cells as they may relate to myelination, and direct quantitative observations from such preparations as well as some information on the genetic control of myelination are described in other chapters. In this chapter, we will focus on some of the studies of oligodendrocytes in "mixed"cultures that have yielded new information on oligodendrocyte development. Three different types of mixed cultures are widely used and are usually designated simply as explant monolayer, or aggregate cultures.

The "explant" culture method has been in use the longest and is well characterized for some CNS tissues, especially spinal cord (e.g. Sobkowitcz *et al.,* 1968) and cerebellum [see the review by Seil (1977)]. In this method, a small piece of tissue is excised and immobilized on a coverslip coated with an adhesive substrate, collagen, and maintained in a complex nutrient medium containing serum and sometimes embryo extract. The simplest such cultures contain two distinct zones, the region of the explant and the outgrowth zone. Within the explant, spatial relationships between neuronal groups are often retained, as are connecting fiber tracts, and functional synapses are formed. Many neurons are lost soon after explantation (often as many as 75%), but those that survive are reasonably stable for several weeks. The outgrowth zone consists of neurites emanating from the explant, some migrating neurons (e.g., granule cells), glial cells, and connective-tissue cells. Much of the neuritic component of the outgrowth zone is lost in the absence of target tissues by several weeks into the culture period. The glial-cell outgrowth continues to expand and often forms a monolayer of cells around the explant. An interesting feature of these cultures is that while central myelin forms predictably in the explant zone, relatively little myelin is formed in the outgrowth, even though both neurites and glial cells are present there. This deficiency stands in marked contrast to the outgrowth areas of explant cultures of peripheral sensory ganglia, where abundant stable myelin is formed by Schwann cells.

Myelination in CNS explants was first observed by Hild (1957) in cultures of newborn cat cerebellum. In retrospect, this observation can be appreciated as the first demonstration that oligodendrocyte maturation in its entirety might proceed *in vitro,* and while the oligodendrocytes themselves could rarely, if ever, be directly visualized, the highly refractile myelin segments denoting maturation were clearly visible by LM even within the depth of the tissue.

Subsequently, explant cultures of cerebellum and spinal cord have been used extensively by Bornstein, Seil, and others in the study of possible immunological mechanisms of demyelinating diseases, such as MS and the experimental animal disease experimental allergic encephalomyelitis (EAE) (reviewed in Seil, 1977). In the course of these studies, it was found (Raine and Bornstein, 1970) that demyelination of cultures by EAE serum was reversible, indicating that the oligodendrocytes or the myelin segments or both lost after treatment with the immune sera were regenerated or renewed. After several such demyelinating episodes, however, no replacement of myelin (or oligodendrocytes) could be observed. These studies suggest that while the oligodendrocyte population might have a reserve or regenerative capacity, this capacity may be limited.

Furthermore, using cultures of embryonic spinal cord, it was discovered that very small concentrations of antiserum in the presence of complement could either prevent remyelination after demyelination or prevent initial myelin formation in developing cultures (Bornstein and Raine, 1970). This phenomenon was also reversible; i.e., washing out the antiserum permitted myelination or remyelination to occur. EM analysis of the inhibited cultures showed a total absence of differentiated oligodendrocytes.

The effects of antiserum just discussed were all complement-dependent phenomena. In a sequential analysis of the myelin breakdown in these cultures, it was observed that an increased birefringence of the sheaths preceded the rapid breakdown of the myelin. The increase in birefringence could be separated from the myelin breakdown by incubating the cultures in antiserum without complement. In such cultures, the width of the myelin lamella was doubled and the intraperiod line became invisible, but the myelin did not break down and could be maintained in this swollen state for several weeks.

When cultures were treated with antiserum without complement at the beginning of myelin formation, mature myelin did not form (Diaz et al., 1978). Instead, the oligodendrocytes produced a large number of processes that appeared to wander aimlessly, without ensheathing axons in their vicinity. This abnormal behavior of the oligodendrocyte was considered evidence that myelination could be blocked between the stages of process growth and axon ensheathment.

The antiserum used in all these studies has recently been shown immunocytochemically to bind specifically to oligodendrocytes at or near the surface of explants of fetal mouse spinal cord (Bonnaud-Toulze et al., 1981). Oligodendrocytes could be stained nearly a full week before the appearance of myelin (i.e., by the 5th day in vitro) and were stained over the entire plasmalemma including the inner and outer mesaxons of the myelin sheaths. Often, reaction product was found in the periaxonal space. Staining could be observed before, during, and after myelination.

There has been considerable controversy over the nature of the antigen(s) with which EAE serum reacts to cause demyelination (for reviews, see Seil, 1977; Saida et al., 1970; Bonnaud-Toulze et al., 1981), but it is believed not to be MBP. It may be of interest to note here that one of the earliest recognized candidates for the antigen was galactocerebroside (GalCer) which has subsequently been shown to be an immunological marker for oligodendrocytes. Fry et al. (1974) reported that rabbit antisera to GalCer inhibited myelination and caused demyelination of cultures. This observation was confirmed by Hruby et al., (1977) with rabbit antisera to synthetic GalCer. Recently, A. Johnson and Bornstein (1978) have confirmed that antisera to GalCer and EAE sera bind to and affect CNS cultures in much the same way. Thus, it seems possible that GalCer is one of the antigens recognized by some EAE antisera.

The experiments just described illustrate that specific and reversible manipulation of the oligodendrocytes can be achieved in explant cultures. The oligodendrocytes destroyed by the antisera were rapidly replaced several times within the same explant, implying the coexistence of a morphologically and antigenically distinct precursor along with the myelinating oligodendrocytes.

Despite the advantages offered by explant cultures, the complexity retained by such preparations presents many obstacles to a complete analysis of cellular behavior. For this reason, "aggregate" and "monolayer" culture methods have become increasingly preferred, but these are relatively younger and less well characterized. In both these methods, the tissue chosen is enzymatically or mechanically dissociated before culturing. In the "aggregate" method (Honegger and Richelson, 1976; Seeds, 1973; Trapp et al., 1979), the cells are prevented from attaching to a substrate and instead are forced to form spherical aggregates of different sizes by gentle rotation on a shaker. Initially, these aggregates appear homogeneous and consist of randomly distributed neurons and glial cells. By a few weeks in culture, neurons, astrocytes, and oligodendrocytes appear well differentiated and are segregated, with neurons and oligodendrocytes occupying the middle of the aggregates and astrocytes and mononuclear cells in the other half of the sphere. Both synapse and myelin formation and changes in biochemical activity reflect progressive differentiation in these cultures. By 5–6 weeks, however, most of the neurons and oligodendrocytes present initially have died and the aggregates appear to become homogeneous once more, consisting predominantly of astrocytes (Trapp et al., 1979).

An interesting feature of these cultures was noted in correlated morphological and biochemical studies (Trapp et al., 1979). In older cultures, when neither neurons, neuronal processes, nor synapses could be found, there was still an undiminished activity of some neurotransmitter enzymes (Matthieu et al., 1978). Furthermore, after the disappearance of myelinated axons, both MBP and 2′,3′-cyclic nucleotide 3′-phosphohydrolase were found in substantial quantities (Trapp et al., 1979). The significance of these biochemical activities in the absence of correlated morphological structure remains to be clarified.

While the study of oligodendrocytes in aggregate cultures has not yielded much new information about the oligodendrocyte, the reproducibility in aggregate organization, the amounts of tissue that can be maintained in vitro, and the production of myelin sheaths are all positive features that make this the preferred approach of many workers.

In the monolayer approach, a mixed population of cells obtained from dissociation of immature rat brain is plated into culture dishes in nutrient medium and allowed to adhere to the substrate (e.g., Yavin and Yavin, 1977;

McCarthy and deVellis, 1980). In some instances, this method does not favor neuronal survival, and over a period of several weeks, the following phenomena occur: A confluent layer of flat cells believed to consist mainly of astrocytes, endothelial cells, and connective tissue cells forms over the entire culture surface. Sometimes this layer is more than one cell thick; i.e., it becomes a multilayer of cells. On top of this layer, small process-bearing cells (believed to be primarily oligodendrocytes) form aggregates or networks that are loosely attached to the underlying layer. Many of these cells may float off into the supernatant medium or be shaken off by gentle agitation of the dish. McCarthy and de Vellis (1980) presented morphological and immunohistochemical evidence that many of these cells were oligodendrocytes and that they could be separated from the underlying cells and subsequently cultured.

Neurons clearly do survive, however, in some types of monolayer cultures (see for example Raju et al., 1981), but the degree of neuronal survival appears to be quite variable, possibly depending on the age and source of the dissociated tissue. In certain of these cultures, the small round process-bearing cells (presumed to be oligodendrocytes) also begin to disappear after several weeks, conceivably through disattachment or cell death (Rioux et al., 1980). After 8–10 weeks, such cultures consist mainly of astrocytes, phagocytic cells, and other more nondescript elements. Although synapses may form in monolayer cultures, myelin is either not formed at all or formed in very small quantities (Yavin and Yavin 1977).

Because the cells in monolayer cultures are readily accessible, this type of culture has been widely used for immunocytochemical studies of oligodendrocytic properties. In nearly all these studies the oligodendrocyte is defined by its reaction to antiserum to GalCer or to MBP, or to both. The specificity of antibody to GalCer for the myelinating oligodendrocyte was suggested by the presence of large amounts of this lipid in myelin and by the ability of the antibody to specifically bind to CNS myelin in explant cultures (A. Johnson and Bornstein, 1978). Raff et al., (1978) reported a study of the staining with antibodies to GalCer and glial fibrillary acidic protein (GFAP) of cells in cultures of enzymatically dissociated optic nerve from 6 to 8-day-old rats. About 5% of the cells in 5-day cultures were stained with the anti-GalCer; these were negative for GFAP. These cells had numerous long, thin, and branching processes and were considered to be oligodendrocytes. Mirsky et al. (1980) provided observations on the sequence of appearance of GalCer and MBP in oligodendrocytes in monolayer cultures prepared from embyronic or neonatal tissue. In 1-week-old cultures of neonatal tissue, 2–5% of the cells were identified as oligodendrocytes by anti-GalCer staining. This number did not change from 1 to 8 weeks in culture, suggestive of little mitotic activity in the oligodendrocyte population in such cultures.

These observations are relevant to an important and unresolved question concerning the control of oligodendrocyte proliferation and maturation, namely, what influences do axons exert on oligodendrocyte development? That axons may be important for oligodendrocyte development was indicated by the profound effect on this development in the optic nerve caused by removal of the eye just before the appearance of recognizable oligodendrocytes in the nerve (Fulcrand and Privat, 1977). When the eye was removed at 2 or 5 days postnatally, a few differentiated oligodendrocytes appeared by the 8th day: however, the dramatic increase in the number of these cells that would normally occur in the intact nerve was almost completely prevented. If the operation was carried out at 8 days postnatally, when well-differentiated oligodendrocytes comprised 20% of the glial population, no further increase occurred in this number postoperatively and the percentage of these cells subsequently decreased. Oligodendrocytes persisting after operations at later stages often appeared reactive, and eventually many of them appeared to become enwrapped in membranes resembling myelin (Fulcrand and Privat, 1977).

Although it is not clear from this study whether axons may be required for continued oligodendrocyte proliferation, or simply permit myelinogenic expression of these cells, the data would seem to justify further exploration along similar lines. It has been clearly demonstrated in the PNS that axons or dorsal-root-ganglion neurons are mitogenic for Schwann cells (Wood and Bunge 1975). In addition, we have observed (Wood, unpublished observations) that retinal axons are mitogenic for Schwann cells in culture, demonstrating the presence of a mitogenic component on axons that exist exclusively in the CNS. This is consistent with reported observations that an axolemmal membrane fraction isolated from CNS white matter is also mitogenic for Schwann cells (DeVries *et al.*, 1982; Cassel *et al.*, 1981). Finally, as noted in Section 5 (Ludwin, 1981), the proliferation of oligodendrocytes that precedes remyelination may be triggered by bare axons at the edges of the demyelinated lesion. Thus, the available evidence points to a possible, but as yet not directly demonstrated, role of axons in inducing division of oligodendrocytes or their precursors.

A rather sophisticated morphometric analysis of the proliferation and maturation of oligodendrocytes in monolayer cultures of dissociated diencephalon and telenephalon of 14-day mouse embryos was reported by Rioux *et al.* (1980). In their cultures, the small round cells that segregated on top of the confluent astrocyte carpet were identified as oligodendrocytes by ultrastructural criteria and were counted and measured at various times *in vitro*. The number per unit area of these cells increased remarkably from about the 9th to the 15th day of culture and then declined. Proliferation of both large (7.5-μm-diameter) and medium (4.8-μm-in diameter) cells of this type was observed. After this proliferation phase, the oligodendrocytelike cells disappeared and were essentially gone by the 27th day *in vitro*. Monolayer cultures prepared in this way from early embryonic tissue are likely to contain (at least initially) considerable numbers of surviving neurons; the presence of neurons might explain the proliferation of oligodendrocytes (or their precursors) that was observed.

Recently, it has been shown that the nonproliferating oligodendrocytes in mixed monolayers of neonatal cerebellum or corpus callosum do not respond either to pituitary extract, which is mitogenic for Schwann cells and astrocytes, or to fibroblast or epidermal growth factors (Pruss *et al.*, 1981). However, after 3–4 weeks, cells that were identified as oligodendrocytes by reacting with antibody to GalCer or MBP could occasionally be floated off into the supernatant of these cultures and replated with good efficiency onto carpets of X-irradiated 3T3 cells. The labeling index of these replated cells was strikingly increased compared to those replated onto glass or plastic, so that as many as 50% of them incorporated [AH]-TdR after 2 days of labeling. A mitogenic stimulation of oligodendrocytes could not be produced by either 3T3-cell-conditioned medium or substrate.

The role of axons in inducing or regulating myelinating activity in oligodendrocytes remains to be clarified. There is evidence that axons are among the factors that regulate myelinating activity in Schwann cells in the PNS (Bray *et al.*, 1981; reviewed in Weinberg and Spencer, 1976; Skoff, 1980). However, there is a growing body of evidence from experiments on oligodendrocytes in culture that the continued expression of specific myelin components does not require the presence of axons.

When Mirsky *et al.* (1980) prepared monolayer cultures from 5 to 8-day-old rat cerebellum, optic nerve, or corpus callosum and stained them after 1–10 weeks in culture with antibodies to MBP and GalCer, they found a perfect overlap in staining; i.e., all the MBP-positive cells were also GalCer-positive and vice versa. However, when cells were cultured from neonatal optic nerve GalCer-positive cells could be found by 1 day *in vitro*, but MBP staining was observed only after 5–6 days in culture.

The immunological staining patterns just described were observed in the absence of neurons (e.g., in cultures of dissociated optic nerve). They suggested to Mirsky *et al.* (1980) that oligodendrocytes did not need a continuing signal from neurons to produce myelin-specific molecules. This was in marked contrast to their observations of the failure of Schwann cells to make myelin-specific molecules when the neurons were absent. The results further seemed to imply that myelin-specific glycolipids were earlier indicators of the cells' commitment to myelination than was the presence of MBP. The time of MBP appearance in the oligodendrocytes from optic nerve was remarkably close to the time when the cells would have been forming myelin had they remained in the animal.

In still more recent experiments to explore developmental parallels between glial cells in dissociated monolayers and *in vivo*, Abney *et al.* (1981) dissociated embryonic rat brain tissue at 10 days of gestation and subsequently compared the age at which cells could be stained with specific antibodies in cultures to that at which their cousins *in situ* could be stained in fresh suspension. They reported a remarkable correspondence in the staining pattern *in vitro* and *in vivo*. Thus, for example, GFAP-positive astrocytes could be first found in fresh suspensions of dissociated brain at 15–16 days of gestation or in 5 to 6-day-old cultures of brain cells prepared from embryos at 10 days of gestation. Similarly, GalCer-positive cells (oligodendrocytes) were first found in fresh suspensions of cells from brains of 2 to 3-day-postnatal animals and in 13 to 14-day-old cultures of brains dissociated at 10 days of gestation (gestation = 21.5 days in rat). Results such as these have been interpreted to mean that the developmental expression of some of the cell-specific properties of glial cells, including oligodendrocytes, are controlled by some sort of internal "clock," rather than by interactions between cells. However, because some neurons were present in these cultures, interactions of glial cells with axons may have occurred; thus, the possibility that axons may have influenced glial maturation was not ruled out.

Roussel *et al.* (1981) reported that oligodendrocytes in mixed monolayer (or multilayer) cultures of newborn rat brain hemispheres progressively developed the capacity to react with antisera to MBP and to Wolfgram protein. A few of the cells they identified as oligodendrocytes were stained by antibodies to MBP by the 8th day in culture. After 4 weeks, most of the oligodendrocytes were stainable with both MBP and Wolfgram protein. Roussel *et al.* (1981) observed that while the synthesis of the myelin proteins did occur in their cultures, myelin sheaths were not formed.

In an extensive study of the staining of oligodendrocytes by antibodies to both GalCer and MBP antisera from several different laboratories were compared (Bologa-Sandru *et al.*, 1981). A total of 20 different antisera to GalCer and 8 different antisera to MBP were used. All these antisera gave similar staining in the cultures tested on successive days of incubation (at 7, 14, 21, and 28 days *in vitro*). At 7 days *in vitro,* only staining with anti-GalCer sera was found, but by 14 days *in vitro,* cells stained with both anti-MBP and anti-GalCer were seen. By 28 days *in vitro* the number of MBP and GalCer-positive cells was only 3% of the number of cells staining with anti-GalCer alone. Thus 97% of the oligodendrocytes identified with anti-GalCer never developed a detectable MBP content. A slow increase in the number of GalCer-positive oligodendrocytes occurred in these cultures over the 4-week culture period. Because neuronal survival, and thus the possibility of axon–glial interaction, was not evaluated in the last two studies, they did not resolve the issue of neuronal influence on myelin-component expression by oligodendrocytes.

The developmental expression of antigens by oligodendrocytes in mono-layers was also studied by Schachner et al. (1981) and by Berg and Schachner (1981). The antigens studied were those defined by monoclonal antibodies O1, O2, O3, and O4 the specificity of which had been characterized by their lack of reactivity with neurons, astrocytes, or fibroblasts in vitro, by morphological studies of tissue sections of intact brain, and by identification of the stained cells by EM criteria. The antibody designated O1 was found to stain only cells that also stained with GalCer antibodies, but O2, O3, and O4 antibodies stained other unclassified cells. Schachner et al. (1981) felt that antibodies O3 and O4 were staining an early form of oligodendrocyte that could not be stained with anti-GalCer. In monolayer cultures of 13-day embryonic mouse cerebellum, O3 and O4 staining could be found by the 3rd day in vtiro, which would correspond to the 16th embryonic day. O1 staining was definite by the 5th day in vitro, corresponding to the 18th embryonic day. Considering the immaturity of the cerebellum in vivo at embryonic day 18, these studies indi-cate the earliest development of cells with oligodendrocyte characteristics yet reported. These cells made up approximately 2–3% of the total cell population by 1 week in culture.

To summarize these results from studies of monolayer cultures, oligoden-drocytes appear to be capable of a continued synthesis of the myelin-specific substances GalCer and MBP without synthesizing myelin sheaths, and even in the absence of neurons. Furthermore, GalCer appears to be present in or on oligodendrocytes before MBP can be detected. Finally, the continued prolif-eration of oligodendrocytes is poor when neurons are absent, as in optic-nerve cultures, but some increase in number of oligodendrocyte-like cells does occur in cultures in which neurons are more likely to be present (e.g., cultures of dissociated embryonic brain). Nonetheless, the numbers of oligodendrocytes in these cultures remain low (a few percent or less). In one instance, their prolif-eration was stimulated by the presence of nondividing 3T3 cells. In general, the morphological relationships between oligodendrocytes and persisting axons in these cultures have not been studied systematically.

The variable survival of CNS neurons in monolayer cultures has detracted from the usefulness of such cultures in assessing the potential role of neurons to induce or stimulate oligodendrocyte proliferation and myelin synthesis. To conclude this discussion of observations on oligodendrocytes in culture, we would like to briefly describe a new approach in which the sine qua non for the formation of myelin sheaths, a stable axonal population capable of inducing myelination, is ensured (Wood et al., 1980). In this approach glial cells are added to networks of dissociated dorsal-root-ganglion (DRG) neurons (Figure 6a, b) after the suppression of endogenous Schwann cells and fibroblasts by fluorodeoxyuridine. Because axons of the DRG cells normally grow into the CNS, where many of them are myelinated by oligodendrocytes, normal axon–

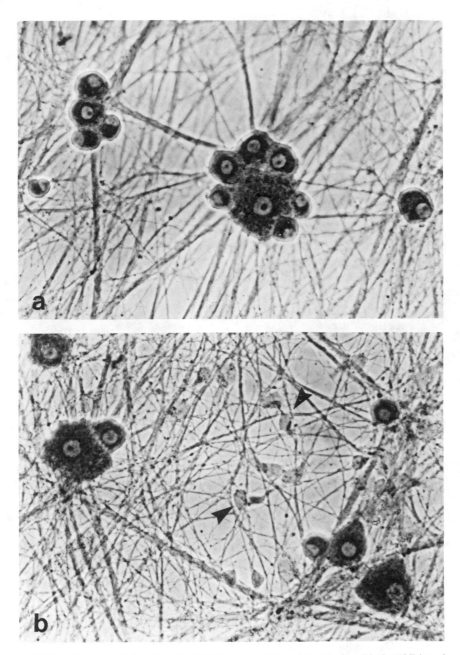

FIGURE 6. Network of dissociated rat DRG neurons before (a) and after (b) the addition of glial cells from embryonic spinal cord. Endogenous Schwann cells and fibroblasts were suppressed by treatment with 10^{-5} M fluorodeoxyuridine for 2 weeks prior to the addition of glial cells. (a) Networks prepared from older embryos (days 19–21 of gestation) and containing both large and small neuronal somata and an extensive outgrowth of naked axons that have some tendency to form thick fascicles. (b) A similar network 5 days after the addition at low density of mechanically dissociated spinal cord cells taken from embryos on day 15 of gestation. Two glial cells. Stained with Sudan black. ×340.

oligodendrocyte interactions might be expected in such cultures. We have observed a dramatic proliferation of glial cells obtained by mechanical dissociation of embryonic spinal-cord fragments and seeded at low density (Figure 6b) onto the extensive fascicles of naked axons (Figure 6a) contained in these cultures. Axons became extensively myelinated in areas of either high or low cell density. The myelin sheaths were visible by LM and the myelinating oligodendrocytes could be easily stained by antibodies (Figure 7a, b). Myelination in larger fascicles was remarkably complete, as shown in Figure 8, which is an electron micrograph of such a fascicle 8 weeks after the addition of glia obtained from the spinal cord of a rat embryo at day 15 of gestation. Often, such fascicles were completely surrounded by astrocyte processes. Axons within the fascicles were partitioned into smaller groups by astrocytes processes that were easily recognized in electron micrographs by their content of filaments. It should be emphasized that the entire course of oligodendrocyte development was encompassed in these cultures, including proliferation, maturation, and the formation of intact myelin sheaths.

A major advantage of this approach is that the neurons and glial cells can be obtained separately, and various recombinations of these cells can be undertaken in the cultures. Similar experiments have proven to be fruitful in the study of cellular interactions among neurons, Schwann cells, and fibroblasts from the PNS (Wood and Bunge, 1975; Salzer and Bunge, 1980; Salzer *et al.*, 1980*a,b;* M. B. Bunge *et al.*, 1980, 1982; Carey *et al.*, 1981). Since methods have been devised for obtaining pure oligodendrocytes from both developing and adult tissue and pure astrocytes from developing tissue, the prospects for evaluating the importance of cell–cell interactions and humoral factors for oligodendrocyte development seem particularly encouraging.

7. CONCLUSION

It is possible to construct a brief (and in part speculative) life history of the oligodendrocyte (in rodents) based on the available information as reviewed in the foregoing sections. At an as yet undetermined point in the embryonic period, ventricular or subventricular cells are induced to enter the oligodendrocyte lineage; the inducing factors are not yet known. Following their recruitment, these cells continue to proliferate slowly while migrating to occupy positions throughout the developing and expanding neuropil. These migrating cells, relatively few in number, contain only a small amount of organelle-poor cytoplasm characterized by the presence of many free ribosomes and polysomes, and they exhibit few processes. Just before myelination begins, these cells cease migrating but undergo accelerated proliferation to form the interfascicular rows of oligodendrocytes that begin to exhibit cytoplasmic characteristics that

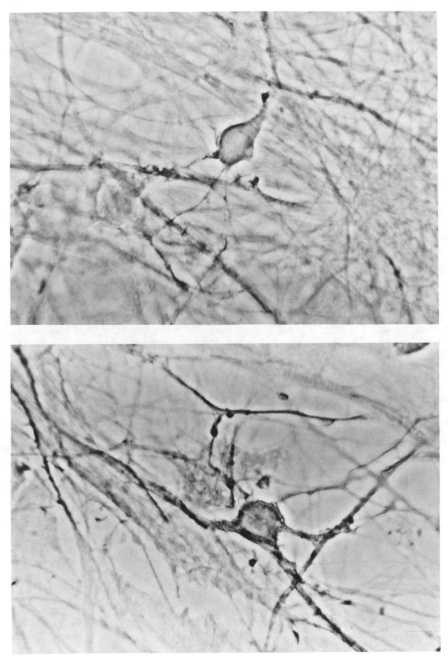

FIGURE 7. Myelinating oligodendrocytes in cultures of dissociated DRG neurons stained by antibodies to proteolipid protein. These cultures were prepared as described in the Figure 6 caption. The antibody stains the cell soma, the processes, and the myelin segments in the cells shown. The culture was fixed for staining 5 weeks after the addition of glial cells to the network. ×1130. (Courtesy of Dr. F. Mithen, using antibodies supplied by Dr. H. Agrawal.)

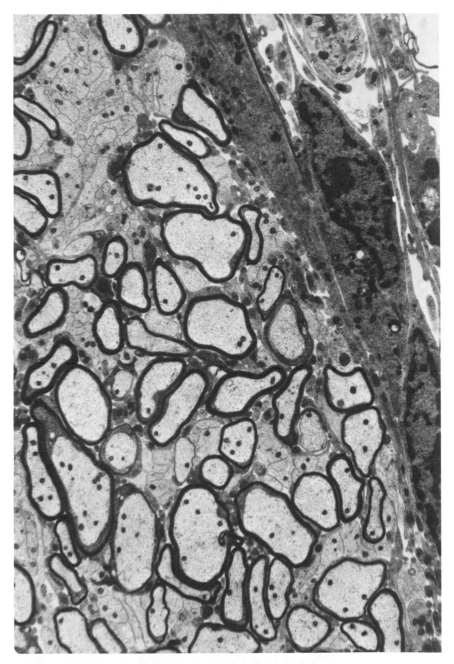

FIGURE 8. Electron micrograph of a portion of an extensively myelinated fascicle in a DRG network prepared as in Figure 6. The culture was fixed 8 weeks after the addition of glial cells at a density similar to that shown in Figure 6b. While most of the large axons have become myelinated, the small-diameter axons remain unmyelinated. A glial sheath composed of astrocyte-cell bodies and their processes completely surrounds this fascicle and is seen here along the right margin of the photograph. ×11,000.

distinguish them as oligodendrocytes. It is during the final round of cell division that these oligodendrocytes begin to exhibit many processes that enwrap neighboring axons; myelin-sheath formation then begins with the cessation of cell division. A given oligodendrocyte would require several weeks for the synthesis of complete myelin membranes and the consolidation of its several myelin sheaths. At the end of this period, the mature oligodendrocyte retains the capability to restore components of the myelin sheath that are lost through normal turnover mechanisms, but as a terminally differentiated cell does not have the capability to construct new myelin sheaths. In the mature state, the cell is relatively unresponsive to drastic changes in its environment. Remyelination, which requires construction of entirely new myelin segments, is dependent on a prior proliferation of undifferentiated stem cells that are retained in relatively small numbers among the mature cells.

The speculative aspects of this view of the life history of the oligodendrocyte result from at least three significant gaps in our knowledge of oligodendrocytes. These gaps center around the following questions: (1) What is the nature of the cells from which new oligodendrocytes (or their distinctive precursors) arise, either during development or during remyelination? (2) What intrinsic and extrinsic factors direct oligodendrocyte recruitment, proliferation, and maturation? (3) What are the capabilities of the fully expressed mature oligodendrocyte, especially with regard to myelin repair or remyelination or both? The answers to these questions appear to be crucial for understanding the process of normal myelination in the CNS, as well as the induction of and recovery from demyelinating lesions.

ACKNOWLEDGMENTS

We would like to acknowledge the helpful comments of Dr. Robert P. Skoff, as well as his kind donation of the electron-microscopic autoradiograph used in Figure 4. We also wish to thank Ms. Susan Mantia for preparing the manuscript. This work was supported by National Multiple Sclerosis Society Grant RG 1118 and NIH Grant NS 09923.

8. REFERENCES

Abercrombie, M., and Johnson, M., 1946, Quantitative histology of Wallerian degeneration. I. Nuclear population in rabbit sciatic nerve, *J. Anat.* **80**:37–50.
Abney, E. R., Bartlett, P., and Raff, M. C., 1981, Astrocytes, ependymal cells, and oligodendro-

cytes develop on schedule in dissociated cell cultures of embryonic rat brain, *Dev. Biol.* 83:301–310.

Asbury, A., 1975, The biology of Schwann cells, in: *Peripheral Neuropathy*, Vol. I (P. Dyck, P. K. Thomas, and E. H. Lambert, eds.), W. B. Saunders, Philadelphia, pp. 201–212.

Berg, G., and Schachner, M., 1981, Immuno-electron microscopic identification of O-antigen-bearing oligodendroglial cells *in vitro*, *Cell Tissue Res.* 21:313–325.

Bischoff, R., 1979, Tissue culture studies on the origin of myogenic cells during muscle regeneration in the rat, in: *Muscle Regeneration* (A. Mauro, ed.), pp. 13–29, Raven Press, New York.

Blakemore, W. F., 1976, Invasion of Schwann cells into the spinal cord of the rat following local injection of lysolecithin, *Neuropathol. Appl. Neurobiol.* 2:21–39.

Bologa-Sandru, L., Siegrist, H. P., Zgraggen, H., Hofmann, K., Wiesmann, U., Dahl, D., and Herschkowitz, N., 1981, Expression of antigenic markers during the development of oligodendrocytes in mouse brain cultures, *Brain Res.* 210:217–229.

Bonnaud-Toulze, E., Johnson, A., Bornstein, M., and Raine, C., 1981, A marker for oligodendrocytes and its relation to myelinogenesis: An immunocytochemical study with experimental allergic encephalomyelitis serum and C. N. S. cultures, *J. Neurocytol.* 10:645–657.

Bornstein, M., and Raine, C., 1970, Experimental allergic encephalomyelitis: Antiserum inhibition of myelination *in vitro*, *Lab. Invest.* 23:536–542.

Bray, G. M., Rasminsky, M. and Aguayo, A., 1981, Interactions between axons and their sheath cells, *Annu. Rev. Neurosci.* 4:127–162.

Bunge, M. B., Bunge, R. P., and Ris., H., 1961, Ultrastructural study of remyelination in an experimental lesion in adult cat spinal cord, *J. Biophys. Biochem. Cytol.* 10:67–94.

Bunge, M. B., Bunge, R. P., and Pappas, G. D., 1962, Electron microscopic demonstrations of connections between glia and myelin sheaths in the developing mammalian central nervous system, *J. Cell Biol.* 12:448–453.

Bunge, M. B., Williams, A. K., Wood, P. M., Uitto, J., and Jeffrey, J., 1980, Comparison of nerve cell and nerve cell plus Schwann cell cultures, with particular emphasis on basal lamina and collagen production, *J. Cell Biol.* 84:184–202.

Bunge, M. B., Williams, A. K., and Wood, P. M., 1982, Neuron–Schwann cell interaction in basal lamina formation, *Dev. Biol.* 92:449–460.

Bunge, R. P., 1968, Glial cells and the central myelin sheath, *Physiol. Rev.* 48:197–251.

Caley, D., and Maxwell, D. S., 1968, An electron microscopic study of the neuroglia during postnatal development of the rat cerebellum, *J. Comp. Neurol.* 133:45–70.

Carey, D. J., and Bunge, R. P., 1981, Factors influencing the release of proteins by cultured Schwann cells, *J. Cell Biol.* 91:666–672.

Cassel, D., Wood, P., Bunge, R. P., and Glaser, L., 1982, Mitogenicity of brain axolemma membranes and soluble factors for dorsal root ganglion Schwann cells, *J. Cell Biochem.* 18:443–445.

Colman, D. R., Kreibich, G., Frey, A. B., and Sabatini, D. D., 1982, Synthesis and incorporation of myelin polypeptides into CNS myelin, *J. Cell Biol.* 95:598–608.

Dal Canto, M. C., and Lipton, H. L., 1980, Schwann cell remyelination and recurrent demyelination in the central nervous system of mice infected with attenuated Theiler's virus, *Am. J. Pathol.* 98:101–122.

Del Cerro, M., and Schwarz, J., 1976, Prenatal development of Bergmann glial fibers in rodent cerebellum, *J. Neurocytol.* 5:669–676.

Del Rio Hortega, P., 1921, Estudios obre la neuroglia: La glia de escasas radiaciones (oligodendroglia), *Bol. R. Soc. Esp. Hist. Nat.* 21:63–92.

Del Rio Hortega, P., 1922, Son homologables la glia de escasas radiaciones y la celula de Schwann?, *Bol. R. Soc. Esp. Hist. Nat.* 10:25–29.

Del Rio Hortega, P., 1924, La glie a radiations peu nombreuses et la cellule de Schwann sont elles homologables?, *C. R. Soc. Biol.* **91:**818–820.

Del Rio Hortega, P., 1928, Tercera aportación al conocimiento morfologico e interpretación funcional de la oligodendroglia, *Mem. R. Soc. Esp. Hist. Nat.* **14:**5–122.

DeVries, G. H., Salzer, J. L., and Bunge, R. P., 1982, Axolemma-enriched fractions isolated from PNS and CNS are mitogenic for Schwann cells, *Dev. Brain Res.* **3:**295–299.

Diaz, M., Bornstein, M., and Raine, C. S., 1978, Disorganization of myelinogenesis in cultures by anti-CNS antisera, *Brain Res.* **154:**231–239.

Fry, J., Weissbarth, S., Lehrer, G., and Bornstein, M., 1974, Cerebroside antibody inhibits sulfatide synthesis and myelination and demyelinates in cord tissue cultures, *Science* **183:**540–542.

Fugita, H., and Figita, S., 1964, Electron microscopic studies on the differentiation of the ependymal cells and the glioblast in the spinal cord of domestic fowl, *Z. Zellforsch.* **64:**262–272.

Fugita, S., 1963, The matrix cell and cytogenesis in the developing central nervous system, *J. Comp. Neurol.* **120:**37–42.

Fugita, S., 1965, An autoradiographic study on the origin and fate of the sub-pial glioblast in the embryonic chick spinal cord, *J. Comp. Neurol.* **124:**51–60.

Fulcrand, J., and Privat, A., 1977, Neuroglial reactions secondary to Wallerian degeneration in the optic nerve of the postnatal rat: Ultrastructural and quantitative study, *J. Comp. Neurol.* **176:**189–224.

Gebicke-Harter, P., Althaus, H., Schwartz, P., and Neuhoff, V., 1981, Oligodendrocytes from postnatal cat brain in cell cultures. 1. Regeneration and maintenance, *Brain Res.* **227:**497–518.

Hall, S., and Gregson, N., 1975, The effects of mitomycin C on the process of regeneration in the mamalian peripheral nervous system, *Neuropathol. Appl. Neurobiol.* **1:**149–170.

Hardesty, I., 1904, On the development and nature of the neuroglia, *Am. J. Anat.* **3:**229–268.

Hardesty, I., 1905, On the occurrence of sheath cells and the nature of the axone sheaths in the central nervous system, *Am. J. Anat.* **4:**329–354.

Harkness, R. P., 1957, Regeneration of the liver, *Br. Med. Bull.* **13:**87–93.

Henrikson, C., and Vaughn, J., 1974, Fine structural relationships between neurites and radial glial processes in developing mouse spinal cord, *J. Neurocytol.* **3:**659–675.

Herndon, R. M., Price, D. L., and Weiner, P. P., 1977, Regeneration of oligodendroglia during recovery from demyelinating disease, *Science* **195:**693–694.

Hild, W., 1957, Myelinogenesis in cultures of mammalian nervous tissue, *Z. Zellforsch.* **46:**71–95.

Hinds, J. W., and Ruffett, T. L., 1974, Cell proliferation in the neural tube: An electron microscopic and Golgi analysis in the mouse cerebral vesicle, *Z. Zellforsch.* **115:**226–264.

Honegger, P., and Richelson, E., 1975, Biochemical differentiation of mechanically dissociated mammalian brain in aggregating cell cultures, *Brain Res.* **109:**335–354.

Hruby, S., Alvord, E., and Seil, F., 1977, Synthetic galactocerebrosides evoke myelination inhibiting antibodies, *Science* **195:**173–175.

Imamoto, K., Paterson, J., and Leblond, C., 1978, Radioautographic investigation of gliogenesis in the corpus callosum of young rats. I. Sequential changes in oligodendrocytes, *J. Comp. Neurol.* **180:**115–138.

Johnson, A., and Bornstein, M., 1978, Myelin-binding antibodies *in vitro:* Immunoperoxidase studies with experimental allergic encephalomyelitis, antigalactocereroside and multiple sclerosis sera, *Brain Res.* **159:**173–189.

Johnson, E. S., and Ludwin, S. K., 1981, The demonstration of recurrent demyelination and remyelination of axons in the central nervous system, *Acta Neuropathol. (Berlin)* **53:**93–98.

Koenig, H., Bunge, M. B., and Bunge, R. P., 1962, Nucleic acid and protein metabolism in white matter—Observations during experimental demyelination and remyelination: A histochemical and autoradiographic study of spinal cord of the adult cat, *Arch. Neurol.* **6:**17–33.

Kruger, L., and Maxwell, D. S., 1966, Electron microscopy of oligodendrocytes in normal rat cerebrum, *Am. J. Anat.* **118:**411–436.

Levitt, R., Cooper, M. L., and Rakic, P., 1981, Coexistence of neuronal and glial precursor cells in the cerebral ventricular zone of the fetal monkey: An ultrastructural immunoperoxidase analysis, *J. Neurosci.* **1:**27–39.

Ling, E. A., and Leblond, C. P., 1973, Investigation of glial cells in semithin sections. II. Variation with age in the numbers of the various glial cell types in rat cortex and corpus callosum, *J. Comp. Neurol.* **149:**73–82.

Ling, E., Paterson, J., Privat, A., Mori, S., and Leblond, C. P., 1973, Investigation of glial cells in semithin sections. I. Identification of glial cells in the brain of young rats, *J. Comp. Neurol.* **149:**43–72.

Lisak, R., Pleasure, D., Silberberg, D., Manning, M., and Saida, T., 1981, Long term cultures of bovine oligodendroglia isolated with a Percoll gradient, *Brain Res.* **223:**107–122.

Ludwin, S. K., 1978, Central nervous system demyelination and remyelination in the mouse: An ultrastructural study of cuprizone toxicity, *Lab. Inves.* **39:**597–612.

Ludwin, S. K., 1979a, An autoradiographic study of cellular proliferation in remyelination of the central nervous system, *Am. J. Pathol.* **95:**683–690.

Ludwin, S. K., 1979b, The perineuronal satellite oligodendrocyte—A possible role in myelination, *Acta Neuropathol.* **47:**49–53.

Ludwin, S. K., 1980, Chronic demyelination inhibits remyelination in the central nervous system: An analysis of contributing factors, *Lab Invest.* **43:**382–387.

Ludwin, S. K., 1981, Pathology of demyelination and remyelination, *in: Demyelinating Disease: Basic and Clinical Electrophysiology* (S. G. Wasman and J. M. Ritchie eds.), pp 123–168, Raven Press, New York.

Matthieu, J. J., Honegger, P., Trapp, B. D., Cohen, S. R., and Webster, H. de F., 1978, Myelination in rat brain aggregating cell cultures, *Neuroscience* **3:**545–572.

McCarthy, K., and deVellis, J., 1980, Preparation of separate astroglial and oligodendroglial cell cultures from rat cerebral tissue, *J. Cell Biol.* **85:**890–902.

McKenna, O., Arnold, G., and Holtzman, E., 1976, Microperoxisome distribution in the central nervous system in the rat, *Brain Res.* **117:**181–194.

Mirsky, R., Winter, J., Abney, E., Pruss, R., Gavrilovic, J., and Raff, M., 1980, Myelin specific proteins and glycolipids in rat Schwann cells and oligodendrocytes in culture, *J. Cell Biol.* **84:**483–494.

Mori, S., and Leblond, C. P., 1969, Electron microscopic features and proliferation of astrocytes in the corpus callosum of the rat, *J. Comp. Neurol.* **137:**197–226.

Mori, S., and Leblond, C. P., 1970, Electron microscopic identification of three classes of oligodendrocytes and a preliminary study of their proliferative activity in the corpus callosum of young rats, *J. Comp. Neurol.* **139:**1–30.

Paterson, J., Privat, A., Ling, E., and Leblond, C., 1973, Investigation of glial cells in semithin sections. III. Transformation of subependymal cells into glial cells, as shown by radioautography after ³H-thymidine injection into the lateral ventricle of the brain of young rats, *J. Comp. Neurl.* **149:**83–102.

Penfield, W., 1932, *Cytology and Cellular Pathology of the Nervous System,* Hoeber, New York.

Peters, A., 1964, Observations on the connexions between myelin sheaths and glial cells in the optic nerves of young rats, *J. Anat.* **98:**125–134.

Peters, A., and Vaughn, J. E., 1970, Morphology and development of the myelin sheath, in: Myelination (A. N. Davison and A. Peters, eds.), pp. 3–79, Charles C. Thomas, Springfield, Illinois.

Peters, A., Palay, S. L., and Webster, H. de F., 1976, *The Fine Structure of the Nervous System: The Neurons and Supporting Cells,* W. B. Saunders, Philadelphia.

Philips, D., 1973, An electron microscopic study of macroglia and macroglia in the lateral funiculus of the developing spinal cord in the fetal monkey, *Z. Zellforsch.* **140**:145–167.

Poduslo, S. E., Miller, L., and Wolinsky, J., 1982, The production of a membrane by purified oligodendroglia maintained in culture, *Exp. Cell Res.* **137**:203–215.

Privat, A., and Leblond, C. P., 1972, The subependymal layer and neighboring region in the brain of the young rat, *J. Comp. Neurol.* **146**:277–301.

Pruss, R. M., Bartlett, P., Gavrilovic, J., Lisak, R., and Rattray, S., 1981, Mitogens for glial cells: A comparison of the response of cultured astrocytes, oligodendrocytes and Schwann cells, *Brain Res.* **254**:19–35.

Raff, M. C., Mirsky, R., Fields, K. L., Lisak, R., Dorfmann, S., Silberberg, D., Gregson, N., Liebowitz, S., and Kennedy, M., 1978, Galactocerebroside is a specific cell surface antigenic marker for oligodendrocytes in culture, *Nature (London)* **274**:813–816.

Raine, C., and Bornstein, M., 1970, Experimental allergic encephaloyelitis: A light and electron microscope study of remyelination and sclerosis *in vitro, J. Neuropathol Exp. Neurol.* **29**:552–574.

Raju, T., Bignami, A., and Dahl, D., 1981, *In vivo* and *in vitro* differentiation of neurons and astrocytes in the rat embryo, *Dev. Biol.* **85**:344–357.

Rioux, F., Derbin, C., Margules, S., Joubert, R., and Bisconte, J., 1980, Kinetics of oligodendrocyte-like cells in primary cultures of mouse embryonic brain, *Dev. Biol.* **76**:87–99.

Robertson, W., 1899, On a new method of obtaining a black reaction in certain tissue-elements of the central nervous system (platinum method), *Scott. Med. Surg. J.* **4**:23–30.

Roussel, G., Labourdette, G., and Nussbaum, J. L., 1981, Characterization of oligodendrocytes im primary cultures of brain hemispheres of new born rats, *Dev. Biol.* **81**:372–378.

Saida, T., Saida, K., Silberberg, D. H., 1979, Demyelination produced by experimental allergic neuritis serum and anti-galactocerebroside antiserum in CNS cultures, *Acta Neuropathol.* **48**:19–25.

Salzer, J., and Bunge, R. P., 1980, Studies of Schwann cell proliferation. I. An analysis in tissue culture of proliferation during development, Wallerian degeneration and direct injury, *J. Cell Biol.* **84**:739–752.

Salzer, J., Bunge, R. P., and Glaser, L., 1980*a*, Studies of Schwann cell proliferation. III. Evidence for the surface localization of the neurite mitogen, *J. Cell Biol.* **84**:767–778.

Salzer, J., Williams, A. K., Glaser, L., and Bunge, R. P., 1980*b*, Studies of Schwann cell proliferation. II. Characterization of the stimulation and specificity of the response to a neurite membrane fraction, *J. Cell Biol.* **84**:753–766.

Sauer, F. C., 1935, Mitosis in the neural tube, *J. Comp. Neurol.* **62**:377–405.

Schachner, M., Kim, S., and Zehnli, R., 1981, Developmental expression in central and peripheral nervous system of oligodendrocyte cell surface antigens (O antigens) recognized by monoclonal antibodies, *Dev. Biol.* **83**:328–338.

Schmechel, D., and Rakic, P., 1979, A Golgi study of radial glial cells in developing monkey telecephalon: Morphogenesis and transformation into astrocytes, *Anat. Embryol.* **156**:115–152.

Sears, T. A., 1982, *Neuronal–glial Cell Interrelationships,* Dahlem Konferenzen 1982, Springer-Verlag, New York.

Seeds, N., 1973, Differentiation of aggregating brain cell cultures *in: Tissue Culture of the Nervous System* (G. Sato, ed.), pp. 35–55, Plenum Press, New York.

Seil, F., 1977, Tissue culture studies of demyelinating disease: A critical review, *Ann. Neurol.* **2:**345–355.

Seil, F., 1979, Cerebellum in tissue culture, *Rev. Neurosci.* **4:**105–177.

Skoff, R. P., 1975, The fine structure of pulse labelled (^{3}H-thymidine) cells in degenerating rat optic nerve, *J. Comp. Neurol.* **161:**595–612.

Skoff, R. P., 1980, Neuroglia: A reevaluation of their origin and development, *Pathol. Res. Pract.* **168:**279–300.

Skoff, R. P., and Vaughn, J. E., 1971, An autoradiographic study of proliferation in degenerating rat optic nerve, *J. Comp. Neurol.* **141:**133–156.

Skoff, R., Price, D., and Stocks, A., 1976a, Electron microscopic autoradiographic studies of gliogenesis in rat optic nerve. I. Cell proliferation, *J. Comp. Neurol.* **169:**291–312.

Skoff, R., Price, D., and Stocks, A., 1976b, Electron microscopic autoradiographis studies of gliogenesis in rat optic nerve. II. Time of origin, *J. Comp. Neurol.* **179:**313–333.

Smart, I., and Leblond, C. P., 1961, Evidence for division and transformation of neuroglial cells in the mouse brain, as derived from autoradiography after injection of thymidine-H^3, *J. Comp. Neurol.* **116:**349–367.

Sobkowicz, H., Guillery, R., and Bornstein, M., 1968, Neuronal organization in long term cultures of the spinal cord of the fetal mouse, *J. Comp. Neurol.* **132:**365–395.

Stensaas, L. J., and Stensaas, S. S., 1968, Astrocytic neuroglial cells, oligodendrocytes and microgliacytes in the spinal cord of the toad. II. Electron microscopy, *Z. Zellforsch. Mikrosk. Anat.* **86:**184–213.

Sternberger, N., Itoyama, Y., Kies, M., and Webster, H de F., 1978, Myelin basic protein demonstrated immunocytochemically in oligodendroglia prior to myelin sheath formation, *Proc. Natl. Acad. Sci. U.S.A.* **75:**2521–2524.

Sturrock, R. R., 1976, Light microscopic identification of immature glial cells in semithin sections of the developing mouse corpus callosum, *J. Anat.* **122:**521–537.

Szuchet, S., Stefansson, K., Wollmann, R., Dawson, G., and Arnason, B. G., 1980, Maintenance of isolated oligodendrocytes in long-term culture, *Brain Res.* **200:**151–164.

Tennekoon, G., Cohen, S., Price, D., and McKhann, G., 1977, Myelinogenesis in optic nerve: A morphological, autoradiographic and biochemical analysis, *J. Cell Biol.* **72:**604–616.

Tennekoon, G. I., Kishimoto, Y., Singh, I., Nonaka, A., and Bourre, J., 1980, The differentiation of oligodendrocytes in the rat optic nerve, *Dev. Biol.* **79:**149–158.

Trapp, B., Honegger, P., Richelson, E., and Webster, H de F., 1979, Morphological differentiation of mechanically dissociated fetal rat brain in aggregating cell cultures, *Brain Res.* **160:**117–130.

Vaughn, D., and Peters, A., 1974, Neuroglial cells in the cerebral cortex of rats from young adulthood to old age: An electron microscopic study, *J. Neurocytol.* **3:**405–429.

Vaughn, J. E., 1969, An electron microscopic analysis of gliogenesis in rat optic nerve, *Z. Zellforsch.* **94:**292–324.

Vaughn, J., 1971, The morphology and development of neuroglial cells, in: *Cellular Aspects of Neural Growth and Differentiation* (D. C. Pease, ed.), pp. 103–134, University of California Press, Berkeley, California.

Vaughn, J. E., and Pease, D. C., 1970, Electron microscopic studies of Wallerian degeneration in rat optic nerves. II. Astrocytes, oligodendrocytes and adventitial cells, *J. Comp. Neurol.* **140:**207–226.

Weinberg, H. J., and Spencer, P. S., 1976, Studies on the control of myelinogenesis. II. Evidence for the neuronal regulation of myelin production, *Brian Res.* **113:**363–378.

Wood, P., and Bunge, R. P., 1975, Evidence that sensory axons are mitogenic for Schwann cells, *Nature (London)* **256:**662–664.

Wood, P., Okada, E., and Bunge, R. P., 1980, The use of networks of dissociated dorsal root ganglion neurons to induce myelination by oligodendrocytes in culture, *Brain Res.* **196:**247–252.

Yavin, Z., and Yavin, E., 1977, Synaptogenesis and myelinogenesis in dissociated cerebral cells from rat embryo or polylysine-coated surfaces, *Exp. Brain Res.* **29:**137–147.

CHAPTER 2

IN VIVO METABOLISM OF OLIGODENDROGLIAL LIPIDS

PIERRE MORELL and ARREL D. TOEWS

1. INTRODUCTION

A basic assumption for studies of *in vivo* lipid metabolism in oligodendroglial cells is that the metabolism of lipids in myelin reflects the activity of these glial cells. This is not a trivial assumption. The cytoplasmic connection between the oligodendroglial cell perikaryon and myelin can be visualized in the developing CNS (Bunge, 1968). However, "connections between these elements have never been demonstrated in a normal adult animal, unlike the PNS counterpart, the Schwann cell" (Raine, 1981). Nevertheless, it is generally assumed that metabolism of the mature myelin sheath (which, as will be documented below, is reasonably vigorous) requires extensive contact with elements of the oligodendroglial-cell perikaryon through cytoplasmic channels. These connections may not be easy to visualize; due to their tortuous courses, it is unlikely

PIERRE MORELL and ARREL D. TOEWS • Department of Biochemistry and Nutrition and Biological Sciences Research Center, University of North Carolina at Chapel Hill, Chapel Hill, North Carolina 27514

that a thin section prepared for electron microscopy will include the complete channel (see Chapter 1 for further discussion).

In general, the assumption that most of the lipid components of myelin are synthesized *de novo* and combined with myelin proteins into some precursor fraction, all within the oligodendroglial-cell perikaryon, has not been seriously challenged, although as noted later, some lipid-synthetic enzymes appear to be present in myelin itself. The idea that the eventual degradation of myelin lipids takes place primarily in oligodendroglial-cell organelles is also generally accepted. Our interpretation of the literature is also based on these same assumptions.

In addition to the oligodendroglial perikaryon, metabolic support of myelin by the axon has also been considered, since there are some indications of transfer of compounds from the axon to myelin. Although several studies have failed to demonstrate an axonal origin for myelin proteins and glycoproteins (Autilio-Gambetti *et al.*, 1975; Droz *et al.*, 1973; Bennett *et al.*, 1973; Matthieu *et al.*, 1978), there is evidence that some intact lipids do diffuse across the axonal membrane into the surrounding myelin (Rawlins, 1973; Droz *et al.*, 1978, 1979, 1981; Haley and Ledeen, 1979; Brunetti *et al.*, 1981; Ledeen and Haley, 1983). It has also been noted that certain phospholipid precursors, derived from the degradation of axonal phospholipids, may be transferred from the axon to myelin phospholipids (Droz *et al.*, 1978, 1979, 1981; Haley and Ledeen, 1979; Brunetti *et al.*, 1981; Ledeen and Haley, 1983), but in this case, autoradiographic evidence indicates the participation of the oligodendroglial-cell perikaryon in the actual synthetic process. There is no indication that either of these mechanisms constitutes a quantitatively significant supply of precursors involved in metabolism of myelin lipids. However, it is worthwhile to keep in mind the possibility that interchange of metabolic products, possibly even including lipid components, between the oligodendroglial-cell-myelin compartment and the axon might conceivably play a role in the control of myelinogenesis.

2. LIPID COMPOSITION OF MYELIN

Although a detailed discussion of the isolation of myelin is beyond the scope of this chapter, there are available several protocols, utilizing combinations of differential and density-gradient centrifugation steps coupled with osmotic shocks, that allow isolation of this membranous material from tissue homogenates with a high degree of purity and a relatively high yield (Norton, 1974, 1977*a*). The high lipid protein ratio of myelin, which is what makes it relatively easy to separate from other membranes in the first place, is a dominant chemical feature (Table 1). In considering functions of the oligodendrog-

TABLE 1. Composition of Mature Central Nervous System Myelin from Several Species[a]

Components	Human	Bovine	Rat
	(% of dry weight)		
Protein	30.0	24.7	29.5
Lipid	70.0	75.3	70.5
	(% of lipid weight)		
Cholesterol	27.7	28.1	27.3
Total galactolipid	27.5	29.3	31.5
Cerebroside	22.7	24.0	23.7
Sulfatide	3.8	3.6	7.1
Total phospholipid	43.1	43.0	44.0
Ethanolamine PG[b]	15.6	17.4	16.7
Choline PG[c]	11.2	10.9	11.3
Sphingomyelin	7.9	7.1	3.2
Serine PG[c]	4.8	6.5	7.0
Inositol PG	0.6	0.8	1.2

[a] From Norton (1981). [b] (PG) phosphoglyceride; primarily ethanolamine plasmalogen. [c] Contains small amounts of plasmalogen.

lial cell, it is useful to keep in mind the truly enormous amount of lipid these cells must synthesize and maintain. In the rat, some 25% of the dry weight of brain is accounted for by myelin, and because of the relative excess of lipids in this membrane relative to other subcellular fractions of brain, 40% of the total lipid of brain, presumably synthesized by oligodendroglial cells, is accounted for by myelin. In humans, where 35% of the dry weight of brain is composed of myelin, more than half the brain lipid is formed by oligodendroglial cells (Norton, 1981).

It has been calculated that during the period of maximal myelin accumulation, oligodendroglial cells synthesize an amount of myelin more than three times the weight of their cell bodies each day (Norton, 1981). The quantitatively most significant lipid components of isolated myelin (Table 1) include cholesterol (a general component found in almost all plasma membranes), cerebroside (a galactolipid that, although not exclusively localized in myelin, is greatly enriched in this structure and is often referred to as the most "myelin-typical" lipid), and ethanolamine plasmalogen (this lipid is not specific to myelin, but is relatively enriched in membranous fractions from certain organs, including brain sulfatide (cerebroside-3-sulfate). Although present at a lower concentration than cerebroside, is also much more concentrated in myelin than in other membranes. Lipids less prominent in myelin than in many other plasma membranes include phosphatidylethanolamine, phosphatidylserine, and the choline-containing lipids, phosphatidylcholine (lecithin) and sphingomyelin. Several minor lipid constituents of myelin have attracted increasing attention lately, in part because it has been suggested that they may have some dynamic function as opposed to the presumably primarily structural significance of the lipids mentioned above. Some gangliosides (sialic-acid-containing glycosphingolipids once thought to be specific to neurons) are found in myelin. Of the order of 0.2% of myelin lipid is composed of gangliosides, primarily the major monosialoganglioside G_{M1} (Suzuki *et al.*, 1968; Ledeen *et al.*, 1980). Interestingly, myelin from higher primates and birds contains, in addition to G_{M1}, sialosylgalactosylceramide (G_{M4} or G_7) (Ledeen *et al.*, 1973, 1980; Cochran *et al.*, 1982). This lipid, presumably produced by modification of cerebroside, appears to be myelin-and oligodendroglial-cell-specific. The postulated role of sialic acid in cell-to-cell recognition and communication phenomena suggests that these gangliosides may serve some similar function during development (see Porcellati *et al.*, 1976; Wiegandt, 1982).

As an aside, it is worth noting that although myelin has traditionally been viewed as a functionally inert structure (acting primarily as an insulator to facilitate saltatory conduction along the axon), there have been recent suggestions in the literature that myelin may also be actively involved, to a certain extent, in controlling the ionic milieu in the vicinity of axons. For example, the enzymes carbonic anhydrase (Cammer *et al.*, 1976; Yandrasitz *et al.*, 1976; Sapirstein *et al.*, 1978), 5'-nucleotidase (Cammer *et al.*, 1980), and Na^+, K^+-ATPase (Reiss *et al.*, 1981; Wood *et al.*, 1977; Schwartz *et al.*, 1981), which are responsible for membrane transport of carbon dioxide, adenosine, and monovalent cations, respectively, have all been reported to be intrinsic to myelin (see Chapter 6). In addition, changes in the permeability of isolated myelin vesicles toward some cations can be induced by the presence of ATP and Mg^{2+} (Wüthrich and Steck, 1981). Certain lipids related to these dynamic functions, and possibly to others as well, might be expected to undergo rather active metabolism. In this connection, the polyphosphoinositides (phosphatidylinositol-4-phosphate and phosphatidylinositol-4,5-*bis*-phosphate), which are predominantly localized in myelin, where they may account for about 6% of the total myelin lipid phosphorus (Eichberg and Dawson, 1965; Eichberg and Hauser, 1973), are of interest. The high metabolic activity of the phosphate groups on the 4 and 5 positions of inositol (Eichberg and Dawson, 1965; Deshmukh *et al.*, 1978*a*, 1981; however see Gonzalez-Sastre *et al.*, 1971), coupled with the observation that these phosphate groups have a high affinity for free Ca^{2+} (Hendrickson and Reinertsen, 1971), raises the possibility that some dynamic control mechanism exists whereby release or retention of Ca^{2+} may make accessible or block certain sites on the myelin sheath.

Finally, in addition to the major galactolipids, cerebroside and sulfatide, myelin also contains small amounts of several fatty acid esters of cerebroside and several glycerol-based galactolipids. The latter include the mono- and digalactosyldiglycerides, some corresponding aklylacyl analogues, and some sulfated derivatives (Norton and Brotz, 1963; Norton and Autilio, 1966; R. A. Pieringer *et al.*, 1973; J. Pieringer *et al.*, 1977).

3. ACCUMULATION OF MYELIN AND "MYELIN-SPECIFIC" LIPIDS DURING DEVELOPMENT

A large portion of the myelin in the CNS accumulates during a relatively brief period during development, and as noted, this is a time of very intense metabolic activity for oligodendroglial cells. In rat brain, myelin deposition begins at about 10–12 days. The rate of myelin deposition increases rapidly to a maximum at about 20 days, after which it declines (Norton and Poduslo, 1973*b*). Although the actual time of the period of rapid myelin accumulation varies somewhat, this same general pattern also occurs in other species, including humans.

It has long been assumed that accumulation of "myelin-specific" lipids in brain correlates with the period of time when oligodendroglial cells are most active in manufacturing myelin. Cerebroside and sulfatide accumulation are the lipid markers most often used. Accumulation of these lipids presumably represents a balance between their synthesis and degradation. These factors can be isolated from each other by studying the incorporation of a radioactive precursor into a "myelin-specific" lipid, since incorporation of the radioactive precursor is probably proportional to the rate of synthesis of that lipid over a time–course of the order of hours. The amount of degradation is generally not significant, since the time–course of these experiments is usually short relative to the turnover times of the lipids being examined. In theory, comparison of the rate of synthesis for a given lipid at different ages might be difficult to interpret because of possible changes in the pool size of the precursor. However, interpretation of data concerning synthesis of cerebroside and sulfatide *in vivo* is consistent with measurements of accumulation of these lipids and of myelin itself; incorporation of precursors into these "myelin-specific" lipids increases as myelination begins, remains high during the period of active myelination, and then decreases as the rate of myelination decreases (Moser and Karnovsky, 1959; Burton *et al.*, 1958; Kishimoto *et al.*, 1965; McKhann and Ho, 1967). Also relevant are temporal studies of the levels of enzyme activity for committed steps in the synthesis of "myelin-specific lipids." Galactosylation of ceramide and sulfation of cerebroside, as measured by *in vitro* assays of partially purified enzyme preparations from brain, correlate with the other data mentioned above; that is, the peak of enzyme activity corresponds to the peak rate of myelin accumulation (Shah, 1971; Brenkert and Radin, 1972; Costantino-Ceccarini and Morell, 1972).

It should be noted that the temporal peaks of incorporation of radioactive precursors into these lipids and the peak of enzyme activity for their synthesis are proportional to the rate of myelin accumulation. This is not a trivial observation, since it would be just as logical to assume that enzyme activity and biosynthesis of these lipids should initially be proportional to the rate of accumulation of myelin, but stay at high levels as accumulation of myelin levels off. The fact that the biosynthesis of these lipids declines as myelin accumulation reaches a plateau at a high level suggests that cerebroside and sulfatide are relatively metabolically stable [as is indeed the case (see Section 6)]. If, on the contrary, they turned over relatively rapidly, the enzyme activity needed to support this metabolism would need to be proportional to the amount of accumulated myelin.

Monogalactosyldiglycerides have also been studied as "myelin-specific" lipids, since approximately two thirds of the total monogalactosyldiglycerides in brain are associated with myelin (Inoue *et al.*, 1971). Synthesis of these lipids in rat brain is very low prior to 10 days of age, increases rapidly to a peak at 17–18 days of age, and then decreases (Wenger *et al.*, 1968, 1970). This pattern is similar to that found for cerebroside and sulfatide. However, unlike cerebroside and sulfatide, which remain at high levels in brain even after their synthesis rates decrease, the level of monogalactosyldiglyceride decreases as the synthesis rate decreases (Inoue *et al.*, 1971). This pattern appears to be unique for these lipids and suggests a possible specialized role for them in the process of myelination, as opposed to a structural role in mature compact myelin.

4. BIOSYNTHESIS OF MYELIN LIPIDS

With relatively minor exceptions, the biosynthetic pathways for brain lipids do not differ significantly from those in other tissues. Since at least during myelinogenesis, much of the synthesis of brain lipids involves oligodendroglial cells, it is assumed that lipid synthesis in these specific cells also does not involve unique metabolic pathways. However, these pathways must be extraordinarily active in these cells, and there are some unique aspects dealing with topics such as the localization of enzymes and their metabolic controls that are worth noting. The general topic of brain lipid synthesis has been reviewed by Ansell (1973) and Wykle (1977).

4.1. Glycerolipids

The major pathways for glycerolipid biosynthesis are outlined in Figure 1. The glycerol backbone of the diacyl phospholipids is derived from phospha-

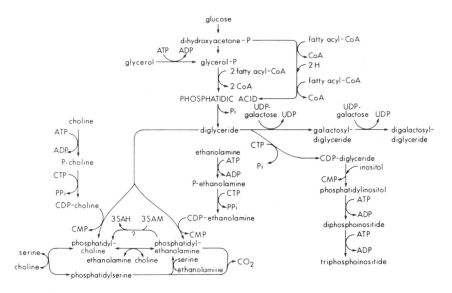

FIGURE 1. Major pathways for glycerolipid biosynthesis. (SAH), S-adenosylhomocysteine; (SAM), S-adenosylmethionine.

tidic acid, which is synthesized either by the acylation of glycerol-3-phosphate or via the dihydroxyacetone-phosphate pathway (the latter involves acylation of dihydroxyacetone-phosphate in the 1 position followed by reduction of the keto group in the 2 position and a subsequent acylation). The salvage pathway, phosphorylation of glycerol, is also present, and this is important for metabolic studies in which radioactive glycerol is used to examine phospholipid synthesis and turnover. Phosphatidylethanolamine and phosphatidylcholine are synthesized primarily by the cytidine pathway discovered by Kennedy and co-workers (See Kennedy, 1961) and first demonstrated in brain by McMurray *et al.* (1957). This pathway involves the phosphorylation of the base moiety at the expense of ATP (to form phosphocholine or phosphoethanolamine), followed by reaction with CTP to give CDP-choline or CDP-ethanolamine. These activated base moieties then react with 1,2-diacylglycerol to give the final product, phosphatidylcholine or phosphatidylethanolamine.

The enzyme activities mentioned above are enriched in the microsomal fraction (Porcellati *et al.*, 1970; E. K. Miller and Dawson, 1972a; Possmayer *et al.*, 1973; Jungalwala, 1974a; Toews *et al.*, 1976), presumably on particles derived from endoplasmic reticulum. Autoradiographic studies also indicate the endoplasmic reticulum as the major site of phospholipid biosynthesis (Droz and Boyenval, 1975; Rambourg and Droz, 1980). Lipids are added first to the cytoplasmic face of the endoplasmic reticulum (or at least on the outside face of microsomal vesicles from brain) and then presumably equilibrate across the membrane by some type of "flip-flop" process that has a half-time of about 30 min (Butler and Morell, 1982). The CDP-ethanolamine:diacylglycerol ethanolaminephosphotransferase and the equivalent enzyme for phosphatidylcholine biosynthesis have also been shown to be associated with highly purified myelin (Wu and Ledeen, 1980), and there is a report that CTP:phosphoethanolamine cytidylyltransferase, the enzyme that precedes the phosphotransferase step in the synthesis pathway, is also present in purified myelin (Kunishita and Ledeen, 1984). The physiological significance of the presence of these enzymes in myelin is not clear, since the other enzymes necessary for glycerophospholipid synthesis have not been demonstrated to be present and it is not clear whether significant amounts of the highly polar base-containing substrates can be present in myelin. The question of capacity for some localized synthesis of myelin phospholipids remains open. These enzymes may be responsible for the labeling of myelin lipids observed following axonal transport of labeled macromolecules.

It should be noted that the pathway for phosphatidylcholine synthesis involving methylation of phosphatidylethanolamine is present only at very low levels in brain (Morganstern and Abdel-Latif, 1974). Although this reaction may be of great significance in local control of membrane properties, especially at the synaptic junction (for a review, see Hirata and Axelrod, 1980), it is probable that most of the choline for bulk lipid synthesis comes from dietary choline or liver production of this compound and must be carried into the brain (possibly in the form of lysophosphatidylcholine).

The synthesis of plasmalogens (glycerophospholipids with an enol-ether-linked hydrophobic chain in the first position and an acyl group in the second position of glycerol) involves the acyldihydroxyacetone-phosphate pathway mentioned above (Hajra, 1969; Wykle and Snyder, 1969). An acyl group in the 1 position (derived from the reaction of acyl-CoA with dihydroxyacetone-phosphate) exchanges with a long-chain alcohol to give alkyldihydroxyacetone-phosphate. Other steps are analogous to the synthesis of diacyl phospholipids; there is a reduction of the keto group in the 2 position and an acyl transferase reaction to give 1-alkyl-2-acylglycerol-3-phosphate. This is followed in turn by hydrolysis of the phosphate. The alkylacylglycerol product reacts with CDP-ethanolamine or CDP-choline to give the alkyl analogue of the common glycerophospholipids (for a review, see Snyder, 1972). These alkylacylglycero-phospholipids are converted to plasmalogens by an interesting desaturation reaction involving a mixed-function oxidase that converts the alkyl linkage to an enol-ether bond (Wykle et al., 1972; Paltauf and Holasek, 1973). The specific activity of CDP-ethanolamine: alkylacylglycerol ethanolaminephosphotransferase, the enzyme that catalyzes the transfer of the base to alkylacylglycerol, is somewhat higher in isolated oligodendroglia than in neuronal perikarya or astrocytes (Freysz and Horrocks, 1980). It has also been noted that total brain activity increases several fold during the oligodendroglial proliferation that occurs at the beginning of myelination (Freysz *et al.*, 1980). Both these findings are consistent with the hypothesis that most of the plasmalogen synthesized in brain is destined for myelin. For a more detailed review of plasmalogen biosynthesis and metabolism in brain, see Horrocks and Sharma (1982).

The base-exchange pathway (the energy-independent, Ca^{2+}-dependent exchange of serine, ethanolamine, and choline for the polar moieties of preexisting phospholipids) is probably operative in brain *in vivo* (Arienti *et al.*, 1976). Although this reaction does not result in the net production of phospholipid, it is probably the major pathway for synthesis of phosphatidylserine and its plasmalogen analogue (Hübscher, 1962; Porcellati *et al.*, 1971). However, it has also been suggested that an energy-dependent pathway is available for synthesis of some phosphatidylserine in brain (Yavin and Zeigler, 1977; Pullarkat *et al.*, 1981). Phosphatidylserine can be decarboxylated to form phosphatidylethanolamine (Abdel-Latif and Abood, 1966); this enzyme activity is localized primarily in mitochondria (Butler and Morell, 1983).

The formation of phosphatidylinositol involves the reaction of CDP-diglyceride with free inositol (Paulus and Kennedy, 1960; Hawthorne and Kai, 1970). Note the difference from the biosynthesis of most other phospholipids in that in this case, it is the diglyceride rather than the polar moiety that is activated. As noted previously, a large fraction of the di- and triphosphoinositides, which are derived from phosphatidylinositol, are localized in myelin. Although the enzyme responsible for the synthesis of phosphatidylinositol is in the microsomal fraction, the subsequent phosphorylation of the inositol moiety at the 4 position (to give diphosphoinositide) involves an enzyme localized primarily in the plasma membrane, while the final phosphorylation at the 5 position of inositol (to give triphosphoinositide) involves an enzyme in the cytosol (Hawthorne and Kai, 1970). The latter two enzymes, both of which require Mg^{2+} and are inhibited by Ca^{2+}, have also been reported to be present in myelin (Deshmukh *et al.*, 1978a).

Mono- and digalactosyldiglycerides, neutral glycerolipids that do not contain a phosphate moiety, are also associated with myelin (Inoue *et al.*, 1971; Deshmukh *et al.*, 1971). Synthesis of these lipids involves reaction of a diglyceride with UDP-galactose, followed by a second galactosylation step, also requiring UDP-galactose, in the case of digalactosyldiglyceride (Wenger *et al.*, 1968, 1970.) Sulfated derivatives of these galactosyldiglycerides, also associated with myelin (J. Pieringer *et al.*, 1977), are formed via a phosphoadenosine-phosphosulfate-mediated reaction (Subba Rao *et al.*, 1977).

4.2. Sphingolipids

The long-chain base sphingosine, from which the sphingolipids derive their name, is formed from palmitic acid (possibly first involving reduction to an alcohol) and serine (Stoffel, 1971; Gatt and Barenholz, 1973). This reaction, as well as subsequent reactions involved in the biosynthesis of sphingolipids, are shown in Figure 2. It appears most likely that the next step in the synthesis of myelin sphingolipids involves acylation of the amide moiety to form ceramide. A pathway involving condensation of acyl-CoA and sphingosine has been studied in several laboratories using brain preparations (Sribney, 1966; Morell and Radin, 1970). Another pathway for synthesis, the reverse reaction of ceramidase to bring together a free fatty acid and sphingosine, can be demonstrated *in vitro* (Yavin and Gatt, 1969), although its *in vivo* significance, if any, is not clear. Recently, a new reaction for the synthesis of ceramide from lignoceric acid and sphingosine has been demonstrated (Singh and Kishimoto, 1980). Although originally reported to be pyridine-nucleotide-dependent, this requirement is as a substrate for ATP production (Singh, 1983). This reaction, as well as the acyl-CoA-dependent reaction, exhibit specificity in line with what is expected of a system that is in large part dedicated to cerebroside production, in that the 24-carbon (lignocerate) chain is a better substrate than is the 16-carbon (palmitoyl) chain. The pyridine-nucleotide-dependent and acyl-CoA-requiring reactions for ceramide synthesis both show increased activity during the period of active myelination (Singh and Kishimoto, 1982).

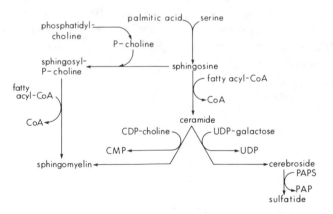

FIGURE 2. Major pathways for sphingolipid biosynthesis. Some of the reactions (e.g., the formation of sphingosine from palmitic acid and serine) actually involve several intermediate steps; the various cofactors required for these steps are not shown. (PAPS), 3'-phosphoadenosine 5'-phosphosulfate; (PAP) 3',5'-diphosphoadenosine.

Much of the ceramide produced in oligodendroglial cells is destined for synthesis of cerebroside, although some is utilized for the synthesis of sphingomyelin as well as for a number of quantitatively less significant sphingolipids. It should be noted that hydroxy fatty acids are prominent components of myelin cerebroside. The alpha-hydroxy fatty acids are formed from their corresponding nonhydroxy fatty acids in brain (Hajra and Radin, 1963; Hoshi and Kishimoto, 1973; Murad and Kishimoto, 1975). This hydroxylase activity is decreased in the brains of myelin-deficient mutants (Murad and Kishimoto, 1975). These hydroxylated fatty acids are incorporated into ceramide (Ullman and Radin, 1972) and then into cerebrosides (see below).

The galactosylation of ceramide by UDP-galactose to form cerebroside is a well-studied and active reaction in brain. The developmental pattern and activity of the enzyme involved (UDP-galactose:ceramide galactosyltransferase) correlate with myelination and are thus presumably primarily oligodendroglial in nature (Shah, 1971; Brenkert and Radin, 1972; Costantino-Ceccarini and Morell, 1972). A puzzling point is that *in vitro,* this reaction has specificity such that hydroxy-fatty-acid-containing ceramide is vastly more active than nonhydroxy-fatty-acid-containing ceramide with respect to activity of the substrate for cerebroside formation. Another point of interest is that at least *in vitro,* sphingosine is readily galactosylated (by UDP-galactose) to form psychosine (Cleland and Kennedy, 1960; Morell and Radin, 1969; Neskovic *et al.,* 1969; J. Hildebrand *et al.,* 1970). Therefore, it has been suggested that a possible pathway for formation of cerebroside might involve acylation of psychosine. Although initial reports of this reaction were subsequently shown to be due to nonenzymatic artifacts (Hammarström, 1971a), there is one report of the enzymatic synthesis of cerebroside by this pathway under specialized conditions (Curtino and Caputto, 1974). However, the ceramide pathway probably constitutes the quantitatively most significant pathway for cerebroside synthesis in brain (Hammarström, 1972b; Hammarström and Samuelsson, 1972).

Some of the cerebroside is converted to sulfatide by a phosphoadenosine-phosphosulfate-dependent reaction. Although the cerebroside sulfotransferase enzyme involved in this sulfation is well characterized (McKhann *et al.,* 1975; Balasubramanian and Bachhawat, 1965; McKhann and Ho, 1967; Farrell and McKhann, 1971), both *in vitro* (Poduslo *et al.,* 1978; Benjamins and Iwata, 1979) and *in vivo* (Hayes and Jungalwala, 1976; Shoyama and Kishimoto, 1978) metabolic studies suggest that the pool of recently synthesized cerebroside is not readily available for sulfation.

Activities of the enzymes that catalyze the final steps in the synthesis of cerebrosides and sulfatides are enriched in isolated oligodendroglia, relative to isolated neuronal perikarya (Benjamins *et al.,* 1974). In addition, these enzymes have a relatively low activity in the myelin-deficient jimpy and quaking mice mutants (Neskovic *et al.,* 1972; Yahara *et al.,* 1981). Both of these findings are consistent with the presence of most of the cerebroside and much of the sulfatide in myelin. There is some evidence that some of the galactosyltransferase activity responsible for cerebroside synthesis may also be associated with myelin itself (Neskovic *et al.,* 1973; Costantino-Ceccarini and Suzuki, 1975).

A pathway for synthesis of sphingomyelin from ceramide and CDP-choline is well known (Sribney and Kennedy, 1958; Kopaczyk and Radin, 1965; Fujino *et al.,* 1968). However, the *in vitro* specificity of the enzyme with respect to the fatty acyl moiety does not correspond to the fatty acid composition of sphingomyelin found *in vivo*. Other possible synthetic routes include acylation of sphingosylphosphorylcholine (Brady *et al.,* 1965) and the pathway mediated by the enzyme activity that transfers the phosphocholine moiety of phosphatidylcholine directly to ceramide (Diringer *et al.,* 1972; Marggraf and Anderer, 1974). Ullman and Radin (1974) noted evidence of the latter reaction in several organs, but not in brain. Thus, the synthetic pathway for this important myelin component is not yet completely understood.

Gangliosides, complex glycosphingolipids containing sialic acid, are present in low amounts in myelin (for a review of general synthesis pathways, see Wiegandt, 1982). Of particular interest is the ganglioside sialosylgalactosylceramide (G_7 or G_{M4}), which is a major ganglioside of human, chimpanzee, monkey, and avian CNS myelin (Ledeen *et al.,* 1973, 1980). This ganglioside, which appears to be specific for myelin (and presumably oligodendroglial cells) in the aforenamed species, is probably synthesized by reaction of CMP-sialic acid with galactosylceramide (cerebroside), since its fatty acid composition is very similar to that of myelin cerebroside (Ledeen *et al.,* 1973). *In vitro* biosynthesis of G_7 by this pathway has been demonstrated in brain microsomes (Yu and Lee, 1976); this *in vitro* biosynthetic activity in brain appears to be restricted to oligodendroglial cells (Stoffyn *et al.,* 1981).

Like the phospholipids, the sphingolipids are probably synthesized, at least partially, at the level of the smooth endoplasmic reticulum (for example, Morell and Radin, 1969; Morell *et al.,* 1970; Basu *et al.,* 1971; Farrell and McKhann, 1971). However, they are also probably processed to some extent at the level of the Golgi apparatus (Fleisher, 1977; Desmukh *et al.,* 1978*b;* Benjamins *et al.,* 1982). The synthesis of sulfatide is more highly localized in Golgi membranes than is the synthesis of galactocerebroside (Benjamins *et al.,* 1982). These lipids must then somehow be assembled into a myelin precursor membrane that is in the process of becoming specialized to form myelin (see Section 5).

4.3. Cholesterol

The synthesis and metabolism of cholesterol in the nervous system have recently been reviewed by Horrocks and Harder (1984). The enzymatic pathway for the synthesis of cholesterol in brain (Figure 3) is generally similar to that in other organs (Wykle, 1977). The established sequence is followed from acetate to lanosterol. Two alternate pathways from lanosterol to cholesterol are present in brain (Ramsey, 1977). Despite the general overall similarities in the synthetic pathways, there are several unique aspects of substrate utilization and metabolic control for cholesterol biosynthesis in the CNS. Although these specialized aspects of cholesterol metabolism may not be specific to oligodendroglial cells, as compared to other brain-cell types, myelin deposition certainly accounts for the great bulk of cholesterol synthesis during the postnatal developmental period. It should be noted that in addition to *in situ* synthesis, some cholesterol in brain may be obtained via transfer from the plasma (Davison *et al.*, 1958; Dobbing, 1968; Serougne *et al.*, 1976). The transfer of cholesterol from plasma to brain is much greater during development, when active myelination is present, than in adults (Dobbing, 1963).

Circulating mevalonate is a relatively poor precursor for brain cholesterol (Edmond, 1974). This is somewhat surprising, since mevalonate is already in the synthesis pathway primarily committed to cholesterol biosynthesis. However, Edmond and Popjak (1974) have desribed a shunt, present in some organs, whereby mevalonate is cycled back through hydroxy-methylglutaryl (HMG)-CoA and then to acetoacetate (see Figure 3). The final enzyme in this shunt HMG-CoA acetoacetate lyase, is not present in brain (Edmond, 1974). Thus, in other tissues, most circulating mevalonate not incorporated into cholesterol is converted into acetoacetate, which may itself be used for cholesterol and fatty acid synthesis in a number of organs, including brain (see below). This shunt, along with a possible blood–brain barrier to entry of mevalonate,

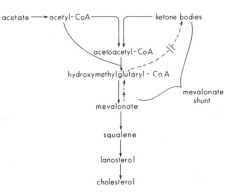

FIGURE 3. General pathway for cholesterol biosynthesis. In peripheral tissues, some mevalonate is recycled back to acetoacetate (a ketone body) through the mevalonate shunt (---→); the presence of a complete shunt in peripheral tissue is at least partially responsible for the poor utilization of circulating mevalonate for brain cholesterol synthesis. The last reaction in this shunt, the conversion of hydroxymethylglutaryl-CoA to acetoacetate, does not occur in brain.

may account for the relatively poor direct utilization of circulating mevalonate by brain. However, mevalonate is still the preferred cholesterol precursor relative to acetate when these compounds are injected intracerebrally (Ramsey *et al.,* 1971).

It is also noteworthy that the brain (including presumably the oligodendroglial cells) efficiently utilizes ketone bodies for cholesterol synthesis (for references see Koper *et al.,* 1981). As noted by Edmond (1974), acetoacetate is metabolically inert in the liver because of the absence of enzyme activity to convert it to the CoA derivative (acetoacetyl-CoA synthetase is low in the liver of newborn rats, although this activity may increase slightly after weaning). However, in brain, acetoacetate and β-hydroxybutyrate are especially good precursors for cholesterol because they can be converted directly to acetoacetyl-CoA in the cytosol. In contrast, glucose must first be metabolized to acetyl-CoA in the mitochondria; this acetyl-CoA in turn must be transported out of the mitochondria into the cytosol before its incorporation into cholesterol (Webber and Edmond, 1979). This efficient utilization of ketone bodies for sterol synthesis may not be unique to the CNS, since another organ of ectodermal origin, skin, also falls into this category. In any case, the physiological advantages of using ketone bodies for synthesis of myelin cholesterol are clear in light of the ketogenic balance of the suckling mammal. During this period, concentrations of ketone bodies are relatively high while glucose concentrations are relatively low. In addition, the uptake of ketone bodies by brain during this period is high (Hawkins *et al.,* 1971) and the activities of the enzymes involved in ketone-body utilization are also increased (Robinson and Williamson, 1980; Page *et al.,* 1971). Relative to whole brain, isolated oligodendrocytes are enriched in ketone-body-metabolizing enzymes (Pleasure *et al.,* 1979). The alternative to utilization of ketone bodies would be to use glucose (the only other readily available source of carbon to enter brain in large amounts), which under many circumstances is better spared for other essential pathways.

In addition to the different quantitative aspects of substrate utilization mentioned above, there may also be differences in the control of cholesterol synthesis in brain, relative to other tissues. The major control point in most nonneural tissues is at the level of HMG-CoA reductase, which is regulated by levels of circulating low-density lipoproteins. However, regulation of cholesterol synthesis by low-density lipoproteins does not appear to be significant in brain (see Chapter 5 for a more detailed discussion), and in fact, the quantitative significance of feedback inhibition of HMG-CoA reductase in brain is itself a matter of controversy. Interpretations of available data range from no feedback regulation all the way to suggestions that this is the major control point in brain, as it is in liver (for discussion and references see Bowen *et al.,* 1974). A recent study by Shah (1981) presents data suggesting that brain HMG-CoA reductase activity is controlled via "protein mediated interconversion of phosphorylated and dephosphorylated forms of the enzyme which have different catalytic activity." However, possibly an even more important control point of cholesterol synthesis in brain lies between squalene and cholesterol; this conversion sequence operates rapidly in liver, but much more slowly in brain. Ramachandran and Shah (1977) have suggested that the decarboxyla- tion of pyro-phosphomevalonate may be a regulatory point in cholesterol bio- synthesis in developing brain. Possible control steps in this sequence are dis- cussed in more detail by Wykle (1977).

It should be noted that control of cholesterol synthesis is of particular importance, since, unlike the case with other lipids, no rapid degradative path- way is available as a control step or fine-tuning device to match the availability of cholesterol with its requirement. Unlike the other major body lipids, choles- terol cannot be degraded by mammalian tissue (except for minor pathways involved in hormone and bile acid metabolism), and cholesterol is removed from the body only by equilibration with the enterohepatic shunt whereby some cholesterol or its products (primarily bile acids) are lost in the feces. The only way cholesterol can be removed from brain is via exchange with the plasma, and this process is relatively slow (Serougne *et al.,* 1976).

An interesting aspect of cholesterol metabolism is acylation and deacyla- tion. There are several cholesterol ester hydrolases present in brain, one of which is uniquely localized in the myelin sheath (Eto and Suzuki, 1973; Igar- ashi and Suzuki, 1977). It appears that the hydrolase activity is reversible so that this enzyme is potentially synthetic in the sense of combining two sub- strates to give a larger molecule. However, in a broader sense, this acylation may be connected with myelin degradation. The appearance of cholesterol esters during myelinogenesis (Adams and Davison, 1959; Alling and Svenner- holm, 1969; Eto and Suzuki, 1972; Hildebrand and Berthold, 1977; Berthold and Hildebrand, 1979) is presumably related to the myelin remodeling that is part of normal postnatal nervous-system maturation (Berthold, 1973, 1974; Berthold and Hildebrand, 1979). Cholesterol esters also accumulate in certain demyelinating disorders (see Norton, 1977*b;* Morell *et al.,* 1981).

5. ASSEMBLY OF LIPIDS INTO MYELIN

Since the bulk of myelin lipids appear to be synthesized in the endo- plasmic reticulum and Golgi apparatus (although, as previously noted, there is limited enzyme activity for the synthesis of some lipids in mature myelin), the question arises as to how they reach their final location in mature compact myelin. Among the obvious possibilities are: (1) the assembly of complete pieces of myelin membrane at the level of the endoplasmic reticulum or Golgi apparatus, with transfer to the plasma membrane in the form of vesicles, and

(2) transfer of individual lipid molecules by lipid-carrier or -exchange proteins (possibly directed by elements of the cytoskeletal network) from the intracellular membranes where they are synthesized to that portion of the plasma membrane that is differentiating to form mature myelin. As we discuss below, the assembly of myelin probably involves a combination of both these processes (and perhaps others as well). Several possible mechanisms involved in the assembly of myelin are illustrated schematically in Figure 4. Note that the process of myelin assembly during development (when myelin is accumulating rapidly) may involve mechanisms different from those responsible for maintenance of mature myelin. In this section, we will confine our discussion to myelin assembly during development; maintenance of mature myelin is discussed in Section 6.

The general concept of plasma-membrane synthesis as currently understood—namely, that membrane components are packaged as precursor vesicles destined by directed transport to be incorporated into growing plasma membranes via fusion of the vesicles with preexisting membrane (Palade, 1975; for a review, see Morré *et al.,* 1979)—probably applies to myelinating oligodendroglial cells. Fusion of these vesicles would increase the surface of the oligodendrocyte and, through the process of membrane flow, might provide the driving force for the extension of oligodendroglial processes and for the eventual spiraling of these processes around the axons to produce myelin, as suggested by Rumsby (1978, 1980). As depicted in Figure 4, these precursor vesicles may be those responsible for general plasma-membrane formation in the oligodendroglial cell (A in Figure 4). However, in myelinating oligodendroglia, there may also be vesicles, with a composition more like that of myelin than the plasma membrane itself, that are specifically directed to fuse with the surface membrane only in specialized regions of the cell where the myelin is actually being formed (B in Figure 4). Formation of the latter vesicles should be especially active during the period of active myelination. The actual fusion of precursor vesicles with the growing oligodendroglial plasma-membrane–myelin complex has not been observed. However, small vesicles have been shown to accumulate in oligodendroglial cytoplasm and in the inner and outer cytoplasmic loops of the myelin-forming processes when myelination proceeds at low temperature (Cullen and Webster, 1977), lending support for this hypothesis of membrane synthesis in myelinating oligodendrocytes. Braun *et al.* (1980*a,b*) have demonstrated the presence of a discrete population of microsomal-sized vesicles, containing certain myelin-specific proteins, in mouse brain during early stages of myelinogenesis, further implicating specific myelin precursor vesicles in the process of myelinogenesis.

However, the process of myelin assembly is considerably more complicated than the mere fusion of membrane precursor vesicles with the growing oligodendroglial plasma membrane. For one thing, the compositions of mature

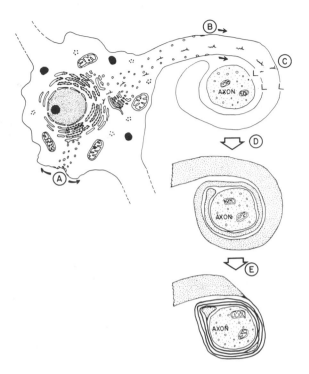

FIGURE 4. Diagram of possible mechanisms of CNS myelin assembly and maturation. A myelinating oligodendrocyte is shown with one process beginning to spiral around an axon. Some newly synthesized proteins and lipids are transferred from the endoplasmic reticulum and Golgi apparatus, where they are synthesized and processed, to the growing plasma membrane via precursor vesicles. These vesicles, which bud off the endoplasmic reticulum and Golgi apparatus, are directed to the plasma membrane by mechanisms possibly involving cytoskeletal elements. (A, B) Two somewhat different possibilities for extension of the plasma membrane via this mechanism are illustrated. (A) Precursor vesicles, similar in composition to the preexisting plasma membrane, fuse with the surface membrane and cause an overall increase in membrane surface area. The membrane flow away from this region (indicated by the solid arrows) indirectly leads to formation and extension of the myelinating process. If this scheme occurs, additional mechanisms must exist to retain relatively more of the protein (and probably also specific proteins) in the plasma membrane portion of the plasma membrane–myelin unit (see the text). (B) Specialized myelin precursor vesicles already similar in composition to myelin, are directed to fuse only with the surface membrane of the myelinating process of the cell. In this case, membrane flow (solid arrows) from this area directly accounts for extension of the myelinating process. In addition to fusion of precursor vesicles, specific lipids and proteins are also added to the myelin membrane as maturation occurs (see the text). This process is depicted only for lipids. These lipids are presumably complexed with some type of carrier or transfer protein, possibly directed to the desired location by microtubules or other cytoskeletal elements; this transported complex is denoted as ~L in the figure. Incorporation of these lipids into the maturing myelin (C) presumably occurs at a site in the process past the region were vesicle fusion occurs. Continued extension of the myelinating process of the oligodendrocyte, with subsequent spiraling around the axon (D), followed by extrusion of most of the cytoplasm and close apposition (or possibly even fusion) of the adjacent membrane surfaces (E) eventually gives rise to compact mature myelin, which is depicted in the bottom drawing.

myelin and oligodendroglial plasma membrane differ somewhat, with the latter having a higher proportion of protein (Poduslo, 1975). Thus, as Rumsby (1980) has suggested, a gradient of chemical composition exists from the oligodendroglial plasma membrane along the processes (of varying length) extending to the compact myelin. The manner in which this gradient is formed during myelinogenesis and later maintained is not known, but some type of special mechanisms must exist either to direct the transport of specific lipids and proteins to specific membrane-assembly sites (see below) or, alternatively, to retain molecules required for specific plasma-membrane functions in the plasma membrane itself. Cytoskeletal elements such as tubulin may be involved in either or both of these processes.

In addition to the aforedescribed complication, there is considerable metabolic evidence that mature myelin is not assembled synchronously as a unit. When protein synthesis is inhibited with puromycin or cycloheximide, the appearance of newly synthesized protein in isolated myelin is blocked; however, lipid synthesis, as well as the appearance of newly synthesized lipid in myelin, continues at a normal rate for 3–6 hr (Benjamins *et al.*, 1971; Smith and Hasinoff, 1971). These results indicate that the addition of newly synthesized lipid to myelin is not dependent on the synchronous addition of newly synthesized protein.

These findings do not eliminate the possibility that preexisting protein is required for addition of newly synthesized lipids to myelin, since there could be more than one intracellular pool of these myelin components. However, the observations discussed above, coupled with the fact that the composition of myelin changes somewhat during the process of maturation and compaction (Horrocks *et al.*, 1966; Norton and Poduslo, 1973), suggest that at least some of the components of the mature myelin membrane may be incorporated by mechanisms other than those involved in the bulk synthesis of membranes in general. Individual lipid molecules may be added to the maturing myelin membrane via soluble lipid-exchange proteins (C in Figure 4). Soluble lipoproteins that bind sulfatide have in fact been reported in brain (Hershkowitz *et al.*, 1968), and there is metabolic evidence suggesting the involvement of these soluble lipoproteins in myelin assembly (Hershkowitz *et al.*, 1968, 1969; Pleasure and Prockop, 1972; Jungalwala, 1974a; Pasquini *et al.*, 1975). However, there is also metabolic evidence that sulfatide may be transferred from its site of synthesis to myelin in vesicles that are at least partially associated with lysosomes (Burkart *et al.*, 1982). Soluble proteins that bind cerebroside are also present in brain (Mallia and Radin, 1977), and there is some evidence that the transfer of newly synthesized cerebrosides to myelin may be mediated by a cytosolic component (Yahara *et al.*, 1980). Soluble lipoproteins that bind phospholipids have also been demonstrated in brain (Benjamins and McKhann, 1973b; Harvey *et al.*, 1973). There is *in vitro* evidence both for (Brammer,

1978; Carey and Foster, 1977) and against (E. K. Miller and Dawson, 1972*b;* Pasquini *et al.,* 1975) the transfer of these lipids from their sites of synthesis to myelin via a cytosolic factor. Studies on the kinetics of entry of individual lipid species into myelin are discussed in more detail below.

Because of the physical continuity between the oligodendroglial plasma membrane and the myelin sheath, numerous investigators have attempted to isolate membrane fractions that might represent a "transition membrane" stage between the undifferentiated oligodendroglial plasma membrane and mature myelin. The assumption is that this "immature myelin" and possibly some oligodendroglial plasma-membrane fragments may be attached to, or associated with, mature myelin during the initial isolation steps. A "myelin like" fraction has been isolated from crude myelin following osmotic shock (Agrawal *et al.,* 1970; Fischer and Morell, 1974). This "myelin like" fraction has a composition intermediate between the compositions of microsomes and mature myelin and consists of vesicles larger than microsomes but smaller than myelin vesicles, suggesting that it may consist of any or a combination of oligodendroglial plasma membrane, cytoplasmic loops, and immature uncompacted myelin (Agrawal *et al.,* 1970; Fischer and Morell, 1974). In general, the components of the myelinlike fraction show more rapid incorporation and turnover than those of mature myelin, but it is not known whether this fraction actually represents myelin precursor membranes, a mixture of myelin and microsomes, or possibly even a completely unrelated fraction.

A refinement of the approach described above has been to separate a crude myelin fraction into arbitrary subfractions on the basis of differences in size and density of the myelin vesicles (for references, see Benjamins *et al.,* 1973; Zimmerman *et al.,* 1975; Quarles, 1978). The densest subfraction has a composition similar to that of the myelin-like fraction, with increasing amounts of myelin-enriched lipids and proteins present in progressively less dense subfractions (Eng and Bignami, 1972; Benjamins *et al.,* 1973; Matthieu *et al.,* 1973; Agrawal *et al.,* 1974).

At short times following radioactive-precursor injection, the specific activity of sulfatide (Benjamins *et al.,* 1973), phospholipids (Benjamins *et al.,* 1976*b*), and proteins (Agrawal *et al.,* 1974; Benjamins *et al.,* 1976*a*) is higher in the dense subfractions than in the lighter subfractions, suggesting that the denser subfractions may be precursors to the less-dense subfractions.

In addition, at longer times after precursor injection, the least-dense fractions have the highest specific activities (Benjamins *et al.,* 1973, 1976*a,b;* Daniel *et al.,* 1972), suggesting a possible transfer of components from the dense to the lighter subfractions. All these results suggest that these arbitrarily defined subfractions may actually have some functional significance with regard to myelin assembly. However, as noted previously, the situation is very complex and it should be emphasized that these data are only consistent with, but do not prove, precursor–product relationships, since other kinetic explanations are also possible.

Time-staggered injections of precursors labeled with different isotopes (^{3}H and ^{14}C) have been utilized in an attempt to better define possible precursor–product relationships among subfractions. The idea is to determine whether the various components of myelin are added simultaneously to all the subfractions or whether they enter one subfraction and then move sequentially through the others (Benjamins *et al.*, 1976*a,b*) (See Figure 5). If a given lipid is added simultaneously, the ^{3}H/^{14}C ratio for that lipid at short times following a time-staggered injection sequence should be the same in all fractions. However, if newly synthesized lipids are added to the densest subfraction and then proceed through increasingly lighter subfractions, the isotope ratio should decrease as one examines progressively lighter subfractions (Figure 5).

In one series of experiments, [^{14}C]glycerol was injected intracranially, then 30 min later [^{3}H]glycerol was injected. Rats were killed 15 min after the second injection and myelin subfractions were isolated. Thus, lipids were labeled for 45 min with [^{14}C]glycerol and 15 min with [^{3}H]glycerol (Benjamins *et al.*, 1976*b*). Isotope ratios for choline phosphoglycerides were relatively similar in the subfractions, suggesting simultaneous or nonordered addition of these molecules. (Similar results were also obtained for cerebrosides and sulfatides, using [^{3}H] and [^{14}C]galactose.) However, isotope ratios for ethanolamine phosphoglycerides (both the diacyl and plasmalogen species) decreased from the bottom to the top of the gradient, consistent with a sequential addition. These results suggest that ethanolamine phosphoglycerides are inserted in the maturing membrane at a specific stage (and perhaps at a specific location along the myelinating cell process), while most other major myelin lipids can

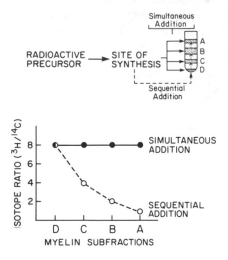

FIGURE 5. *Top:* Diagram illustrating simultaneous vs. sequential entry of lipids into myelin subfractions, which are represented as bands on a discontinuous gradient. The four subfractions shown (A–D) differ from one another in particle density and size, with the least dense particles in subfraction A and the most dense in subfraction D. *Bottom:* Illustration of isotope ratio patterns among myelin subfractions that might be expected following a time-staggered injection protocol (in which a ^{14}C-labeled precursor is injected first, and the same precursor labeled with ^{3}H is injected some time later) if the kinetics of entry for a given lipid were simultaneous (●———●) or sequential (o· · · ·o). Modified from Benjamins *et al.* (1976*b*).

be inserted in a less specific manner at any stage. Again, there are a number of reservations regarding interpretation of these data (for example, the kinetics of addition of individual lipid species was never completely sequential or simultaneous); at best, the data are consistent with, but do not prove, the aforestated hypothesis. Thus, it is also possible that these subfractions are actually metabolically unrelated.

The "simultaneous" entry of cerebrosides, sulfatides, and choline phosphoglycerides may be accomplished by the soluble lipid-exchange proteins mentioned earlier. It is also possible that some myelin lipid arises from its *in situ* synthesis in myelin, since some enzymes of lipid synthesis have been reported to be components of purified myelin (see Section 4).

For additional discussions and reviews of the possible relationships of myelin subfractions and myelin assembly, see Benjamins and Smith (1977), Benjamins and Morell (1977), and Danks and Matthieu (1979). Some data are also available concerning the processing of myelin proteins through vesicular fractions prior to their incorporation into myelin (Pereyra and Braun, 1983; Pereyra *et al.,* 1983).

6. METABOLIC TURNOVER OF MYELIN LIPIDS

The rate at which different lipid components of the myelin sheath turn over, and the relationship of this metabolism to the perikaryon of the oligodendroglial cell, are matters under active investigation in many laboratories. In fact, 15 years ago, an article by Marion Smith (1968) started with the sentence, "The turnover of the lipid components of myelin labeled with radioactive precursors has been extensively investigated," and an already formidable number of papers were referred to. The second sentence summarized what was, at that time, a revisionistic minority view, namely, that "a spectrum of turnover rates exists within the myelin membrane"; this latter statement referenced two papers, Smith and Eng (1965) and Smith (1967), that showed that myelin phospholipids turned over at different rates. When myelinating rats were injected intracranially with [^{14}C]glucose, radioactivity initially incorporated into phosphatidylinositol and lecithin was removed more rapidly than that in phosphatidylserine or sphingomyelin. Also, in agreement with earlier studies from Davison's laboratory, cerebroside and cholesterol were metabolically quite stable.

It soon became clear that the interpretation of continued metabolic turnover of myelin phospholipid was correct. However, it was (and still is) difficult to quantitatively correlate data from different laboratories. For example, the reported half-life of phosphatidylcholine in myelin varies from less than 10 days (Sun, 1973) to 167 days (Lapetina *et al.,* 1970). The experimental design appropriate for such studies, the actual results and the interpretation of the results are all matters of some contention. Even a brief survey of the literature makes it clear that the apparent half-life of a particular lipid in myelin is a function of the class of lipid, the subclass (components of a given lipid class may have different turnover rates depending on their fatty-acid chain lengths), the method of myelin isolation, the radioactive precursor used, the age at which the animal is injected, and the period of time over which decay of radioactivity is followed. Some of these variables are discussed in the following paragraphs.

Dependence of the apparent half-life of brain lipids on the radioactive precursor injected into brain has been known for some time; e.g., the half-time for radioactivity in phosphatidylcholine isolated from brain microsomes was reported as 1.9 days using [^{14}C]glycerol, 11.7 days with [^{14}C]choline, and 18.6 days with [^{32}P]phosphate (Abdel-Latif and Smith, 1970). An important methodological advance was made with the observation by Benjamins and McKhann (1973a) that [2-^{3}H]glycerol was a good pulse label for brain phospholipid. Reutilization of label from this precursor is inefficient because once the phospholipid is catabolized to the level of glycerol-3-phosphate, the isotope is rapidly lost to form water by action of either cytoplasmic glycerol phosphate dehydrogenase (EC 1.1.1.8, an NADPH$^+$-linked enzyme) or the mitochondrial enzyme (EC 1.1.99.5, a respiratory-chain enzyme). Using [2-^{3}H]glycerol as a reference, S. L. Miller *et al.*, (1977) compared the turnover time of various myelin phospholipids using several different radioactive precursors. The results for the labeling of three lipids by any of three radioactive precursors are presented in Table 2, these three examples being sufficient to emphasize the variation of results dependent on precursor.

A reasonable interpretation of these data is that over the time period studied, the aforenamed myelin lipids are catabolized with a half-life of the order of weeks as measured by [2-^{3}H]glycerol turnover, that the phosphate moiety is reutilized to a certain extent, and that the long-chain hydrophobic moieties

TABLE 2. Apparent Half-Lives of Myelin Lipids as Determined Using Different Labeled Precursors[a]

Precursors	Phosphatidyl-choline	Phosphatidyl-ethanolamine	Ethanolamine plasmalogen
[2-^{3}H]Glycerol	25	25	34
Base moiety[b]	39	33	58
[^{14}C]Acetate	54	125	Stable

[a] Data from S. L. Miller *et al.* (1977). Rats were injected intracranially at 17 days of age; half-lives (in days) are for slow-turnover pools and are based on data obtained 15 or more days after injection.
[b] [^{14}C]Choline for phosphatidylcholine; [^{14}C]ethanolamine for phosphatidylethanolamine and ethanolamine plasmalogen.

(into which the radioactive acetate is directed) are preferentially reutilized for synthesis of the different phospholipids. The recycling of acyl moieties of phospholipids has been directly demonstrated (Kishimoto *et al.,* 1965; Sun and Horrocks, 1973). Note that although glycerophospholipid turnover is easily demonstrated, the early reports of the considerably greater metabolic stability of cholesterol, cerebroside, and sulfatide have been confirmed (for references and discussions, see Davison, 1970; Benjamins and Smith, 1977). The metabolic turnover of at least some of the sphingomyelin appears to be intermediate between that of the glycerophospholipid and that of the galactolipids (Jungalwala, 1974*b;* Freysz and Mandel, 1980).

In examining data in the literature for turnover of myelin lipids, it is evident that immediately following the period of maximal incorporation of a precursor in a given lipid, there is a relatively fast metabolic decay. With increasing time after injection, the apparent half-life increases.

Most of these studies have been carried out with animals injected with a radioactive precursor during the time of active myelinogenesis. One interpretation of these results is that for several days after injection and synthesis of lipids, the lipids are not yet buried deep within the myelin sheath and are more accessible to the systems involved in membrane lipid turnover (see Figure 6). This hypothesis receives some support from the observation that when older animals (only slowly accumulating myelin) are injected with a radioactive precursor for myelin lipids, it is primarily the more rapid turnover phase that is observed (S. L. Miller and Morell, 1978). Since myelin is being formed less rapidly (the rate of myelin accumulation is greatly decreased in older animals relative to younger ones) the period of time during which myelin is accessible to lipid-turnover systems prior to being deeply buried under successive layers of myelin is greatly extended.

Another hypothesis (Horrocks *et al.,* 1976; S. L. Miller *et al.,* 1977; Hennacy and Horrocks, 1978; Freysz and Mandel, 1980) is that the rapidly turning over pool represents the lipids at the major dense line (cytoplasmic face), which are more likely to come into contact with cytoplasm. In contrast, the more metabolically stable pool would consist of lipid at the intraperiod line (extracellular face) separated from the cytoplasmic face by the energy barrier to "flip-flop" across the lipid bilayer. In young animals, both metabolic pools would be labeled as myelin is rapidly accumulating. In older animals, the cytoplasmic-face lipids would be preferentially labeled, but would also decay rapidly. A further refinement of this hypothesis is based on a study showing that in myelin of mature rats, sphingomyelin containing short-chain fatty acids (C18:sphingomyelin) turned over at a significant rate (of the order of 2 months), while the long-chain lipid (C24:sphingomyelin) was much more stable metabolically (Freysz and Mandel, 1980; for a contradictory report, see also LeBaron *et al.,* 1981). It has been suggested that the more rapidly turning

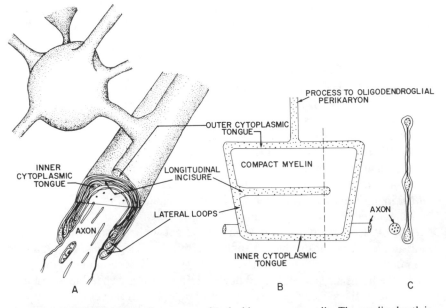

FIGURE 6. (A) Cutaway view of an axon ensheathed by compact myelin. The myelin sheath is connected to the supporting oligodendrocyte by a cytoplasmic process. Note the specialized areas of the myelin sheath that contain oligodendroglial cytoplasm. (B) Diagrammatic view of mature CNS myelin as it would appear if unrolled from the axon. Note that the specialized structures of myelin that contain cytoplasm are all continuous with each other and with the cytoplasm of the oligodendroglial cell, although the latter is located a considerable distance from the sheath itself. (C) Side view of the unrolled compact myelin sheath depicted in (B). Individual lipid species in compact myelin presumably must diffuse laterally within the lipid bilayers of the myelin lamellae until they reach a region of cytoplasm before they can be removed. If actual catabolism takes place predominantly in lysosomes in the cell body (as opposed to degradation in lysosomes in cytoplasmic regions of the myelin sheath), lipids must also be transported by some means back to the cell body. Modified from Bunge (1968) and Hirano and Dembitzer (1967.)

over sphingomyelin may be on the cytoplasmic face while the longer-chain-containing lipid may be on the extracellular face (Freysz and Mandel, 1980; Freysz and Horrocks, 1980).

7. CATABOLISM OF MYELIN LIPIDS

It is generally assumed that the bulk of the myelin lipids are degraded by various hydrolases in lysosomes in the perikaryon of the oligodendrocyte since, with a few notable exceptions (see below), enzymes responsible for lipid catabolism are not present in purified myelin. However, the compact multilamellar nature of mature myelin and its location a considerable distance from the oligodendroglial perikaryon presents some special problems with regard to the turnover of myelin lipids, and the mechanisms by which lipids are transferred from myelin back to the perikaryon are not well understood. Possibilities include removal and transfer by soluble transfer proteins or removal as part of vesicles destined to return to the perikaryon and fuse with lysosomes. These possibilities are essentially the reverse of the processes postulated for myelin assembly. However, it should be noted that the turnover of myelin components must involve more than just random formation of vesicles that are transported back to the cell body and degraded as a unit, since, as noted in Section 6, individual lipids (and proteins as well) show a spectrum of apparent turnover rates. Differences in the actual rates at which lipids in myelin are replaced may be related to their asymmetric location within the lipid bilayer, to different physicochemical interactions with nearby membrane components, to the presence or absence (or differing concentrations) of specific exchange proteins, or to some combination of these factors.

If lipids deep within the compact multilamellar structure of myelin do indeed turn over, lateral diffusion to a specialized region of the sheath (e.g., the lateral loops, inner and outer cytoplasmic tongue, or longitudinal incisures) is probably a prerequisite (see Figure 6), since the alternative movement of lipid molecules radially through consecutive myelin layers is rather unlikely due to the large thermodynamic barrier that exists against such movement. Even after a given lipid molecule reaches one of the specialized myelin structures containing cytoplasm, it still has a long distance to travel before reaching the lysosomes in the perikaryon of the oligodendrocyte. It is possible that a small amount of lipid catabolism may also occur in these specialized cytoplasmic structures themselves, since some of them appear by electron microscopy to have some lysosomal properties (Woelk and Porcellati, 1978), but there is no evidence that this is quantitatively significant. Thus, in view of the complex structure of mature myelin and its spatial relationship to the supporting oligodendrocyte, it is not surprising that much of the lipid turnover in this membrane is somewhat slower than that in other membranes.

Developmental studies on enzymes involved in oligodendroglial lipid metabolism are relatively sparse, in part possibly due to the relatively nonspecific nature of many of the hydrolases. However, the activity of cerebroside galactosidase, the enzyme responsible for catabolism of cerebroside, has been examined in brain during development (Bowen and Radin, 1969*a*). In contrast to the synthetic enzyme, the activity of which corresponds to the rate of myelin accumulation, the hydrolytic activity corresponds to the total amount of myelin present in brain. Activity is initially quite low, but increases rapidly during the period of active myelin accumulation and then remains at a relatively high level. Alterations in the characteristics of cerebroside galactosidase have been noted in myelin-deficient mutant mice (Bowen and Radin, 1969*b*). The amoung of enzyme activity released by sonication is somewhat higher in jimpy mice than in controls, and it has been suggested that the myelin deficiency in these mutants may be related to this factor. Activity of arylsulfatase, presumably involved in sulfatide catabolism, also increases during development, reaching a maximum at 15 days and then remaining at a relatively high level (Bowen and Radin, 1969*a*). It is possible that these and other catabolic enzymes are present in excess in oligodendroglial lysosomes and that the rates of catabolism of the various myelin lipids are limited by their delivery from myelin to the lysosomes. For example, mice that are heterozygous for the twitcher mutation (a genetic deficiency of cerebroside galactosidase in which homozygotes do not survive beyond 3 months) have only half the normal levels of cerebroside galactosidase, but appear normal and do not show any other biochemical or clinical abnormalities (Kobayashi *et al.*, 1980).

Only one enzyme involved in lipid catabolism, a cholesterol ester hydrolase with a pH optimum of 7.1 (Eto and Suzuki, 1973; Igarashi and Suzuki, 1977), has been specifically localized to myelin. This enzyme may be involved in the process of myelination since, as noted previously, there is a transient increase in cholesterol esters in myelin during the period of active myelination that might possibly be involved with the myelin degeneration that is a part of the normal postnatal maturation process.

The activity of plasmalogenase, the enzyme responsible for initiating the degradation of ethanolamine plasmalogens, is much higher in isolated oligodendrocytes than in isolated neurons or astrocytes (Dorman *et al.*, 1977), consistent with the localization of large amounts of plasmalogen in myelin. Plasmalogenase activity is increased early in a number of different demyelinating lesions, leading to the suggestion that it may be involved in the initiation of demyelination (Horrocks *et al.*, 1978).

8. METABOLIC PERTURBATIONS

Although a detailed review is beyond the scope of this chapter, it is worth noting that some of our knowledge regarding the metabolism of myelin and oligodendroglia has been derived from the examination of perturbed systems. A brief discussion with several illustrative examples follows.

It has been known for some time that the myelin sheath and its supporting oligodendrocyte constitute a single metabolic entity. Furthermore, the metabolic integrity of this entity is dependent on the integrity of the ensheathed axon, and an insult to any part of this oligodendrocyte–myelin–neuron–axon unit may lead to metabolic alterations of the entire unit. For example, degeneration of myelin occurs subsequent to either axonal injury (Wallerian degeneration) or injury to the oligodendrocyte perikaryon caused by viruses or anti-bodies to CNS antigens. It is also apparent that unlike their PNS counterparts, the Schwann cells, oligodendrocytes are not able to recover significantly from serious injury. Furthermore, the complex structure of myelin does not allow a large imbalance of its lipid components, as evidenced by the reduced levels of myelin seen in various lipid-storage diseases such as metachromatic leukodys-trophy and Krabbe's disease (globoid-cell leukodystrophy). For more detailed discussions of and references concerned with these aspects of perturbed myelin metabolism, see Norton (1977*b*) and Smith and Benjamins (1977).

Genetic mutants have also been useful in gaining a better understanding of the processes involved in myelin metabolism (for detailed reviews, see Hogan, 1977; Baumann, 1980). The jimpy, myelin-synthesis-deficient, and quaking strains of mutant mice, all of which have genetic defects that appear to be limited to the formation of myelin, have proved especially valuable. The deficiency of numerous myelin components in these mutants suggests that the mutations occur at the level of regulation or coordination of processes involved in myelin assembly.

Numerous drugs and toxins adversely affect myelin, and some of these have been used as tools to examine various aspects of myelin metabolism. For example, administration of hypocholesteremic agents that inhibit cholesterol synthesis (AY9944 or 20, 25-diazocholesterol) to developing animals results in decreased amounts of myelin (Fumigalli *et al.,*1969; Smith *et al.,* 1970; Banik and Davison, 1971). Incorporation of precursors into lipids and proteins is depressed by similar degrees, suggesting that a deficiency in a given lipid com-ponent can limit the assembly of the myelin membrane. In addition to decreased amounts of myelin, much of the cholesterol normally present is replaced by other sterols. If the drug treatments are suspended, these sterols are replaced by cholesterol within several weeks, suggesting a rather active exchange of myelin sterols, even in mature animals.

Exposure of developing animals to heavy-metal toxins, such as inorganic lead, triethyl lead, or triethyl tin, leads to CNS myelin deficits, some of which appear to persist even after exposure to the toxins is terminated. Chronic expo-sure of adult animals to triethyl tin or hexachlorophene produces alterations in myelin, including the presence of a "dissociated myelin" fraction, presumably resulting from the abnormal myelin metabolism associated with these pertur-bations. Other conditions known to alter myelin and myelin metabolism include exposure to cuprizone or diphtheria toxin, deficiencies in copper or vita-min B_{12}, and certain genetic diseases of amino acid metabolism. For a more detailed discussion and references, see Smith and Benjamins (1977).

The importance of adequate nutrition during the period of rapid myelin accumulation (for example, see Wiggins *et al.,* 1976; Wiggins, 1982; Krigman and Hogan, 1976) and the role of thyroid hormones in controlling the developmental pattern of myelinogenesis (for a discussion and references, see Walters and Morell, 1981) have also been demonstrated.

9. CONCLUSIONS AND FUTURE DIRECTIONS

Most of the information that we assume to pertain to lipid metabolism in oligodendroglial cells has been extrapolated from *in vivo* studies. There is general acceptance of the hypothesis that lipids are synthesized primarily on intracellular membranes and, during the period of active myelin accumulation, are transported to a region of the cell where they are combined with proteins to form the specialized membrane that eventually becomes mature myelin. The concept of a continuum of intermediate steps in the maturation of myelin has also received much support. Oligodendroglial cells produce both the "common" and "myelin-specific" lipids that are components of this specialized membrane. There are controls on the activity of both synthetic and, to a lesser extent, catabolic enzymes so that production and turnover of myelin lipids are matched to allow rapid accumulation of myelin early in development and slower accumulation and maintenance of myelin later on.

Many of these concepts will presumably receive an even firmer basis when the long-sought goal is attained of having available readily manipulatable oligodendroglial cell cultures that accumulate myelin. The ability to synchronize myelin formation in culture will allow the elucidation of many details of myelin assembly that are difficult to study in the intact nervous system, in which different cells are at different stages of their program of myelinogenesis at a given time. Nevertheless, it should be kept in mind that most conclusions from *in vitro* studies eventually require confirmation from appropriately designed *in vivo* studies to ensure that the tissue-culture system carries out specialized functions in the same manner as *in vivo*.

Furthermore, there are still many types of questions that, even assuming the availability of well-behaved cell-culture systems, are still best studied *in vivo*. The next few years will most likely see the introduction of recombinant DNA technology and nucleic acid probes to study mechanisms of control of myelinogenesis. Probes to study the precise localization of RNA messages for myelin proteins are currently being developed (e.g., Colman *et al.*, 1982). The study of expression and localization of RNA messages coding for enzymes of myelin lipid synthesis and catabolism is further off because of the lack of pure enzyme preparations that can be sequenced so that the information is available for synthesis of nucleic acid probes. The details of the coordinate control of synthesis and catabolism of many different lipids (and how this is related to expression of the RNA messages and the synthesis of myelin proteins) should eventually be studied *in situ*, since it would then be possible to correlate these results with morphological and biochemical events in other adjacent cells of different types. It is, in fact, the vastly complex interrelationships of the different cell types, which are integral to most nervous-system developmental events, that guarantee a central role for *in vivo* studies in furthering our understanding of how lipid metabolism in oligodendroglial cells is regulated with respect to the task of forming and maintaining myelin.

Acknowledgments

The authors research described herein was supported in part by USPHS Grants NS-11615, HD-03110, and ES-01104. We are grateful to Dr. Lloyd A. Horrocks for his helpful suggestions regarding revisions of this manuscript.

10. REFERENCES

Abdel-Latif, A. A., and Abood, L. G., 1966, *In vivo* incorporation of L-[^{14}C] serine into phospholipids and proteins of the subcellular fractions of developing rat brain, *J. Neurochem.* **13**:1189–1196.

Abdel-Latif, A. A., and Smith, J. P., 1970, *In vivo* incorporation of choline, glycerol and orthophosphate into lecithin and other phospholipids of subcellular fractions of rat cerebellum, *Biochim. Biophys. Acta* **218**:134–140.

Adams, C. W. M., and Davison, A. N., 1959, The occurrence of esterified cholesterol in the developing nervous system, *J. Neurochem.* **4**:282–289.

Agrawal, H. C., Banik, N. L., Bone, A. H., Davison, A. N., Mitchell, R. F., and Spohn, M., 1970, The identity of a myelin-like fraction isolated from developing brain, *Biochem. J.* **120**:635–642.

Agrawal, H. C., Trotter, J. L., Burton, R. M., and Mitchell, R. F., 1974, Metabolic studies on myelin—Evidence for a precursor role of a myelin subfraction, *Biochem. J.* **140**:99–109.

Alling, C., and Svennerholm, L., 1969, Concentration and fatty acid composition of cholesteryl esters of normal human brain, *J. Neurochem.* **16**:751–759.

Ansell, G. B., 1973, Phospholipids and the nervous system, in: *Form and Function of Phospholipids* (G. B. Ansell, J. N. Hawthorne, and R. M. C. Dawson, eds.), pp. 377–422, Elsevier, New York.

Arienti, G., Brunetti, M., Gaiti, A., Orlando, P., and Porcellati, G., 1976, The contribution of net synthesis and base-exchange reactions in phospholipid biosynthesis, in: *Function and Metabolism of Phospholipids in the Central and Peripheral Nervous Systems* (G. Porcellati, L. Amaducci, and C. Galli, eds.), pp. 63–78, Plenum Press, New York.

Autilio-Gambetti, L., Gambetti, P., and Schafer, B., 1975, Glial and neuronal contribution to proteins and glycoproteins recovered in myelin fractions, *Brain Res.* **84**:336–340.

Balasurbramanian, A. S., and Bachhawat, B. K., 1965, Formation of cerebroside sulphate from 3′-phosphoadenosine-5′-phosphosulphate in sheep brain, *Biochim. Biophys. Acta* **106**:218–220.

Banik, N. L., and Davison, A. N., 1971, Exchange of sterols between myelin and other membranes of developing rat brain, *Biochem. J.* **122**:751–758.

Basu, S., Schultz, A. M., Basu, M., and Roseman, S., 1971, Enzymatic synthesis of galactocerebroside by a galactosyltransferase from embryonic chicken brain, *J. Biol. Chem.* **246**:4272–4279.

Baumann, N. (ed.), 1980, *Neurological Mutations Affecting Myelination,* INSERM Symposium No. 14, Elsevier/North-Holland, Amsterdam.

Benjamins, J. A., and Iwata, R., 1979, Kinetics of entry of galactolipids and phospholipids into myelin, *J. Neurochem.* **32**:921–926.

Benjamins, J. A., and McKhann, G. M., 1973*a*, [2-^{3}H] Glycerol as a precursor of phospholipids in rat brain: Evidence for lack of recycling, *J. Neurochem.* **20**:1111–1120.

Benjamins, J. A., and McKhann, G. M., 1973*b*, Properties and metabolism of soluble lipoproteins containing choline and ethanolamine phospholipids in rat brain, *J. Neurochem.* **20**:1121–1129.

Benjamins, J. A., and Morell, P., 1977, Assembly of myelin, in: *Mechanisms, Regulation and Special Functions of Protein Synthesis in the Brain* (S. Roberts, A. Lajtha, and W. H. Gispen, eds.), pp. 183–197, Elsevier/North-Holland, Amsterdam.

Benjamins, J. A., and Smith, M. E., 1977, Metabolism of myelin, in: *Myelin* (P. Morell, ed.), pp. 233–270, Plenum Press, New York.

Benjamins, J. A., Herschkowitz, N. Robinson, J., and McKhann, G. M., 1971, The effects of inhibitors of protein synthesis on incorporation of lipids into myelin, *J. Neurochem.* **18**:729–738.

Benjamins, J. A., Miller, K., and McKhann, G. M., 1973, Myelin subfractions in developing rat brain: Characterization and sulphatide metabolism, *J. Neurochem.* **20**:1589–1603.

Benjamins, J. A., Guarnieri, M., Sonneborn, M., and McKhann, G. M., 1974, Sulphatide synthesis in isolated oligodendroglial and neuronal cells, *J. Neurochem.* **23**:751–757.

Benjamins, J. A., Gray, M., and Morell, P., 1976*a*, Metabolic relationships between myelin subfractions: Entry of proteins, *J. Neurochem.* **27**:521–575.

Benjamins, J. A., Miller, S. L., and Morell, P., 1976*b*, Metabolic relationships between myelin subfractions: Entry of galactolipids and phospholipids, *J. Neurochem.* **27**:565–570.

Benjamins, J. A., Hadden, T., and Skoff, R. P., 1982, Cerebroside sulfotransferase in Golgi-enriched fractions from rat brain, *J. Neurochem.* **38**:233–241.

Bennett, G., di Giamberardino, L., Koenig, H. L., and Droz, B., 1973, Axonal migration of protein and glycoprotein to nerve endings. II. Radioautographic analysis of the renewal of glycoproteins in nerve endings of chicken ciliary ganglion after intracerebral injection of ^{3}H-fucose and ^{3}H-glucosamine, *Brain Res.* **60**:129–146.

Berthold, C. H., 1973, Local "demyelination" in developing feline nerve fibers, *Neurobiology* **3**:339–345.

Berthold, C.-H., 1974, A comparative morphological study of the developing node–paranode region in lumbar spinal roots. II. OTAN-staining, *Neurobiology* **4**:117–131.

Berthold, C. H., and Hildebrand, C., 1979, Free and esterified cholesterol in developing feline lumbosacral spinal roots, *J. Neurochem.* **32**:237–240.

Bowen, D. M., and Radin, N. S., 1969*a*, Cerebroside galactosidase: A method for determination and a comparison with other lysosomal enzymes in developing rat brain, *J. Neurochem.* **16**:501–511.

Bowen, D. M., and Radin, N. S., 1969*b*, Hydrolase activities in brain of neurological mutants: Cerebroside galactosidase, nitrophenyl galactoside hydrolase, nitrophenyl glucoside hydrolase and sulphatase, *J. Neurochem.* **16**:457–460.

Bowen, D. M., Davison, A. N., and Ramsey, R.B., 1974, The dynamic role of lipids in the nervous system, *Int. Rev. Sci. (Biochem. Ser. 1)* **4**:141–179.

Bardy, R. O., Bradley, R. M., Young, O. M., and Kalles, H., 1965, An alternative pathway for the enzymatic synthesis of sphingomyelin, *J. Biol. Chem.* **240**:3693–3694.

Brammer, M. J., 1978, The protein-mediated transfer of lecithin to sub-fractions of mature and developing rat myelin, *J. Neurochem.* **31**:1435–1440.

Braun, P. E., Pereyra, P. M., and Greenfield, S., 1980*a,* Myelin organization and development: A biochemical perspective, in: *Myelin: Chemistry and Biology* (G. A. Hashim, ed.), pp. 1–17, Alan R. Liss, New York.

Braun, P. E., Pereyra, P. M., and Greenfield, S., 1980*b,* Mechanisms of assembly of myelin in mice: A new approach to the problem, in: *Neurological Mutations Affecting Myelination* (N. Baumann, ed.), INSERM Symposium Vo. 14, pp. 413–421, Elsevier/North-Holland, Amsterdam.

Brenkert, A., and Radin, N. S., 1972, Synthesis of galactocerebroside and glucocerebroside by rat brain: Assay procedures and changes with age, *Brain Res.* **36**:183–193.

Brunetti, M., diGiamberardino, L., Porcellati, G., and Droz, B., 1981, Contribution of axonal transport to the renewal of myelin phospholipids in peripheral nerves. II. Biochemical study, *Brain Res.* **219**:73–84.

Bunge, R. P., 1968, Glial cells and the central myelin sheath, *Physiol. Rev.* **48**:197–251.

Burkart, T., Caimi, L., Siegrist, H. P., Herschkowitz, N. N., and Wiesmann, U. N., 1982, Vesicular transport of sulfatide in the myelinating mouse brain: Functional association with liposomes?, *J. Biol. Chem.* **257**:3151–3156.

Burton, R. M., Sodd, M. A., and Brady, R. O., 1958, The incorporation of galactose into galactolipids, *J. Biol. Chem.* **233**:1053–1059.

Butler, M., and Morell, P., 1982, Sidedness of phospholipid synthesis on brain membranes, *J. Neurochem.* **39**:155–164.

Butler, M., and Morell, P., 1983, The role of phosphatidylserine decarboxylase in brain phospholipid metabolism, *J. Neurochem.* **41**:1446–1454.

Cammer, W., Fredman, R., Rose, A. L., and Norton, W. T., 1976, Brain carbonic anhydrase: Activity in isolated myelin and the effect of hexachlorophene, *J. Neurochem.* **27**:167–171.

Cammer, W., Sirota, S. R., Zimmerman, T. T., Jr., and Norton, W. T., 1980, 5'-Nucleotidase in rat brain myelin, *J. Neurochem.* **35**:367–373.

Carey, E. M., and Foster, P. C., 1977, Protein-mediated transfer of phosphatidyl choline to myelin, *Biochem. Soc. Trans.* **5**:1412–1414.

Cleland, W. W., and Kennedy, E. P., 1960, The enzymatic synthesis of psychosine, *J. Biol. Chem.* **235**:45–51.

Cochran, F. B., Yu, R. K., and Ledeen, R. W., 1982, Myelin gangliosides in vertebrates, *J. Neurochem.* **39**:773–779.

Colman, D. R., Kreibich, G., Frey, A. B., and Sabatini, D. D., 1982, Synthesis and incorporation of myelin polypeptides into CNS myelin, *J. Cell Biol.* **95**:598–608.

Costantino-Ceccarini, E., and Morell, P., 1972, Biosynthesis of brain sphingolipids and myelin accumulation in the mouse, *Lipids* **7**:656–659.

Costantino-Ceccarini, E., and Suzuki, K., 1975, Evidence for presence of UDP-galactose:ceramide galactosyltransferase in rat myelin, *Brain Res.* **93**:358–362.

Cullen, M. J., and Webster, H. de F., 1977, The effects of low temperature on myelin formation in optic nerves of *Xenopus* tadpoles, *Tissue Cell* **9**:1–10.

Curtino, J. A., and Caputto, R., 1974, Enzymic synthesis of cerebroside from glycosylsphingosine and stearoyl-CoA by an embryonic chicken brain preparation, *Biochem. Biophys. Res. Commun.* **56**:142–147.

Daniel, A., Day, E. D., and Kaufman, B., 1972, Studies on central nervous system myelin, *Fed. Proc. Fed. Am. Soc. Exp. Biol.* **31**:490.

Danks, D. M., and Matthieu, J.-M., 1979, Hypotheses regarding myelination derived from comparisons of myelin subfractions, *Life Sci.* **24**:1425–1440.

Davison, A. N., 1970, The biochemistry of the myelin sheath, in: *Myelination* (A. N. Davison and A. Peters, eds.), pp. 80–161, Charles C. Thomas, Springfield, Illinois.

Davison, A. N., Dobbing, J., Morgan, R. S., and Payling-Wright, G., 1958, The deposition and disposal of [4-^{14}C] cholesterol in the brain of growing chickens, *J. Neurochem.* 3:39–94.

Deshmukh, D. S., Inoue, T., and Pieringer, R. A., 1971, The association of the galactosyl diglycerides of brain with myelination. II. The inability of the myelin deficient mutant, jimpy mouse, to synthesize galactosyl diglycerides effectively, *J. Biol. Chem.* 246:5695–5699.

Deshmukh, D. S., Bear, W. D., and Brockerhoff, H., 1978a, Polyphosphoinositide biosynthesis in three subfractions of rat brain myelin, *J. Neurochem.* 30:1191–1193.

Deshmukh, D. S., Bear, W. D., and Soifer, D., 1978b, Isolation and characterization of an enriched Golgi fraction from rat brain, *Biochim. Biophys. Acta* 542:284–295.

Deshmukh, D. S., Kuizon, S., Bear, W. D., and Brockerhoff, H., 1981, Rapid incorporation *in vivo* of intracerebrally injected ^{32}Pi into polyphosphoinositides of three subfractions of rat brain myelin, *J. Neurochem.* 36:594–601.

Diringer, H., Marggraf, W. D., Koch, M. A., and Anderer, F. A., 1972, Evidence for a new biosynthetic pathway of sphingomyelin in SV40 transformed mouse cells, *Biochem. Biophys. Res. Commun.* 47:1345–1352.

Dobbing, J., 1963, The entry of cholesterol into rat brain during development, *J. Neurochem.* 10:739–742.

Dorman, R. V., Toews, A. D., and Horrocks, L. A., 1977, Plasmalogenase activities in neuronal perikarya, astroglia and oligodendroglia isolated from bovine brain, *J. Lipid Res.* 18:115–117.

Droz, B., and Boyenval, J., 1975, Le réticulum endoplasmique des axones: Son rôle probable dans le transport axoplasmique des phospholipides membranaires, *J. Microsc. Biol. Cell.* 23:45–46.

Droz, B., Koenig, H. L., and diGiamberardino, L., 1973, Axonal migration of protein and glycoprotein to nerve endings. I. Radioautographic analysis of the renewal of protein in nerve endings of chicken ciliary ganglion after intracerebral injection of ^{3}H-lysine, *Brain Res.* 60:93–127.

Droz, B., diGiamberardino, L., Koenig, H. L., Boyenval, J., and Hassig, R., 1978, Axon–myelin transfer of phospholipid components in the course of their axonal transport as visualized by radioautography, *Brain Res.* 155:347–353.

Droz, B., Brunetti, M., diGiamberardino, L., Koenig, H. L., and Porcellati, G., 1979, Transfer of phospholipid constituents to glia during axonal transport, *Soc. Neurosci. Symp.* 4:344–360.

Droz, B., diGiamberardino, L., and Koenig, H. L., 1981, Contribution of axonal transport to the renewal of myelin phospholipids in peripheral nerves. I. Quantitative radioautographic study, *Brain Res.* 219:57–71.

Edmond, J., 1974, Ketone bodies as precursors of sterols and fatty acids in the developing rat, *J. Biol. Chem.* 249:72–80.

Edmond, J., and Popjak, G., 1974, Transfer of carbon atoms from mevalonate to *n*-fatty acids, *J. Biol. Chem.* 249:66–71.

Eichberg, J., and Dawson, R. M. C., 1965, Polyphosphoinositides in myelin, *Biochem. J.* 96:644–650.

Eichberg, J., and Hauser, G., 1973, The subcellular distribution of phosphoinositides in myelinated and unmyelinated rat brain, *Biochem. Biophys. Acta* 326:210–223.

Eng, L. F., and Bignami, A., 1972, Myelin proteins in young and adult brains, *Trans. Am. Soc. Neurochem.* 3:75.

Eto, Y., and Suzuki, K., 1972, Cholesterol esters in developing rat-brain: Concentration and fatty acid composition, *J. Neurochem.* 19:109–115.

Eto, Y., and Suzuki, K., 1973, Cholesterol ester metabolism in rat brain: A cholesterol ester hydrolase specifically localized in the myelin sheath, *J. Biol. Chem.* **248**:1986–1991.

Farrell, D. F., and McKhann, G. M., 1971, Characterization of cerebroside sulfotransferase from rat brain, *J. Biol. Chem.* **246**:4694–4702.

Fischer, C. A., and Morell, P., 1974, Turnover of proteins in myelin and myelin-like material of mouse brain, *Brain Res.* **74**:51–65.

Fleischer, B., 1977, Localization of some glycolipid glycosylating enzymes in the Golgi apparatus of rat kidney, *J. Supramol. Struct.* **7**:79–89.

Freysz, L., and Horrocks, L. A., 1980, Regulation of the metabolism of myelin phospholipids, in: *Neurological Mutations Affecting Myelination* (N. A. Baumann, ed.), INSERM Symposium No. 14, pp. 223–230, Elsevier/North-Holland, Amsterdam.

Freysz, L., and Mandel, P., 1980, Turnover of molecular species of sphingomyelin in microsomes and myelin of rat brain, *J. Neurochem.* **34**:305–308.

Freysz, L., Horrocks, L. A., and Mandel, P., 1980, Activities of enzymes synthesizing diacyl, alkylacyl, and alkenylacyl glycerophosphoethanolamine and glycerophosphocholine during development of chicken brain, *J. Neurochem.* **34**:963–969.

Fujino, Y., Nakano, M., Negishi, T., and Ito, S., 1968, Substrate specificity for ceramide in the enzymatic formation of sphingomyelin, *J. Biol. Chem.* **243**:4650–4651.

Fumigalli, R., Smith, M. E., Urna, G., and Paoletti, R., 1969, The effect of hypocholesteremic agents on myelinogenesis, *J. Neurochem.* **16**:1329–1339.

Gatt, S., and Barenholz, Y., 1973, Enzymes of complex lipid metabolism, *Annu. Rev. Biochem.* **42**:61–90.

Gonzalez-Sastre, F., Eichberg, J., and Hauser, G., 1971, Metabolic pools of polyphosphoinositides in rat brain, *Biochim. Biophys. Acta* **248**:96–104.

Hajra, A., 1969, Biosynthesis of alkyl-ether containing lipid from dihydroxyacetone phosphate, *Biochem. Biophys. Res. Commun.* **37**:486–492.

Hajra, A. K., and Radin, N. S., 1963, *In vivo* conversion of labeled fatty acids to the sphingolipid fatty acids in rat brain, *J. Lipid Res.* **4**:448–453.

Haley, J. E., and Ledeen, R. W., 1979, Incorporation of axonally transported substances into myelin lipids, *J. Neurochem.* **32**:735–742.

Hammarström, S., 1972a, On the biosynthesis of cerebrosides: Non-enzymatic N-acylation of psychosine by stearoyl coenzyme A, *FEBS Lett.* **21**:259–263.

Hammarström, S., 1972b, On the biosynthesis of cerebrosides containing non-hydroxy acids. 2. Mass spectrometric evidence for the ceramide pathway, *Biochem. Biophys. Res. Commun.* **45**:468–475.

Hammarström, S., and Samuelsson, B., 1972, On the biosynthesis of cerebrosides containing 2-hydroxy acids: Mass spectrometric evidence for biosynthesis via the ceramide pathway, *J. Biol. Chem.* **247**:1001–1011.

Harvey, M. S., Wirtz, K. W. A., Kamp, H. H., Zegers, B. J. M., and Van Deenen, L. L. M., 1973, A study on phospholipid exchange proteins present in the soluble fractions of beef liver and brain, *Biochim. Biophys. Acta* **323**:234–239.

Hawkins, R. A., Williamson, D. H., and Krebs, H. A., 1971, Ketone-body utilization by adult and suckling rat brain *in vivo*, *Biochem. J.* **122**:13–18.

Hawthorne, J. N., and Kai, M., 1970, Metabolism of phosphoinositides, in: *Handbook of Neurochemistry*, Vol. 3 (A. Lajtha, ed.), pp. 491–508, Plenum Press, New York.

Hayes, L., and Jungalwala, F. B., 1976, Synthesis and turnover of cerebrosides and phosphatidyl serine of myelin and microsomal fractions of adult and developing rat brain, *Biochem. J.* **160**:195–204.

Hendrickson, H. S., and Reinertsen, J. L., 1971, Phosphoinositide interconversion: A model for control of Na^+ and K^+ permeability in the nerve axon membrane, *Biochem. Biophys. Res. Commun.* **44**:1258–1264.

Hennacy, D. M., and Horrocks, L. A., 1978, Recent developments in the turnover of proteins and lipids in the myelin and other plasma membranes in the central nervous system, *Bull. Mol. Biol. Med.* **3**:207–221.

Herschkowitz, N., McKhann, G. M., Saxena, S., and Shooter, E. M., 1968, Characterization of sulphatide-containing lipoproteins in rat brain, *J. Neurochem.* **15**:1181–1188.

Herschkowitz, N., McKhann, G. M., Saxena, S., Shooter, E. M., and Herndon, R M., 1969, Synthesis of sulphatide-containing lipoproteins in rat brain, *J. Neurochem.* **16**:1049–1057.

Hildebrand, C., and Berthold, C.-H., 1977, Free and esterifield cholesterol in developing feline white matter, *Lipids* **12**:711–716.

Hildebrand, J., Stoffyn, P., and Hauser, G., 1970, Biosynthesis of lactosyl-ceramide by rat brain preparations and comparisons with the formation of ganglioside GM_1 and psychosine during development, *J. Neurochem.* **17**:403–411.

Hirano, A., and Dembitzer, H., 1967, Structural analysis of the myelin sheath in the central nervous system, *J. Cell Biol.* **34**:555–567.

Hirata, F. and Axelrod, J., 1980, Phospholipid methylation and biological signal transmission, *Science* **209**:1082–1090.

Hogan, E. L., 1977, Animal models of genetic disorders of myelin, in: *Myelin* (P. Morell, ed.), pp. 489–515, Plenum Press, New York.

Horrocks, L. A. and Harder, H. W., 1983, Fatty acids and cholesterol, in: *Handbook of Neurochemistry,* Vol. 3, 2nd ed. (A. Lajtha, ed.), pp. 1–16, Plenum Press, New York.

Horrocks, L. A., and Sharma, M., 1982, Plasmalogens and O-alkyl glycerophospholipids, in: *Phospholipids* (J. N. Hawthorne and G. B. Ansell, eds), pp. 51–93, Elsevier, Amsterdam.

Horrocks, L. A., Meckler, R. J., and Collins, R. L., 1966, Variations in the lipid composition of mouse brain myelin as a function of age, in: *Variations in the Chemical Composition of the Nervous System as Determined by Development and Genetic Factors* (G. B. Ansell, ed.), p. 46, Pergamon Press, Oxford.

Horrocks, L. A., Toews, A. D., Thompson, D. K., and Chin, J. Y., 1976, Synthesis and turnover of brain phosphoglycerides—Results, methods of calculation and interpretation, in: *Function and Metabolism of Phospholipids in the Central and Peripheral Nervous Systems* (G. Porcellati, L. Amaducci, and C. Galli, eds.), pp. 37–54, Plenum Press, New York.

Horrocks, L. A., Spanner, S., Mozzi, R., Fu, S. C., D'Amato, R. A., and Krakowka, S., 1978, Plasmalogenase is activated in early demyelinating lesions, in: *Myelination and Demyelination* (J. Palo, ed.), pp. 423–437, Plenum Press, New York.

Hoshi, M., and Kishimoto, Y., 1973, Synthesis of cerebronic acid from lignoceric acid by rat brain preparation: Some properties and distribution of the α-hydroxylation system, *J. Biol. Chem.* **248**:4123–4130.

Hübscher, G., 1962, Metabolism of phospholipids. VI. The effect of metal ions on the incorporation of L-serine into phosphatidyl-serine, *Biochim. Biophys. Acta* **57**:555–561.

Igarashi, M., and Suzuki, K., 1977, Solubilization and characterization of the rat brain cholesterol ester hydrolase localized in the myelin sheath, *J. Neurochem.* **28**:729–738.

Inoue, T., Deshmukh, D. S., and Pieringer, R. A., 1971, The association of the galactosyl diglycerides of brain with myelination. I. Changes in the concentration of monogalactosyl diglyceride in the microsomal and myelin fractions of brain of rats during development, *J. Biol. Chem.* **246**:5688–5694.

Jungalwala, F. B., 1974*a*, Synthesis and turnover of cerebroside sulfate of myelin in adults and developing rat brain, *J. Lipid Res.* **15**:114–123.

Jungalwala, F. B., 1974*b*, The turnover of myelin phosphatidylcholine and sphingomyelin in the adult rat brain, *Brain Res.* **78**:99–108.

Kennedy, E. P., 1961, Biosynthesis of complex lipids, *Fed. Proc. Fed. Am. Soc. Exp. Biol.* **20**:934–940.

Kishimoto, Y., Davis, W. E., and Radin, N. S., 1965, Turnover of the fatty acids of rat brain gangliosides, glycerophosphatides, cerebrosides, and sulfatides as a function of age, *J. Lipid Res.* **6**:525–531.

Kobayashi, T., Yamanaka, T., Jacobs, J. M., Teixeira, F., and Suzuki, K., 1980, The twitcher mouse: An enzymatically authentic model of human globoid cell leukodystrophy (Krabbe disease), *Brain Res.* **202**:479–483.

Kopaczyk, K. C., and Radin, N. S., 1965, *In vivo* conversions of cerebroside and ceramide in rat brain, *J. Lipid Res.* **6**:140–155.

Koper, J. W., Lopes-Cardozo, M., and Van Golde, L. M. G., 1981, Preferential utilization of ketone bodies for the synthesis of myelin cholesterol *in vivo, Biochim. Biophys. Acta* **666**:411–417.

Krigman, M. R., and Hogan, E. L., 1976, Undernutrition in the developing rat: Effect upon myelination, *Brain Res.* **107**:257–273.

Kunishita, T., and Ledeen, R. W., 1984, Phospholipid biosynthesis in myelin: Presence of CTP: Phosphoethanolamine cytidylyltransferase in purified myelin of rat brain, *J. Neurochem.* **42**:326–333.

Lapetina, E. G., Lunt, G. G., and deRobertis, E., 1970, The turnover of phosphatidylcholine in rat cerebral cortex membranes *in vivo, J. Neurobiol.* **1**:295–302.

LeBaron, F. N., Sanyal, S., and Jungalwala, F. B., 1981, Turnover rate of molecular species of sphingomyelin in rat brain, *Neurochem. Res.* **6**:1081–1089.

Ledeen, R. W., and Haley, J. E., 1983, Axon–myelin transfer of glycerol-labeled lipids and inorganic phosphate during axonal transport, *Brain Res.* **269**:267–275.

Ledeen, R. W., Yu, R. K., and Eng. L. F., 1973, Gangliosides of human myelin: Sialosylgalactosylceramide (G7) as a major component, *J. Neurochem.* **21**:829–839.

Ledeen, R. W., Cochran, F. B., Yu, R. K., Samuels, F. G., and Haley, J. E., 1980, Gangliosides of the CNS myelin membrane, in: *Advances in Experimental Medicine and Biology,* Vol. 125, *Structure and Function of Gangliosides* (P. Mandel and L. Svennerholm, eds.), pp. 167–176, Plenum Press, New York.

Mallia, A. K., and Radin, N. S., 1977, Proteins in the rat brain cytosol which bind cerebrosides, *Trans. Am. Soc. Neurochem.* **8**:187.

Marggraf, W. D., and Anderer, F. A., 1974, Alternative pathways in the biosynthesis of sphingomyelin and the role of phosphatidylcholine, CDPcholine and phosphorylcholine as precursors, *Hoppe-Seyler's Z. Physiol. Chem.* **355**:803–810.

Matthieu, J.-M., Quarles, R. H., Brady, R. O., and Webster, H. de F., 1973, Variation of proteins, enzyme markers and gangliosides in myelin subfractions, *Biochim. Biophys. Acta* **329**:305–317.

Matthieu, J.-M., Webster, H. de F., DeVries, G. H., Corthay, S., and Koellreutler, B., 1978, Glial versus neuronal origin of myelin proteins and glycoproteins studied by combined intraocular and intracranial labelling, *J. Neurochem.* **31**:93–102.

McKhann, G. M., and Ho, W., 1967, The *in vivo* and *in vitro* synthesis of sulphatides during development, *J. Neurochem.* **14**:717–724.

McKhann, G. M., Levy, R., and Ho, W., 1965, Metabolism of sulfatides. I. The effect of galactocerebrosides on the synthesis of sulfatides, *Biochem. Biophys. Res. Commun.* **20**:109–113.

McMurray, W. C., Strickland, K. P., Berry, J. F., and Rossiter, R. J., 1957, Incorporation of ^{32}P-labeled intermediates into the phospholipids of cell-free preparations of rat brain, *Biochem. J.* **66**:634–644.

Miller, E. K., and Dawson, R. M. C., 1972*a*, Can mitochondria and synaptosomes of guinea-pig brain synthesize phospholipids?, *Biochem. J.* **126**:805–821.

Miller, E. K., and Dawson, R. M. C., 1972*b*, Exchange of phospholipids between brain membranes *in vitro, Biochem. J.* **126**:823–835.

Miller, S. L., and Morell, P., 1978, Turnover of phosphatidylcholine in microsomes and myelin in brains of young and adult rats, *J. Neurochem.* **31**:771–777.

Miller, S. L., Benjamins, J. A., and Morell, P., 1977, Metabolism of glycerophospholipids of myelin and microsomes in rat brain: Reutilization of precursors, *J. Biol. Chem.* **252**:4025–4037.

Morell, P., and Radin, N. S., 1969, Synthesis of cerebroside by brain from uridine diphosphate galactose and ceramide containing hydroxy fatty acid, *Biochemistry* **8**:506–512.

Morell, P., and Radin, N. S., 1970, Specificity in ceramide biosynthesis from long chain bases and various fatty acyl coenzyme A's by brain microsomes, *J. Biol. Chem.* **245**:342–350.

Morell, P., Costantino-Ceccarini, E., and Radin, N. S., 1970, The biosynthesis by brain microsomes of cerebrosides containing nonhydroxy fatty acids, *Arch. Biochem. Biophys.* **141**:738–748.

Morell, P., Bornstein, M. B., and Raine, C. S., 1981, Diseases involving myelin, in: *Basic Neurochemistry,* 3rd ed. (G. J. Siegel, R. W. Albers, B. W. Agranoff, and R. Katzman, eds.), pp. 641–659, Little, Brown, Boston.

Morganstern, R. D., and Abdel-Latif, A. A., 1974, Incorporation of [^{14}C]ethanolamine and [^{3}H]methionine into phospholipids of rat brain and liver *in vivo* and *in vitro, J. Neurobiol.* **5**:393–411.

Morré, D. J., Kartenbeck, J., and Franke, W. W., 1979, Membrane flow and interconversions among endomembranes, *Biochim. Biophys. Acta* **559**:71–152.

Moser, H. W., and Karnovsky, M. L., 1959, Studies on the biosynthesis of glycolipides and other lipides of brain, *J. Biol. Chem.* **234**:1990–1997.

Murad, S., and Kishimoto, Y., 1975, α-Hydroxylation of lignoceric acid to cerebronic acid during brain development: Diminished hydroxylase activity in myelin-deficient mouse mutants, *J. Biol. Chem.* **250**:5841–5846.

Neskovic, N. M., Nussbaum, J. L., and Mandel, P., 1969, Enzymatic synthesis of psychosine in "Jimpy" mice brain, *FEBS Lett.* **3**:199–201.

Neskovic, N. M., Sarlieve, L. L., and Mandel, P., 1972, Biosynthesis of glycolipids in myelin deficient mutants: Brain glycosyl transferases in jimpy and quaking mice, *Brain Res.* **42**:147–157.

Neskovic, N. M., Sarlieve, L. L., and Mandel, P., 1973, Subcellular and submicrosomal distribution of glycolipid-synthesizing transferases in jimpy and quaking mice, *J. Neurochem.* **20**:1419–1430.

Norton, W. T., 1974, Isolation of myelin from nerve tissue, in: *Methods in Enzymology,* Vol. 31 (S. Fleischer and L. Packer, eds.), pp. 435–444, Academic Press, New York.

Norton, W. T., 1977*a*, Isolation and characterization of myelin, in: *Myelin* (P. Morell, ed.), pp. 161–200, Plenum Press, New York.

Norton, W. T., 1977*b*, Chemical pathology of diseases involving myelin, in: *Myelin* (P. Morell, ed.), pp. 383–407, Plenum Press, New York.

Norton, W. T., 1981, Formation, structure and biochemistry of myelin, in: *Basic Neurochemistry* (G. J. Siegel, R. W. Albers, B. W. Agranoff, and R. Katzman, eds.), pp. 63–92, Little, Brown, Boston.

Norton, W. T., and Autilio, L. A., 1966, The lipid composition of purified bovine brain myelin, *J. Neurochem.* **13:**213–222.

Norton, W. T., and Brotz, M., 1963, New galactolipids of brain: A monoalkyl-monoacyl-glycerylgalactoside and cerebroside fatty esters, *Biochem. Biophys. Res. Commun.* **12:**198–203.

Norton, W. T., and Poduslo, S. E., 1973*a*, Myelination in rat brain: Method of myelin isolation, *J. Neurochem.* **21:**749–757.

Norton, W. T., and Poduslo, S. E., 1973*b*, Myelination in rat brain: Changes in myelin composition during brain maturation, *J. Neurochem.* **21:**759–773.

Page, M. A., Krebs, H. A., and Williamson, D. H., 1971, Activities of enzymes of ketone-body utilization in brain and other tissues of suckling rats, *Biochem. J.* **121:**49–53.

Palade, G., 1975, Intracellular aspects of the process of protein synthesis, *Science* **189:**347–358.

Paltauf, F., and Holasek, A., 1973, Enzymatic synthesis of plasmalogens: Characterization of the 1-O-alkyl-2-acyl-*sn*-glycero-3-phosphoryl-ethanolamine desaturase from mucosa of hamster small intestine, *J. Biol. Chem.* **248:**1609–1615.

Pasquini, J. M., Gomez, C. J., Najle, R., and Soto, E. F., 1975, Lack of phospholipid transport mechanisms in cell membranes of the CNS, *J. Neurochem.* **24:**439–443.

Paulus, H., and Kennedy, E. P., 1960, The enzymatic synthesis of inositol monophosphatide, *J. Biol. Chem.* **235:**1303–1311.

Pereyra, P. M., and Braun, P. E., 1983, Studies on subcellular fractions which are involved in myelin membrane assembly: Isolation from developing mouse brain and characterization by enzyme markers, electron microscopy, and electrophoresis, *J. Neurochem.* **41:**957–973.

Pereyra, P. M., Braun, P. E., Greenfield, S., and Hogan, E. L., 1983, Studies on subcellular fractions which are involved in myelin assembly: Labeling of myelin proteins by a double radioisotope approach indicates developmental relationships, *J. Neurochem.* **41:**974–988.

Pieringer, J., Rao, G. S., Mandel, P., and Pieringer, R. A., 1977, The association of the sulphogalactosyl-glycerolipids of rat brain with myelination, *Biochem. J.* **166:**421–428.

Pieringer, R. A., Deshmukh, D. S., and Flynn, T. J., 1973, The association of the galactosyldiglycerides of nerve tissue with myelination, *Prog. Brain Res.* **40:**397–405.

Pleasure, D. E., and Prockop, D. J., 1972, Myelin synthesis in peripheral nerve *in vitro:* Sulfatide incorporation requires a transport lipoprotein, *J. Neurochem.* **19:**283–295.

Pleasure, D., Lichtman, C., Eastman, S., Lieb, M., Abramsky, O., and Silberberg, D., 1979, Acetoacetate and D-(−)-beta-hydroxybutyrate as precursors for sterol synthesis by calf oligodendrocytes in suspension culture: Extramitochondrial pathway for acetoacetate metabolism, *J. Neurochem.* **32:**1447–1450.

Poduslo, S. E., 1975, The isolation and characterization of a plasma membrane and a myelin fraction derived from oligodendroglia of calf brain, *J. Neurochem.* **24:**647–654.

Poduslo, S. E., Miller, K., and McKhann, G. M., 1978, Metabolic properties of maintained oligodendroglia purified from brain, *J. Biol. Chem.* **253:**1592–1597.

Porcellati, G., Biasion, M. G., and Pirotta, M., 1970, The labeling of brain ethanolamine phosphoglycerides from cytidine disphosphate ethanolamine *in vitro, Lipids* **5:**734–742.

Porcellati, G., Arienti, G., Pirotta, M., and Giorgini, D., 1971, Base-exchange reactions for the synthesis of phospholipids in nervous tissues: The incorporation of serine and ethanolamine into the phospholipids of isolated brain microsomes, *J. Neurochem.* **18:**1395–1402.

Porcellati, G., Ceccarelli, B., and Tettamanti, G. (eds.), 1976, *Advances in Experimental Medicine and Biology,* Vol. 71, *Ganglioside Function: Biochemical and Pharmacological Implications,* Plenum Press, New York.

Possmayer, F., Meiners, B., and Mudd, J. B., 1973, Regulation by cytidine nucleotides of the acylation of *sn*-[^{14}C]glycerol 3-phosphate: Regional and subcellular distribution of the enzymes responsible for phosphatidic acid synthesis *de novo* in the central nervous system of the rat, *Biochem. J.* **132:**391–394.

Pullarkat, R. K., Sbaschnig-Agler, M., and Reha, H., 1981, Biosynthesis of phosphatidylserine in rat brain microsomes, *Biochim. Biophys. Acta* **663**:117–123.

Quarles, R. H., 1978, The biochemical and morphological heterogeneity of myelin and myelin-related membranes, in: *Biochemistry of Brain* (S. Kumar, ed.), pp. 81–102, Pergamon Press, Oxford.

Raine, C. S., 1981, Neurocellular anatomy, in: *Basic Neurochemistry*, 3rd ed. (G. J. Siegel, R. W. Albers, R. Katzman, and B. W. Agranoff, eds.), pp. 21–47, Little, Brown, Boston.

Ramachandran, C. K., and Shah, S. N., 1977, Studies on mevalonate kinase, phosphomevalonate kinase, and pyrophosphomevalonate decarboxylase in developing rat brain, *J. Neurochem.* **28**:751–757.

Rambourg, A., and Droz, B., 1980, Smooth endoplasmic reticulum and axonal transport, *J. Neurochem.* **35**:16–25.

Ramsey, R. B., 1977, Effect of extended hypocholesterolemic drug treatment on peripheral and central nervous system sterol content of the rat, *Lipids* **12**:841–846.

Ramsey, R. B., Jones, J. P., Naqui, S. H. M., and Nicholas, H. J., 1971, The biosynthesis of cholesterol and other sterols by brain tissue. II. A comparison of *in vitro* and *in vivo* methods, *Lipids* **6**:225–232.

Rawlins, F. A., 1973, A time–sequence autoradiographic study of the *in vivo* incorporation of [1,2-^{3}H] cholesterol into peripheral nerve myelin, *J. Cell Biol.* **58**:42–53.

Reiss, D. S., Lees, M. B., and Sapirstein, V. S., 1981, Is Na$^+$K$^+$-ATPase a myelin-associated enzyme?, *J. Neurochem.* **36**:1418–1426.

Robinson, A. M., and Williamson, D. H., 1980, Physiological roles of ketone bodies as substrates and signals in mammalian tissues, *Physiol. Rev.* **60**:143–187.

Rumsby, M. G., 1978, Organization and structure in central-nerve myelin, *Biochem. Soc. Trans.* **6**:448–462.

Rumsby, M. G., 1980, Myelin structure and assembly—introductory thoughts, in: *Neurological Mutations Affecting Myelination* (N. Baumann, ed.), INSERM Symposium No. 14, pp. 383–388, Elsevier/North-Holland, Amsterdam.

Sapirstein, V. S., Lees, M. B., and Tractenberg, M. C., 1978, Soluble and membrane bound carbonic anhydrase from rat CNS: Regional development, *J. Neurochem.* **31**:283–288.

Schwartz, M., Ernst, S. A., Siegel, G. J., and Agranoff, B. W., 1981, Immunocytochemical localization of (Na$^+$,K$^+$)-ATPase in the goldfish optic nerve, *J. Neurochem.* **36**:107–115.

Serougne, C., Lefevre, C., and Chevallier, F., 1976, Cholesterol transfer between brain and plasma in the rat: A model for the turnover of cerebral cholesterol, *Exp. Neurol.* **51**:229–240.

Shah, S. N., 1971, Glycosyl tranferases of microsomal fractions from brain: Synthesis of glucosyl ceramide and galactosyl ceramide during development and the distribution of glucose and galactose transferase in white and grey matter, *J. Neurochem.* **18**:395–402.

Shah, S. N., 1981, Modulation *in vitro* of 3-hydroxy-3-methylglutaryl coenzyme A reductase in brain microsomes: Evidence for the phosphorylation and dephosphorylation associated with inactivation and activation of the enzyme, *Arch. Biochem. Biophys.* **211**:439–446.

Shoyama, Y., and Kishimoto, Y., 1978, *In vivo* metabolism of 3-ketoceramide in rat brain, *J. Neurochem.* **30**:377–382.

Singh, I., 1983, Ceramide synthesis from free fatty acids in rat brain: Function of NADPH, and substrate specificity , *J. Neurochem.* **40**:1565–1570.

Singh, I., and Kishimoto, Y., 1980, Ceramide synthesis in rat brain: Characterization of the synthesis requiring pyridine nucleotide, *Arch. Biochem. Biophys.* **202**:93–100.

Singh, I., and Kishimoto, Y., 1982, Brain-specific ceramide synthesis activity: Change during brain maturation and in jimpy mouse brain, *Brain Res.* **232**:500–505.

Smith, M. E., 1967, The metabolism of myelin lipids, in: *Advances in Lipid Research,* Vol. 6 (R. Paoletti and D. Kritchevsky, eds.), pp. 241–278, Academic Press, New York.

Smith, M. E., 1968, The turnover of myelin in the adult rat, *Biochim. Biophys. Acta* **164**:285–293.

Smith, M. E., and Benjamins, J. A., 1977, Model systems for the study of perturbations of myelin metabolism, in: *Myelin* (P. Morell, ed.), pp. 447–488, Plenum Press, New York.

Smith, M. E., and Eng. L. F., 1965, The turnover of the lipid components of myelin, *J. Am. Oil. Chem. Soc.* **42**:1013–1018.

Smith, M. E., and Hasinoff, C. M., 1971, Biosynthesis of myelin proteins *in vitro, J. Neurochem.* **18**:739–747.

Smith, M. E., Hasinoff, C. M., and Fumigalli, R., 1970, Inhibitors of cholesterol synthesis and myelin formation, *Lipids* **5**:665–671.

Snyder, F., 1972, The enzymic pathways of ether linked lipids and their precursors, in: *Ether Lipids: Chemistry and Biology* (F. Snyder, ed.), pp. 121–156, Academic Press, New York, and London.

Sribney, M., 1966, Enzymatic synthesis of ceramide, *Biochim. Biophys. Acta* **125**:542–547.

Sribney, M., and Kennedy, E. P., 1958, The enzymatic synthesis of sphingomyelin, *J. Biol. Chem.* **233**:1315–1322.

Stoffel, W., 1971, Sphingolipids, *Annv. Rev. Biochem.* **40**:57–82.

Stoffyn, A., Stoffyn, P., Farooq, M., Snyder, D. S., and Norton, W. T., 1981, Sialosyltransferase activity and specificity in the biosynthesis *in vitro* of sialosylgalactosylceramide (G_{M4}) and sialosylgalactosylceramide (G_{M3}) by rat astrocytes, neuronal perikarya, and oligodendroglia, *Neurochem. Res.* **6**:1149–1157.

Subba Rao, G. Norcia, L. N., Pieringer, J., and Pieringer, R. A., 1977, The biosynthesis of sulphogalactosyldiacylglycerol of rat brain *in vitro, Biochem. J.* **166**:429–435.

Sun, G. Y., 1973, The turnover of phosphoglycerides in the subcellular fractions of mouse brain: A study using [1-^{14}C] oleic acid as precursor, *J. Neurochem.* **21**:1083–1092.

Sun, G. Y., and Horrocks, L. A., 1973, Metabolism of palmitic acid in the subcellular fractions of rat brain, *J. Lipid Res.* **14**:206–214.

Suzuki, K., Poduslo, J. F., and Poduslo, S. E., 1968, Further evidence for a specific ganglioside fraction closely associated with myelin, *Biochim. Biophys. Acta* **152**:576–586.

Toews, A. D., Horrocks, L. A., and King, J. S., 1976, Simultaneous isolation of purified microsomal and myelin fractions from rat spinal cord, *J. Neurochem.* **27**:25–31.

Ullman, M. D., and Radin, N. S., 1972, Enzymatic formation of hydroxy ceramides and comparison with enzymes forming non-hydroxy ceramides, *Arch. Biochem. Biophys.* **152**:767–777.

Ullman, M. D. and Radin, N. S., 1974, The enzymatic formation of sphingomyelin from ceramide and lecithin in mouse liver, *J. Biol. Chem.* **249**:1506–1512.

Walters, S. N., and Morell, P., 1981, The effects of altered thyroid states on myelinogenesis, *J. Neurochem.* **36**:1792–1801.

Webber, R. J., and Edmond, J., 1979, The *in vivo* utilization of acetoacetate, $\beta(-)$-3-hydroxybutyrate, and glucose for lipid synthesis in brain in the 18-day-old rat, *J. Biol. Chem.* **254**:3912–3920.

Wenger, D. A., Pititpas, J. W., and Pieringer, R. A., 1968, The metabolism of glyceride glycolipids. II. Biosynthesis of monogalactosyl diglyceride from uridine diphosphate galactose and diglyceride in brain, *Biochemistry* **7**:3700–3707.

Wenger, D. A., Subba Rao, K., and Pieringer, R. A., 1970, The metabolism of glyceride glycolipids. III. Biosynthesis of digalactosyl diglyceride by galactosyl transferase pathways in brain, *J. Biol. Chem.* **245**:2513–2519.

Wiegandt, H., 1982, The gangliosides, in: *Advances in Neurochemistry,* Vol. 4 (B. W. Agranoff and M. H. Aprison, eds.), pp. 149–223, Plenum Press, New York.

Wiggins, R. C., 1982, Myelin development and nutritional insufficiency, *Brain Res.* **257**:151–176.

Wiggins, R. C., Miller, S. L., Benjamins, J. A., Krigman, M. R., and Morell, P., 1976, Myelin synthesis during postnatal nutritional deprivation and subsequent rehabilitation, *Brain Res.* **107**:257–273.

Woelk, H., and Porcellati, G., 1978, Myelin catabolism, *Proc. Eur. Soc. Neurochem.* **1**:64–77.

Wood, J. G., Jean, D. H. Whitaker, J. N., McLaughlin, B. J., and Albers, R. W., 1977, Immunocytochemical localization of sodium, potassium ATPase in knifefish brain, *J. Neurocytol.* **6**:571–581.

Wu, P.-S., and Ledeen, R. W., 1980, Evidence for the presence of ethanolaminephosphotransferase in rat central nervous system myelin, *J. Neurochem.* **35**:659–666.

Wüthrich, C., and Steck, A. J., 1981, A permeability change of myelin membrane vesicles towards cations is induced by MgATP but not by phosphorylation of myelin basic protein, *Biochim. Biophys. Acta* **640**:195–206.

Wykle, R. L., 1977, Brain, in: *Lipid Metabolism in Mammals,* Vol. 1 (F. Snyder, ed.), pp. 317–366, Plenum Press, New York,.

Wykle, R. L., and Snyder, F., 1969, The glycerol source for the biosynthesis of alkyl glycerol ethers, *Biochem. Biophys. Res. Commun.* **37**:658–662.

Wykle, R. L., Blank, M. L., Malone, B., and Snyder, F., 1972, Evidence for a mixed-function oxidase in the biosynthesis of ethanolamine plasmalogens from 1-alkyl-2-acyl-*sn*-glycero-3-phosphorylethanolamine, *J. Biol. Chem.* **247**:5442–5447.

Yahara, S., Singh, I., and Kishimoto, Y., 1980, Cerebroside and cerebroside III-sulfate in brain cytosol: Evidence for their involvement in myelin assembly, *Biochim. Biophys. Acta* **619**:177–185.

Yahara, S., Singh, I., and Kishimoto, Y., 1981, Levels and syntheses of cerebrosides and sulfatides in subcellular fractions of jimpy mutants, *Neurochem. Res.* **6**:885–892.

Yandrasitz, J. R., Ernst, S. A., And Salganicoff, L., 1976, The subcellular distribution of carbonic anhydrase in homogenates of perfused rat brian, *J. Neurochem.* **27**:707–716.

Yavin, E., and Gatt, S., 1969, Enzymatic hydrolysis of sphingolipids. VIII. Further purification and properties of rat brain ceramidase, *Biochemistry* **8**: 1692–1698.

Yavin, E., and Zeigler, B. P., 1977, Regulation of phospholipid metabolism in differentiating cells from rat brain cerebral hemispheres in culture, *J. Biol. Chem.* **252**:260–267.

Yu, R. K., and Lee, S. H., 1976, *In vitro* biosynthesis of sialosylgalactosylceramide (G_7) by mouse brain microsomes, *J. Biol. Chem.* **251**:198–203.

Zimmerman, A. W., Quarles, R. H., Webster, H. de F., Matthieu, J., and Brady, R. O., 1975, Characterization and protein analysis of myelin subfractions in rat brain: Developmental and regional comparisons, *J. Neurochem.* **25**:749–757.

CHAPTER 3

PROTEIN METABOLISM OF OLIGODENDROGLIAL CELLS IN VIVO

JOYCE A. BENJAMINS

1. INTRODUCTION

The oligodendroglial cell and its associated myelin membranes have provided a unique opportunity to assess the *in vivo* protein metabolism of a given cell type *in situ* among a mixture of cell types. This is because the oligodendroglial cell synthesizes in large amounts several proteins that are virtually specific for oligodendroglia and myelin. Few attempts have been made to measure the overall rate of protein synthesis in oligodendroglia compared to other cell types or to examine individual proteins in the oligodendroglial cell body. Thus, this chapter will emphasize what is known about the metabolism of the oligodendroglial proteins in which myelin is enriched. We can trace our ability to examine these proteins to the development of methods for isolation of myelin and sodium dodecyl sulfate (SDS) gel electrophoresis. These methods, coupled with isotope tracer methods, have enabled us to learn a great deal about the metabolism of those oligodendroglial proteins that are deposited in myelin.

Many aspects of protein metabolism in oligodendroglia can now be investigated in isolated oligodendroglia or in culture systems. However, the *in vivo*

JOYCE A. BENJAMINS ● *Department of Neurology, Wayne State University School of Medicine, Detroit, Michigan 48201* studies must ultimately be the yardstick for determining whether events in a given "simple" system accurately reflect what is occurring in the intact tissue. Thus, a review of our current conclusions from *in vivo* studies and a survey of the questions raised will be of value in designing future experiments both *in vivo* and *in vitro*.

Three areas have been investigated intensively over the past 10–15 years: (1) How does synthesis of myelin proteins change during development? (2) Do the myelin proteins turn over once they are inserted into the membrane? (3) Where in the cell are the proteins synthesized, how are they transported to mature compact myelin, and what mechanisms are involved in assembly of the myelin membrane? The first two questions are relatively direct, but the third has proved more of a challenge. Some of our conclusions about these proteins have derived from studies of brain composition at various ages. A large number of studies have utilized radioactive precursors as tracers to follow the metabolism of proteins. The fate of these tracers has been followed by (1) isolation of individual proteins from myelin or related fractions or (2) autoradiographic analysis of oligodendroglial cell bodies and myelin sheaths. Studies that have addressed the question of rates of overall protein synthesis in oligodendroglia are discussed in Section 2. Section 3 considers criteria for identifying a given brain protein as oligodendroglial. The myelin basic proteins, proteolipid proteins, Wolfgram proteins, and myelin-associated glycoproteins are then discussed with regard to their rates of appearance during development (Section 4) and their subsequent turnover once accumulation has stopped (Section 5). The final topic considered is the intracellular processing of myelin proteins by oligodendroglia, from their synthesis to subsequent deposition into the myelin membrane (Section 6).

2. COMPARISON OF PROTEIN SYNTHESIS IN WHITE MATTER AND GRAY MATTER

Comparison of rates of total protein synthesis of white matter and gray matter using autoradiography indicated higher incorporation in regions enriched in neurons (for example, Droz and Koenig, 1970). More recent studies, which take into account the uptake of amino acid and quantitate the autoradiographic results, show rates of leucine incorporation of 2.5 and 4.9 nmoles leucine/g tissue per min for white and gray matter, respectively, in the conscious adult rat (C. B. Smith *et al.,* 1980). Myelin, which accounts for much of the content of white matter, has no capacity to synthesize proteins. When corrected for myelin content, the remaining glial-cell bodies must have rates of protein synthesis higher than this estimate suggests.

At present, no comparable information is available from *in vivo* studies for myelinating white matter, in which the rates of protein synthesis are presumed to be considerably higher. Evidence for this higher rate has been found *in vitro,* however. In a comprehensive study, M. E. Smith (1973) investigated the capacity of rat-brain slices to synthesize proteins isolated in the myelin fraction compared to nonmyelin proteins. The slices were incubated with [^{14}C]leucine for 2 hr prior to isolation of myelin. A regional survey of five CNS regions (Figure 1) showed a sharp decrease in all regions in radioactivity recovered in myelin protein between 20 and 60 days. For example, radioactivity incorporated into proteins in the myelin fraction per milligram of protein fell 30-fold in spinal cord and 20-fold in cerebrum. When these values are corrected for the 3- to 4-fold increase in myelin yield between 20 and 60 days (Norton and Poduslo, 1973), the results represent a decrease of approximately 5- to 8-fold in the rate of synthesis of myelin proteins by oligodendroglia. Over the same period, incorporation into proteins in the nonmyelin fraction showed

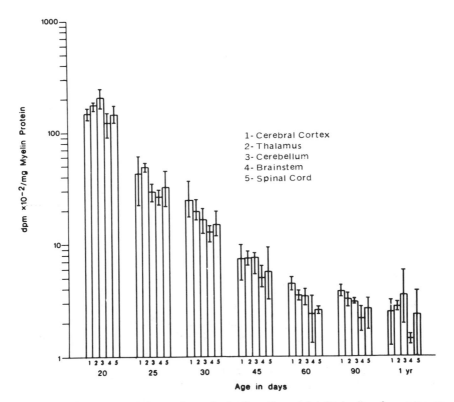

FIGURE 1. Developmental changes in synthesis of myelin proteins. Brain slices from rats were incubated with [^{14}C]leucine for 2 hr prior to isolation of myelin. From M. E. Smith (1973).

little decrease. The proportions of myelin-related protein synthesis at 20 days were 40 and 15% of the total, respectively, in slices from spinal cord and cerebral cortex. By 60 days, these values fell to 15 and 5% of the total. Comparison of brain regions at 20 days demonstrated that the rate of synthesis of myelin proteins was greatest in those regions with highest myelin content and earliest onset of myelination, that is, spinal cord > brainstem > cerebral cortex. These results reflect the capacity of oligodendroglia in various brain regions for synthesis of myelin proteins and are consistent with morphological changes in myelination in these regions (Jacobson, 1963).

3. CRITERIA FOR IDENTIFYING A GIVEN PROTEIN AS OLIGODENDROGLIAL

As with any other differentiated cell type, the oligodendroglial cell synthesizes some proteins that are virtually specific for oligodendroglia and many other proteins that are ubiquitous or at least widely distributed among other cell types. The most rigorous evidence that a given protein is oligodendroglial would be demonstration of the synthesis of that protein by oligodendroglia *in situ* or in culture. Short of that, we are generally safe in assuming that most of the proteins found in a given cell are indeed synthesized there. With establishment that myelin is part of the oligodendroglial cell, we know that proteins in which white matter or isolated myelin is highly enriched are likely to be oligodendroglial, with the caveat that a number of other elements including axons and astroglia are present in white matter and do contribute to the protein pattern. If a given protein appears during myelination and disappears during demyelination, this is generally taken as supporting evidence for its oligodendroglial origin. Again, however, changes accompanying the deposition or loss of myelin may also occur in astroglia or axons.

Most of our information about oligodendroglial proteins has come from analysis of the composition of myelin fractions (see Braun and Brostoff, 1977; Norton, 1981). Every method of myelin isolation and gel separation currently in use clearly shows the major myelin basic proteins (MBPs), two in rodents [molecular weight (M_r) 18,500 and 14,000] and one in other species (M_r 18,500); proteolipid protein (PLP) (M_r 24,000); and the Wolfgram proteins (M_r 43,000–62,000 in myelin. Most investigators also report the presence of DM-20 (M_r 20,000), probably related to PLP; the "prelarge" and "presmall" forms of the basic proteins [M_r 21,000 and 17,000 (Barbarese *et al.,* 1977)]; the myelin-associated glycoprotein(s) (MAG) (M_r 110,000); and numerous uncharacterized high-molecular-weight proteins in myelin. Note that the molecular-weight designations are those in most common use and may not always correspond to the actual molecular weights or apparent molecular weights observed in some gel systems (Magno-Submilla and Campagnoni, 1977; J. F. Poduslo and Rodbard, 1980).

The use of immunoblot methodology has shown recently that the major basic proteins may be part of a family of cross-reactive proteins that presumably share common sequences (Carson, 1981; Carson *et al.*, 1983; Greenfield *et al.*, 1982). The other protein species that cross-react with basic proteins are of high molecular weight, and it is not yet known whether primarily oligodendroglia and myelin are enriched in these proteins or whether the proteins are distributed more generally in other cell types as well. The same statement applies to a number of glycoproteins found in isolated myelin fractions by virtue of their lectin-binding properties (McIntyre *et al.*, 1979; Quarles *et al.*, 1979; J. F. Poduslo *et al.*, 1980). Myelin is enriched in a number of enzyme activities besides 2′,3′-cyclic nucleotide 3′-phosphohydrolase (CNP), but the protein component corresponding to each enzymatic activity has not been clearly identified in most cases. Extensive discussion of this topic is presented in Chapter 6.

Since myelin is a specialized extension of the oligodendroglial plasma membrane, the major proteins of myelin are assumed to be synthesized by the oligodendroglial cell. On the other hand, not all the proteins isolated with myelin need be oligodendroglial in origin. One study suggested that some proteins of the membrane may arise from neurons via axoplasmic flow and subsequent axon–glial transfer (Giorgi *et al.*, 1973). However, numerous studies indicate that none of the major proteins of myelin are transferred from axons (for example, Autilio-Gambetti *et al.*, 1975; Matthieu *et al.*, 1978; Haley and Ledeen, 1979; Giorgi and DuBois, 1981; see Norton, 1983), although the possibility that minor high-molecular-weight proteins could enter myelin by this route has not been ruled out. Another source of nonoligodendroglial proteins in myelin fractions could be contaminating axolemma or other axonal structures, since the myelin sheath and axon are intimately related *in situ*. Although the osmotic shock of crude myelin used in most preparative procedures minimizes axonal contribution, some axonal proteins may still be present (Haley *et al.*, 1981). Further, during myelin isolation, extrinsic proteins could stick artifactually to the membranes from any source in the original homogenate. From the preceding discussion, it is obvious that the method of myelin isolation may determine which proteins are found in the myelin fractions. While this is certainly a problem for proteins present in small amounts, most investigators in the field would agree that the major proteins of myelin are synthesized by oligodendroglia.

Isolation of oligodendroglial cells and analysis of their proteins can provide direct confirmation of their protein composition, provided artifactual loss or adsorption of proteins does not occur during isolation. Analysis of proteins in cultured oligodendroglia may partially overcome this problem; comparison of *in vivo* studies with changes seen in a given culture system is described in

Chapter 7. The protein composition of isolated oligodendroglia has been investigated in several laboratories; the findings are reviewed in Chapter 7 and by Norton (1983). MBPs are found in isolated oligodendroglial fractions, but the true levels have not been determined with certainty, due to the possibility of loss or adsorption of basic protein during isolation. Interestingly, PLP has not been demonstrated by direct chemical measurement in oligodendroglia; the availability of immunoblot and immunoassay methods for this protein should allow its measurement in the near future. The presence of the Wolfgram proteins in the cell body can be inferred from the activity of CNP in isolated oligodendroglia.

All the well-characterized proteins of myelin have now been detected in oligodendroglia by immunocytochemical methods. Immunocytochemical studies tell us that a protein cross-reactive with a given antiserum is present, but not necessarily that a specific protein is present. Problems with fixation, penetration, or sensitivity may prevent identification of a protein actually present, or its conformation may be such that it does not react with a given antiserum. However, this approach is of great value in combination with other approaches in providing a wealth of new information about the localization of specific proteins in the oligodendroglia. This method has provided qualitative evidence that the MBP, PLP, Wolfgram proteins, and major MAG are highly enriched in oligodendroglia. As discussed in detail in Chapter 4, oligodendroglial cell bodies stain intensely during the earliest stages of myelination, then much less intensely as myelination proceeds, indicating a shift of these proteins from the cell body to myelin. A number of other oligodendroglial proteins have yet to be characterized. Several antisera highly specific for oligodendroglia have been described (S. E. Poduslo *et al.*, 1977; Abramsky *et al.*, 1978; Traugott *et al.*, 1978) but the antigens have not been identified. The antisera do not cross-react with myelin or with other cell types, indicating the antigens are unique to oligodendroglial cell bodies.

4. APPEARANCE AND SYNTHESIS OF OLIGODENDROGLIAL PROTEINS DURING DEVELOPMENT

4.1. Basic Proteins

As the oligodendroglial cell begins to produce myelin, we would predict that increased synthesis and deposition of the myelin proteins would be observed. Several studies have measured levels of the MBPs in whole brain; their levels do increase as rate of myelination increases, although the correlation is not exact.

An interesting comparison can be made between the amount of myelin isolated and the levels of MBP in that same region at a given age (Table 1). Little MBP can be detected in brain before myelination begins (Cohen and Guarnieri, 1976). At 15 days in rat cerebrum, basic proteins have reached 30% of adult levels, while only 10% of the adult yield of myelin is isolated by the method of Norton and Poduslo (1973). By 30 days, the values are in closer agreement, with basic proteins at 50% of adult levels and myelin yield at 53%. The difference at 15 days between basic protein content and myelin yield could arise due to low recovery of myelin at this early stage of myelination. However, much of the difference is probably due to the presence of a greater proportion of basic protein in oligodendroglial cell bodies than in myelin sheaths at 15 days as indicated by immunocytochemical studies (Sternberger *et al.*, 1978*a,b*). From the basic protein values, Cohen and Guarnieri (1976) estimated a myelin content of 7.5% of dry weight, while Norton and Poduslo (1973) obtained a theoretical yield of 2.7% by isolation. These results suggest that at early ages, basic protein may give an overestimate of myelin content and isolation of myelin an underestimate. In the adult, myelin constitutes 25% of the dry weight of cerebrum as estimated by basic protein content (if all basic protein were in myelin) and 28% as estimated from myelin yield. Thus, in older brain, the two estimates are in closer agreement and indicate that less basic protein is found in oligodendroglial cell bodies.

These results are in contrast to the data of Barbarese *et al.* (1978). In their study, levels of basic proteins were measured by radioimmunoassay (RIA) in homogenate and isolated myelin from mouse brain. At all ages, from 15 days to adult, about 90% of the total basic protein was recovered in the isolated myelin fraction. The authors concluded that myelin recovery was the same at all ages studied and that most of the basic protein in brain was found in myelin even at the earliest stage of myelination examined (15 days), indicating "no substantial pool of non-myelin basic protein at any age." The species

Table 1. Comparison of Myelin Yield and Basic Protein Content of Rat Cerebrum During Development[a]

	Myelin isolated		Calculated myelin content $\dfrac{\text{mg myelin, dry wt}}{\text{mg tissue, dry wt}} \times 100$	Basic protein measured		Calculated myelin content $\dfrac{\text{mg myelin, dry wt}}{\text{mg tissue, dry wt}} \times 100$
Age	mg/g wet wt	Percentage of adult		mg/g wet wt	Percentage of adult	
15 Days	2.9	9.6%	1.6% (2.7%)	1.4	30%	7.5%
30 Days	16.2	53%	9% (15%)	2.8	60%	15%
Adult[b]	30.2	100%	17% (28%)	4.6	100%	25%

[a] The data for myelin content are from Norton and Poduslo (1973); for MBP, from Cohen and Guarnieri (1976). The numbers in parentheses represent the total myelin yield if a 60% recovery of myelin was obtained at each age. The myelin content is expressed as mg dry weight myelin/mg dry weight tissue, assuming that dry weight of cerebrum is 18% relative to wet weight (Clausen, 1969) and that basic protein constitutes 10% of the dry weight of myelin (Cohen and Guarnieri, 1976).

[b] Adult values are for 144-day-old rats for the myelin data and 120-day-old rats for the basic protein data.

and the methods for myelin isolation and immunoassay differ from those used in the studies discussed above, so direct comparison is difficult. Further, both the myelin yields and total levels of basic protein per gram of tissue are considerably lower than those found in the other two studies. However, the data suggest that the mouse may have less extra-myelin basic protein than the rat at 15 days, perhaps due to slightly earlier maturation. Correlation between quantitative morphometric studies and biochemical measures should provide accurate values for myelin content during early stages of development and allow more detailed assessment of the intracellular distribution of basic protein.

Changes occur during development in the ratios of the four basic protein species found in rodent brain. In myelin, the ratio of 14K protein to 18.5K protein increases with age in both mice (Morell et al., 1972) and rats (Adams and Osborne, 1973; Cammer and Norton, 1976). Between 10 and 30 days after birth in mice, the molar ratios among the four proteins in myelin are 1:5:2:10, in descending order according to molecular weight (Barbarese et al., 1978). Between 30 and 60 days, the proportion of 14K protein continues to accumulate in myelin, while that of the 18.5K protein remains constant and the relative amounts of 21.5K and 17K proteins decrease. The investigators concluded that the increase in the ratio of 14K to 18.5K protein in myelin during development is due to continued accumulation of 14K protein after accumulation of other proteins has stopped. They suggest that this could represent addition of 14K protein to previously formed myelin, replacement of other proteins by 14K protein during repair, or formation of new myelin containing only 14K protein. Thus, the four basic proteins show different patterns of accumulation in myelin. We do not yet know to what extent the differences seen in the basic protein composition of myelin at various ages represent differences in rates of synthesis, assembly into myelin, or relative rates of turnover in the oligodendroglial cells (Barbarese et al., 1978).

Analysis of the rates of synthesis of the 14K and 18.5K basic proteins in mouse brain between 14 and 39 days showed a peak of synthesis for both proteins at 18 days of age, coincident with the period of maximal myelin deposition (C. W. Campagnoni et al., 1978). Throughout development, the smaller basic protein was synthesized at a greater rate than the larger basic protein (Figure 2). This is consistent with the relative enrichment of myelin in the 14K protein compared to the 18.5K protein and indicates that rate of synthesis is a major factor in this enrichment.

4.2. Proteolipid Proteins

Several studies have shown that levels of total brain PLP increase dramatically during the period of myelination (Nussbaum and Mandel, 1973; Lerner et al., 1974; A. T. Campagnoni et al., 1976). These PLP preparations were

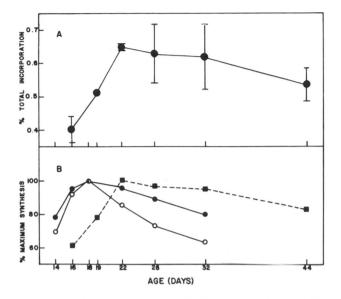

FIGURE 2. Developmental changes in synthesis of basic proteins and proteolipid proteins (PLPs) in mouse. Radioactive precursors were injected intracerebrally, and the proteins were isolated from brain after 2 hr. (A) Synthesis of myelin PLP during brain development. The radioactivity in the PLP band on SDS–polyacrylamide gels was divided by total incorporation into trichloro-acetic-acid-precipitable protein and multiplied by 100. (B) Developmental curves comparing relative synthetic rates of the myelin PLP (■) with the large basic protein (o) and the small basic protein (●). To facilitate comparison, the data for each protein were normalized to the age at which maximal synthesis occurred, 18 days for basic proteins and 22 days for PLP. From A. T. Campagnoni and Hunkeler (1980).

heterogeneous, with myelin PLP a minor component at early stages of myelination, then becoming more prominent as myelination progressed. Although specific methods to measure PLP are now available (Trotter *et al.,* 1981; Macklin and Lees, 1982), a developmental survey of various regions using these assays has not yet been reported.

A. T. Campagnoni *et al.* (1976) examined the content and composition of total PLP from several brain regions in mice between 10 and 33 days. The PLP content of each region increased 6- to 10-fold during this period. Two proteins of M_r 26,000 and 21,500 (corresponding to myelin PLP and the DM-20 protein) increased dramatically in quantity during myelination, with the highest concentrations in the most heavily myelinated regions (basal ganglia and hippocampus). In cerebral cortex between 15 and 33 days, total PLP increased 2-fold per gram tissue, similar to the 2-fold increase found for basic protein in cerebrum during this period (Cohen and Guarnieri, 1976). Subsequent studies demonstrated that synthesis of PLP in brain increases during myelination (A.

T. Campagnoni and Hunkeler, 1980). Compared to synthesis of basic protein, PLP synthesis begins somewhat later and does not reach its maximal rate until 22 days, 4 days later than the peak for basic proteins (Figure 2).

4.3. Wolfgram Proteins

The third major class of myelin proteins that have been examined during development is the Wolfgram proteins (Wolfgram, 1966). With the recent finding that the Wolfgram proteins of M_r 43,000–48,000 in myelin contain the enzyme CNP (Sprinkle *et al.,* 1980; Drummond and Dean, 1980; Muller *et al.,* 1981), information about the content of these Wolfgram proteins can be inferred from enzymatic activity, in addition to direct measurement of amounts of protein present. Unlike basic proteins and PLP, CNP can be detected in brain at birth in the rat (Sprinkle *et al.,* 1978*a*) and is found in tissues other than brain and nerve (Sprinkle *et al.,* 1978*b*). However, both biochemical and immunocytochemical data indicate that oligodendroglia and myelin are highly enriched in these proteins (see Chapters 4 and 6).

Sprinkle *et al.* (1978*a*) measured CNP activity in several regions of rat brain during development. In all regions examined, total activity increased between 4 and 120 days with the greatest rate of increase at two to three weeks after birth. The increase correlated with the onset of myelination and with increases in levels of MBP and activity of cerebroside sulfotransferase in each region. Between 10 and 60 days, there was a close correlation between CNP and MBP levels. However, after 60 days, basic protein levels increased more rapidly than CNP activity. The authors suggest that this may be due to more rapid turnover of CNP or distribution of CNP only in certain regions of the myelin sheath. In another study comparing regions of developing rat CNS, Banik and Smith (1977) isolated microsomal fractions with the density of myelin from five regions beginning at 3–5 days after birth. The isolation of multi-lamellar myelin and appearance of basic protein and PLP in these myelin fractions coincided well with morphological studies. Thus, myelin could be isolated first from spinal cord, then brainstem, cerebellum, and forebrain. Enzymatic activity of CNP was first found primarily in microsomal fractions with a density greater than myelin, then later appeared to a greater extent in fractions with the density of myelin, so that in the adult, 40–60% of the total CNP activity in all regions was recovered in myelin.

The results of these two studies indicate that the level of CNP is a good indicator of myelination during the period of most active deposition of myelin. However, at very early stages, CNP levels may reflect primarily activity in the oligodendroglial cell body or possibly in other cell types. Myelin isolated at these early stages has a higher proportion of Wolfgram proteins than that isolated from more mature brains. At later stages of myelination, a given oligo-dendroglial cell may produce myelin with less Wolfgram protein than initially, or those oligodendroglia that differentiate later may produce myelin less enriched in Wolfgram proteins than those that differentiate earlier.

4.4. Myelin-Associated Glycoproteins

Histochemical studies (Wolman and Hestrin-Lerner, 1960), chemical analysis (Margolis, 1967), and lectin-binding studies (Matus *et al.*, 1973) have provided evidence for the presence of glycoproteins in CNS myelin. However, specific glycoproteins were first demonstrated by sensitive *in vivo* labeling studies using [^{3}H]fucose and other radioactive sugar precursors (Quarles *et al.*, 1973*a*, 1980*b*). The most prominent and best characterized of these is a glycoprotein (or glycoproteins) of M_r 110,000 designated myelin-associated glycoprotein (MAG). Levels of MAG increase with myclination (Druse *et al.*, 1974), and heavier myelin subfractions appear to bc enriched in the protein (Matthieu *et al.*, 1973). Like CNP, MAG reaches its adult level at an earlier age than basic protein (Johnson *et al.*, 1980). The protein has a slightly higher apparent molecular weight in immature myelin than in mature myelin (Quarles *et al.*, 1973*b*), a change that appears to involve peptide-bond cleavage rather than oligosaccharide modifications (McIntyre *et al.*, 1978). Immuno-cytochemical studies suggest that the protein is concentrated in the innermost and outermost wraps of myelin, in regions of uncompacted myelin, and in the oligodendroglial-cell body (Sternberger *et al.*, 1979).

A number of other glycoproteins have been identified as minor constituents of purified CNS myelin by lectin binding (Quarles *et al.*, 1979; J. F. Poduslo *et al.*, 1980). There is indirect evidence, based on periodic acid–Schiff (PAS) staining and lectin binding, that CNP may be a glycoprotein (Muller *et al.*, 1981). Sixteen lectin-binding constituents of CNS myelin have been examined for developmental changes (J. F. Poduslo, 1981). Both increases and decreases in binding for specific proteins were observed for each of several lectins; with development, levels of glycoproteins increase, and oligosaccharide branches become modified and more elaborately branched.

4.5. Summary of Changes

From *in vivo* studies on the appearance and synthesis of myelin proteins, we can conclude that the oligodendroglial cell greatly increases its production of myelin proteins during the period of myelination. The magnitude of this increase can be deduced from the estimate of Norton and Poduslo (1973) that each oligodendroglial cell makes three times its weight in membrane each day during this period. However, we know very little about the metabolism of the myelin proteins within the glial-cell body compared to their metabolism in myelin. We know even less about the metabolism of oligodendroglial proteins that are not enriched in myelin.

A number of studies have addressed the question of whether oligodendroglia *in situ* begin synthesizing the myelin proteins in a synchronous manner or whether some proteins appear before others. Norton (1983) has recently discussed the difficulty of addressing this question in developing brain regions with a heterogeneous population of oligodendroblasts, differentiating oligodendroglia, and actively myelinating oligodendroglia. We know that myelin as isolated shows a change in composition as myelination progresses, and we know that some myelin proteins are detected in brain before others. However, we cannot determine with certainty from *in vivo* studies whether a single oligodendrocyte produces myelin that changes in composition from early to late stages of myelination or whether oligodendroglia that arise earlier produce myelin of a different composition than those that appear later.

When homogenates of brain regions or optic nerve are analyzed for myelin proteins, the composition reflects the results of net synthesis of the oligodendroglial cell, that is, the total of the content of the cell body plus the myelin sheaths. As discussed in the preceding sections, the available data *in vivo* indicate that CNP appears early in differentiation, followed by MAG, MBP, then PLP. Analyses of optic nerve (Detering and Wells, 1976; Tennekoon *et al.,* 1977) have supported these observations in a system in which events are more synchronous than in large brain regions (Figure 3).

Analysis of myelin fractions rather than homogenates at very early stages of myelination may provide clues about the sequence of events in myelin deposition. Thus, myelin fractions isolated from brains of young animals and heavier myelin subfractions have a higher content of higher-molecular-weight proteins, suggesting that these are the earliest components of myelin. (Matthieu *et al.,* 1973; Quarles, 1980*a*). With regard to specific lower-molecular-weight proteins, the relative proportion of small basic protein increases with maturation, while the relative proportions of large basic protein, DM-20, and Wolfgram proteins decrease. For these proteins, results for myelin isolated from optic nerve (Lane and Fagg, 1980) agree well with results from other, more heterogeneous brain regions. The changes in MAG and PLP are not so clearcut. One study in rat brain has found that the proportion of MAG, as measured by PAS staining, remained constant between 14 and 60 days (Druse *et al.,* 1974). However, in myelin isolated from optic nerve, the proportion of MAG, as measured by concanavalin A binding, decreased between 15 and 60 days (Lane and Fagg, 1980). Analysis with more specific methods should resolve whether this discrepancy is due to methodological or regional differences.

The issues of whether PLP appears in myelin before basic protein and whether it increases in myelin relative to basic proteins during development are

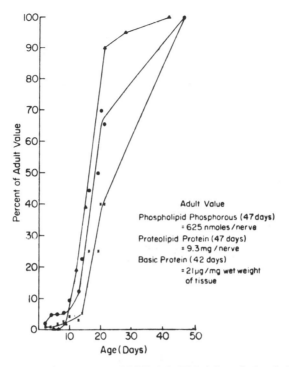

FIGURE 3. Developmental appearance of MBP (▲), PLP (●), and phospholipid phosphorus (×) in rat optic nerves. The values are expressed as percentages of the values found in a 42- and a 47-day-old animal. From Tennekoon *et al.*, (1977).

still unresolved. Some studies of myelin isolated at very early stages of myelination have found little or no PLP relative to basic protein (Morell *et al.*, 1972; Fishman *et al.*, 1975; Detering and Wells, 1976), while others have found early enrichment in PLP relative to basic protein (Einstein *et al.*, 1970; Banik *et al.*, 1974). Results for homogenates compared to myelin show that oligodendroglia begin to synthesize basic protein before PLP. If PLP appears in myelin at the same time or before basic protein, this would suggest that basic protein accumulates in the cell until synthesis of PLP begins. Synthesis of PLP in the cell body and its subsequent deposition in myelin would then trigger deposition of basic protein. Hartman *et al.* (1982) have recently reported that large-diameter fibers in some regions stain more intensely for basic protein than small-diameter fibers in the same regions. Again, this suggests that as more and more lamellae are laid down, the content of basic protein may increase and that of PLP decrease. Alternatively, different axons may signal deposition of myelin of slightly different composition throughout. This finding again emphasizes the difficulty discussed by Norton (1983) in drawing conclusions about the sequence of events in a single axon–oligodendroglial unit from studies on whole brain or even regions in which there may be heterogeneity with regard to both axons and glia and with regard to stage of myelination. Thus, differences found with maturation in the earlier studies of composition may reflect contributions of some later-developing myelin sheaths in that region, rather than changes in each sheath.

5. LONG-TERM TURNOVER STUDIES

The question of how oligodendroglia metabolize proteins once they are inserted into myelin has been investigated by following long-term isotopic decay of these proteins in myelin after injection of radioactive amino acids. The problems with this approach and the conclusions reached have been summarized in several reviews (Benjamins and Smith, 1977; Benjamins and Morell, 1978). Most studies are in agreement that PLP has a very long half-life in rat myelin, more than 100 days. Thus, once assembled into myelin, PLP does not leave readily. This implies that the protein is anchored tightly to the membrane and cannot exchange for newly synthesized protein in cytoplasmic loops or other regions with access to the cell body. Further, it must be resistant to any proteolytic enzymes present in myelin or its cytoplasmic inclusions. Basic protein appears to have a more appreciable turnover in some studies, with values for half-lives ranging from 20 to more than 100 days, depending on the methods used. Thus, basic protein in myelin exchanges with newly synthesized basic protein to some extent and is most likely susceptible to degradation by proteases that may be either in the regions where exchange is occurring or in lysosomes elsewhere in the cell. The mechanism by which basic protein leaves myelin and gets transported to the site of degradation is not known. The differences in turnover of these two proteins are consistent with their respective integral and peripheral locations within the lipid bilayer.

Among the higher-molecular-weight proteins, the turnover of the Wolfgram proteins is greater than that of basic protein or PLP (Fischer and Morell, 1974; Lajtha et al., 1977). One study of fucose incorporation as a function of age suggests that myelin glycoproteins are relatively stable (Glasgow et al., 1972). However, the high-molecular-weight proteins as a group appear to have a more rapid turnover than the major myelin proteins (Fischer and Morell, 1974; M. E. Smith, 1972; Sabri et al., 1974).

When both short and long intervals after injection of isotope are examined, the major proteins of myelin exhibit at least two rates of isotopic decay, one with a half-life around 5–7 days, the other around 100 days or greater (Singh and Jungalwala, 1979). The shorter half-lives may represent turnover of those proteins nearest metabolically active regions of the sheath, with the longer half-lives ascribed to those proteins that end up in less active areas of the sheath. Since the animals in this study were 65 days old at injection, almost all oligodendroglia should be relatively mature, so the results probably reflect what is happening in any given oligodendrocyte, rather than two populations of oligodendroglia, one less mature than the other, with more rapid turnover. [Biphasic decay curves have also been found for myelin lipids (see Chapter 2).]

An alternative approach to short-term pulse-labeling is that used by Lajtha *et al.* (1977); in these studies, a pellet of labeled tyrosine was implanted in adult mice to keep the specific radioactivity of precursor constant over several days. In this way, several problems of labeling with a single injection may be circumvented. First, a pulse may not label all proteins in a uniform manner, since those most metabolically active will be most highly labeled. Second, reutilization of label may occur, especially in myelin. With the constant-precursor method, the investigators found that the rate of protein turnover was about 40% of that of whole brain proteins, and about one fifth of the myelin proteins were replaced within 10 days. Each of the major myelin proteins showed some turnover, in the order Wolfgram > DM-20 > basic = PLP. Thus, by 10 days, about 29% of the Wolfgram proteins had been replaced, compared to 12–13% of the basic protein and PLP. The similarity in half-lives of these last two proteins with this method compared to the relatively shorter half-life for basic protein found in most studies using a pulse of precursor may be due to the longer labeling period.

Myelin proteins labeled in young animals have a somewhat slower turnover rate than those labeled in older animals. Fischer and Morell (1974) examined the long-term turnover of myelin proteins in mouse brain and found that proteins labeled at 14 days had longer half-lives than those labeled at 60 days (Table 2). These results suggest that myelin deposited during the period of active myelination represents a stable core of membrane, probably the innermost lamellae in areas farthest from cytoplasmic loops, nodes, or oligodendroglial cytoplasm. The proteins labeled at 60 days may be deposited in outer wraps and near these more active metabolic regions and thus show a higher rate of turnover. Support for this concept comes from a recent study in which Shapira *et al.* (1981) examined long-term turnover of proteins in fractions of myelin from rat brain separated on a continuous density gradient. The animals were injected at 14 days of age. These investigators concluded that the lighter membranes represented a "stable core" of myelin membranes with little turnover, whereas the heavier membranes continued to accumulate with development and demonstrated appreciable turnover.

Few attempts have been made to examine the turnover of extramyelin pools of basic protein, PLP, and other myelin proteins. One study that addresses this question is that of Fischer and Morell (1974), in which the long-term turnover of proteins was examined in myelinlike fractions as well as mye-

Table 2. Half-Lives of Proteins of Myelin and Myelin-Like Material[a]

| | Injected at 14 days | | Injected at 60 days | |
Protein	Myelinlike	Myelin	Myelinlike	Myelin
Proteolipid	22	stable	21	102
Wolfgram	20	70	19	40
Basic (fast)	16	stable	19	96
Basic (slow)	14	stable	19	83

[a] From Fischer and Morell (1974). Mice were injected intraperitoneally with [³H]leucine, divided into four injections at 12-hour intervals. Myelin and myelin-like fractions were isolated by the initial steps in the method of Norton and Poduslo (1973), then further purified on CsCl gradients. Proteins were separated by SDS gel electrophoresis. Half lives were determined from the decay of radioactivity in the major myelin proteins, measured at 10, 20, 40, and 80 days, after injection of isotope.

lin (Table 2). The half-life of a given protein in the myelinlike fractions was shorter than its counterpart in myelin. Also, the half-lives were similar whether the animals were injected at 15 days or 60 days. The myelin proteins in the myelinlike fraction still exhibit markedly longer half-lives than the average microsomal or supernatant proteins (Singh and Jungalwala, 1979). How much of this represents contribution from myelin fragments in this fraction and how much represents a unique oligodendroglial membrane is not known. Further, we do not know how much of the decay of label in this fraction represents degradation of protein and how much represents slow transport into myelin.

Several studies have suggested the presence of extramyelin membranes in oligodendroglia with very slow turnover (Druse *et al.,* 1974; see the review in Benjamins and Morell, 1978 and Quarles, 1980*a*). This may represent a plasma-membrane fraction or some unique membrane that is protected from the usual degradation processes for other membranes in the cell. This pool of protein or lipid could be synthesized in some portion of the cell, such as a long oligodendroglial process, in which the usual lysosomal and membrane recycling processes are not occurring. Does the oligodendrocyte have a metabolically stable reservoir of myelin components available throughout the life of the animal? What happens to these reservoirs during an insult to myelin, or during demyelination? Again, we cannot definitively rule out the possibility that the finding of a stable nonmyelin pool is an artifact arising from myelin fragments in the fractions under study.

Further attempts to examine the turnover of these proteins in membranes other than myelin will require the use of more complex subcellular fractionation methods (Braun *et al.,* 1980; Pereyra *et al.,* 1983). These studies will be difficult, since the identity and purity of a given membrane fraction will have to be assessed carefully to define its cellular and subcellular origin.

The mechanisms for degrading the myelin proteins are not known. Breakdown may occur via proteases intrinsic to myelin itself. Alternatively, proteins may move slowly through the myelin lamellae by lateral diffusion, so that some proteins end up exposed to cytoplasmic loops or glial cytoplasm where proteases might act. Axonal–glial specializations have been noted, primarily in Schwann cells (Berthold, 1978). These specializations consist of highly interdigitated regions of axonal and glial membrane, primarily at nodal regions. Do axonal processes pinch off portions of myelin and digest them? Immunocytochemical studies might indicate whether this occurs. Day (1981) suggests that there may be a continual shedding of myelin constituents, specifically myelin basic protein, into the extracellular space, thus accounting for the low levels of basic protein immunoreactive material detected in serum. In other cells, there is continual recycling of proteins in the plasma membrane, with internalization of vesicles and subsequent fusion with lysosomal vesicles. The myelin membrane may equilibrate slowly with plasma membrane or exhibit such internalization at regions nearest the oligodendroglial process or cell body.

The most striking property of myelin turnover is the very slow rate observed for the majority of the proteins, rather than the small amount of turnover that does occur. This suggests that most of the proteins are protected from the usual degradative mechanisms either by virtue of sequestration within the tightly wrapped myelin lamellae or by the isolation of the myelin sheath from the cell body proper, at the end of a long process. Comparison with long-term turnover of proteins in PNS myelin may help evaluate the role of the geometry of the oligodendroglial cell in protecting the myelin proteins from degradation (M. E. Smith, 1983).

6. PROCESSING OF MYELIN PROTEINS BY OLIGODENDROGLIA

6.1. Sites of Synthesis

The subcellular location of synthesis of the major myelin proteins has been investigated primarily by two experimental approaches. The first is isolation of free and membrane-bound ribosome fractions from brain and subsequent *in vitro* translation, either with the intact ribosomes or with messenger RNA (mRNA) extracted from the ribosmal fractions. The second approach has involved injection of radioactive amino acids into the animal, then preparation of subcellular fractions at short intervals to determine the origin of the newly synthesized proteins.

Most of the studies to date on sites of synthesis have examined the MBPs. In an early study by Lim *et al.* (1974), polyadenylate [poly(A)]-RNA from rat brain microsomal fractions was injected into frog oocytes. Proteins were synthesized that immunoprecipitated with antisera to MBPs and comigrated with the basic proteins following gel electrophoresis. Although data for free ribosomes were not presented, the authors reported preliminary findings suggesting that basic proteins were synthesized predominantly on membrane-bound rather than free polysomes.

Our laboratory subsequently investigated synthesis of MBP using free and membrane-bound polysomes from 17-day-old rat brainstem prepared by the high-salt method of Ramsey and Steele (1977). The polysomes were translated with supernatant fractions from liver or brain; the free and membrane-bound polysomes synthesized protein at comparable rates. MBPs were isolated from the incubation mixtures by acid extraction and electrophoresis in two gel systems. In this system, MBPs were synthesized to a nearly equal extent on both classes of ribosomes (Townsend and Benjamins, 1979). Similar findings in 25-day-old rats have been reported by Hall and Lim (1981) and Hall *et al.* (1982), also using the method of Ramsey and Steele for polysome isolation, but extracting poly(A)-RNA and translating wtih reticulocyte lysates. Products were identified by chromatography on carboxymethyl (CM)-cellulose and by immunoprecipitation.

Two other studies have reported synthesis of basic protein predominantly on free ribosomes, with little evidence for synthesis on membrane-bound ribosomes. In their initial studies, C. W. Campagnoni *et al.* (1978) demonstrated synthesis of basic protein by brain homogenates. In subsequent studies, they demonstrated the capacity of postmitochondrial and postmicrosomal supernatants and of mRNA from brains of 3-week-old mice to synthesize MBPs (A. T. Campagnoni *et al.,* 1980; Mathees and Campagnoni, 1980). When free and bound polysomes were translated in the presence of brain cell sap, basic proteins were synthesized by the free polysomes at a rate 10-fold greater than by the membrane-bound polysomes. The proteins were identified by their comigration properties with MBPs on CM-cellulose, acid urea gels, and SDS gels. Subsequent studies using immunoprecipitation showed that the four major basic proteins were synthesized, with no evidence for a precursor–product relationship between the four species (Yu and Campagnoni, 1982).

Another recent study with 8-day-old rat brainstem has also found MBP synthesized predominantly on free polysomes (Colman *et al.,* 1982). After isolation of free ribosomes and microsomes, the investigators extracted mRNA, translated it in a wheat germ system, and identified the basic proteins by immunoprecipitation and gel electrophoresis. The efficiency of translation for each class of polysomes was not reported. As above, the four major basic proteins found in rodent myelin were identified as products. Of special interest was the finding of an mRNA fraction isolated with myelin. The polysomes in this fraction synthesized basic proteins more efficiently than the bulk of the free ribosomes. The authors concluded that ribosomes in the cytoplasmic processes associated with myelin were highly enriched in message for basic proteins. In an extension of these studies, [^{35}S]methionine was injected intracerebrally into 12-day-old rats, and labeling of basic protein was examined at intervals between 2 and 90 min. At 2 min, no labeled basic protein was found in the microsomal fraction but was found in myelin, consistent with synthesis on free ribosomes and rapid transfer to meylin.

The question of where basic proteins destined for myelin are synthesized has yet to be finally answered. A variety of methodological factors can influence the results obtained from the *in vitro* translation studies—degradation or inactivation of some mRNA species during ribosome isolation or mRNA extraction, extent of cross-contamination between free and membrane-bound polysomcs, copurification of other proteins with the protein of interest, and other factors. Two conclusions can be made with some certainty, however: all the studies find that free ribosomes can synthesize basic proteins, and the proteins appear to be synthesized in mature form, with no evidence for precursors (Carson *et al.*, 1983; Yu and Campagnoni, 1982; Colman *et al.*, 1982). Messenger mRNA that codes for basic proteins is isolated in membrane-bound polysomes under some condiditons. Synthesis of basic protein could begin on free polysomes, then, after completion of a certain sequence, bind to membrane. Other questions to be explored are whether synthesis shifts between free and membrane-bound polysomes during development, whether one or both sites contribute to myelin formation, and whether some species of basic proteins are synthesized preferentially at one site vs. another. The lack of detection of labeled basic protein in microsomal fractions 2 min after administration of amino acid is a convincing demonstration that basic protein is made primarily on free polysomes in rat brain at 12 days (Colman *et al.*, 1982). Both reports of extensive synthesis of basic protein on membrane-bound polysomes utilized the procedure of Ramsey and Steele (1977), in which little cross-contamination of free and membrane-bound polysomes occurs. However, the method should be examined to determine whether mRNA for basic protein is specifically adsorbed to the membrane-bound fraction. Finally, the possible role of polysomes in cytoplasmic loops of myelin in providing basic proteins merits further investigation. The immunocytochemical localization of MBP shifts with development from the oligodendroglial cell body to the myelin sheath (Sternberger *et al.*, 1978*a,b*), and this may be accompanied by enrichment of mRNA for basic protein in the oligodendroglial processes.

Several studies indicate that myelin PLP is synthesized on membrane-bound ribosomes, as predicted from its location as an integral membrane protein. Studies by Townsend and Benjamins (1979) showed that membrane-bound polysomes preferentially synthesized proteins that comigrated with PLP and were extracted with chloroform–methanol. Colman *et al.* (1982) definitively showed synthesis of PLP on membrane-bound polysomes; in this case, the protein was identified by immunoprecipitation and comigration with PLP.

6.2. Kinetics of Assembly into Myelin

Examination of the time–course of appearance of newly synthesized proteins in myelin has provided information about the ways in which the oligodendroglial cells process these proteins. Obviously, by looking only at the last stage of the process, appearance of the proteins in myelin, we cannot reconstruct the entire sequence of events occurring within the oligodendroglial cell, but this approach has provided a starting point for subsequent studies on intracellular events. The conclusions from these studies depend on several assumptions. First is the assumption that the proteins are synthesized not within the myelin membrane itself, but in the cytoplasm of the oligodendroglial cell. Since ribosomes are not present in compacted myelin *per se,* and since isolated myelin shows no capacity for protein synthesis, this appears to be a valid assumption. Second, these studies assume that the various ribosomes within the oligodendroglial cell that synthesize proteins destined for myelin have equal access to amino acid pools. Finally, the radioactive proteins isolated with myelin are assumed to be true constituents of the membrane, and not adsorbed proteins or proteins contributed by contaminating membranes. Insofar as these conditions hold, the time–course of appearance of various proteins in myelin will indicate the length of time that elapses between synthesis of a given protein and its assembly into myelin.

When radioactive amino acids are injected intracerebrally, a pulse of radioactivity is presented to the brain tissue. Under these conditions, labeling of total protein increases rapidly for several minutes, then begins to decline. The specific radioactivity of individual proteins in isolated myelin increases for several hours, then levels off, reflecting accumulation of proteins in myelin. The first studies describing the properties of labeled proteins in myelin looked at time points days or weeks after administration of isotope, and thus examined the fate of proteins once in myelin (see Section 5). In 1971, two studies were published that presented data on the entry of newly synthesized proteins into myelin. D'Monte *et al.* (1971) injected radioactive lysine intracisternally into 40- to 50-day old rats and determined the specific radioactivity of the three major classes of myelin proteins, separated by solubility properties, at 1–3 h after injection. They concluded that the high-molecular-weight proteins showed the most rapid rate of appearance in myelin at this age, followed by basic proteins, then PLP. In an *in vitro* system of brain slices, M. E. Smith and

Hasinoff (1971) obtained similar results, using leucine and glycine as precursors in 38-day-old rats. In a later study (Benjamins *et al.*, 1975), [³H]leucine was injected intracranially into 17-day rats and myelin proteins were separated by SDS gel electrophoresis (Figure 4). The basic and Wolfgram proteins reached maximal specific activity by 2 h, then remained constant up to 24 hr. By contrast, PLP continued to accumulate radioactivity for 6 hr, then leveled off, indicating a delay in appearance of PLP in myelin relative to the other proteins. At 1 hr, the specific radioactivity was highest in the Wolfgram proteins, followed by large and small basic protein, then lowest in PLP. This indicates that relative to the pool of each protein in myelin, the high-molecular-weight and basic protein were initially being added more rapidly than PLP. However, by 6 hr, the specific activity of PLP was 2- to 3-fold higher than that of the basic and Wolfgram proteins, indicating greater deposition of this protein relative to the PLP already in myelin (Figure 4A,B). When the relative molar ratios of each protein added to myelin were calculated, by 6 hr, equimolar amounts of PLP and small basic protein (also B_F, or fast-moving basic protein) were added, with fewer moles of large basic protein and Wolfgram protein, with relative ratios of about 3:3:2:1, respectively (Figure 4C). Differ-

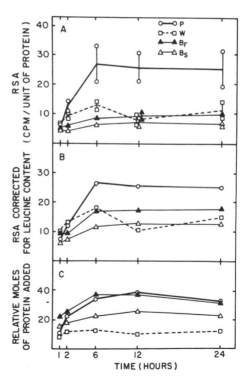

FIGURE 4. Time–course of changes in labeling of myelin proteins. (A) Changes in relative specific activity (RSA) of myelin proteins. Rats were each injected with 200 μCi [³H]leucine at 17 days and killed at the times indicated. Radioactivity and relative protein content were determined after gel electrophoresis. (P) Proteolipid protein; (W) Wolfgram proteins; (B_F) small (fast) basic protein; (B_S) large (slow) basic protein. (B) RSA corrected for leucine content of each protein. (C) Relative moles of each protein added. The radioactivity in each protein band was divided by the number of moles of leucine in 1 mole of that protein. From Benjamins *et al.* (1975).

ent relationships among the proteins entering myelin were found when younger and older animals were studied. At 40 days, the specific activities of Wolfgram and other high-molecular-weight proteins were higher than those of basic protein and PLP at both 1 and 24 hr, in agreement with the D'Monte and Smith studies in animals this age or older.

Subsequent studies in brain slices (Benjamins *et al.,* 1978) used shorter time points and continuous labeling of proteins, rather than a pulse, since a constant level of radioactive amino acids was present in the incubation medium. The basic and Wolfgram proteins appeared in myelin in a nearly linear fashion from 15 min onward, indicating little delay between their synthesis and appearance in myelin. PLP showed a delay in appearance in myelin, entering at a slow rate for 45 min then at a faster rate similar to the other two proteins. Inhibition of protein synthesis and chase studies with nonradioactive amino acids revealed an extramyelin pool of PLP that continued to provide PLP to myelin at a normal rate for 30–60 min after synthesis of newly labeled protein had been stopped. Conversely, entry of basic protein and Wolfgram proteins stopped within several minutes, indicating that only small pools of these proteins were available within the cell for subsequent myelin assembly.

In agreement with these earlier studies in slices, Colman *et al.* (1982) demonstrated similar results *in vivo.* They found labeled PLP in microsomal fractions at 2 and 5 min after intracranial injection of [^{35}S]methionine, but not at 30 min, consistent with transport out of the endoplasmic reticulum. Labeled PLP was not detected in myelin until 30 min after injection of isotope. In contrast, labeled MBP could be detected in myelin as early as 2 min after isotope injection.

While other explanations are possible, one interpretation of these results is that both proteins are synthesized primarily in the cell body, but PLP undergoes more extensive posttranslational processing than basic protein, with PLP moving through a series of intracellular membranes and basic protein transported directly through cytoplasm via vesicles or carrier proteins. Another possibility is that basic protein destined for myelin is synthesized near the site of myelin assembly and travels only short distances through cytoplasm or on vesicles before insertion into the myelin membrane. Conversely, PLP may be synthesized primarily in the cell body proper, then enter a transport system like that in axoplasmic transport. The distance from cell body to the myelinating process has been estimated to be as great as 10–40 μM (Sternberger *et al.,* 1978*b*); however, even the greater distance is too short to allow detection of a transport process like fast axoplasmic transport at a rate of 400 mm/day. At a slow transport of 1 mm/day, about 14 min would be required to move 10 μM. However, in axons, most membrane proteins move at the faster rate of 400 mm/day, with only cytoskeletal elements moving at the slower rate. Thus, the 30- to 45-min delay seen for entry of PLP is most likely due primarily to processing within endoplasmic reticulum and other intracellular membranes such as Golgi, rather than subsequent transport down the oligodendroglial process.

Cycloheximide and puromycin have been used *in vivo* (Benjamins *et al.,* 1971) to study the acute biochemical affects of disruption of myelin assembly *in situ.* In these studies, phosphatidylcholine and sulfatide continued to enter myelin at nearly normal rates for 1 hr when entry of protein into myelin was inhibited by 90%. The slice system has been used more extensively for examining agents that might block entry of proteins or lipids into myelin. In agreement with the *in vivo* experiments, lipid entry occurred at a normal rate when protein entry was blocked, thus indicating independent entry of lipid and protein, at least for short periods (M. E. Smith and Hasinoff, 1971). Triethyl lead (Konat and Clausen, 1980) blocks entry of proteins into myelin, but the effect appears secondary to a depression in synthesis of myelin proteins relative to other proteins. Antiserum to basic protein also blocks entry of proteins into myelin; in this case, synthesis of the myelin proteins was not directly investigated (Pellkofer and Jatzkewitz, 1976). The antiserum used was not heated to remove complement activity, so the effect might be due to serum components other than antibody.

The sodium ionophore monensin has been shown to block secretion and assembly of plasma-membrane proteins in several systems, presumably by disrupting budding of vesicles from the Golgi. When applied to CNS slices, monensin causes disappearance of normal Golgi structures and appearance of dilated vesicles in oligodendroglia (Townsend and Benjamins, 1984), as previously shown for Schwann cells (Rapaport *et al.,* 1982). Monensin inhibits entry of PLP into myelin by about 40%, but has little effect on entry of basic protein (Townsend and Benjamins, 1983). These results suggest that at least some of the PLP destined for myelin is processed through the Golgi or related vesicular structures and that basic protein is processed by another route. Immunocytochemical studies also suggest that PLP may be found in Golgi (Hartman *et al.,* 1982). However, PLP has not yet been directly identified in isolated Golgi fractions. One study indicates that basic protein but not PLP is found in some Golgi-enriched fractions (Pereyra and Braun, 1983). Bizzozero *et al.* (1982) have recently reported that colchicine partially blocks transport of PLP into myelin, but has no effect on entry of basic protein. More detailed investigation of this question is needed to determine conclusively whether PLP is processed through Golgi or via another monensin-sensitive mechanism, perhaps involving other vesicular structures or the cytoskeleton.

6.3. Posttranslational Modification

At present, we know that the peptide backbones of the major myelin proteins can undergo a variety of posttranslational modifications. We do not yet know what role, if any, these modifications play in the metabolism and processing of a given protein. Further, we do not know at what stage between synthesis and assembly these modifications occur.

MBP can be methylated, phosporylated, and sulfated *in vivo*. Details of these reactions have been discussed by Braun and Brostoff (1977) and by Carnegie and Moore (1980). Methylated arginines have been found in all mammalian MBPs examined as well as in the protein from several other species; the unmethylated/mono-/dimethylarginine ratios vary depending on the species (Brostoff and Eylar, 1972; Deibler and Martenson, 1973). Brostoff and Eylar (1972) postulated that the methylated base might play a role in stabilizing the conformation of the protein by cross-chain interactions, since methylated arginine is more hydrophobic than arginine itself. MBPs can be phosphorylated by either endogenous brain enzymes or exogenous protein kinases (Carnegie *et al.*, 1973; Steck and Appel, 1974; Miyamoto and Kakiuchi, 1974). The serine at position 54 is the primary site of phosphorylation by endogenous enzyme(s), while the serine at position 109 is the primary site for exogenous muscle protein kinase. Myelin itself appears to contain an endogenous kinase that can phosphorylate MBP. Basic protein isolated from myelin contains less than 0.2 mole phosphate/mole protein, although it can accept up to 4 moles when phosphorylated *in vitro*. Agrawal *et al.* (1982*a*) have recently reported *in vivo* phosphorylation of all four major basic proteins in rat myelin and have demonstrated convalent linkage of phosphate to serine and threonine residues. The endogenous protein kinase is calmodulin-dependent (Endo and Hidaka, 1980), requiring Mg^{2+} and Ca^{2+} for activity (Petrali *et al.*, 1980). The permeability of myelin vesicles to cations is changed by Mg^{2+}-ATP, but not by phosphorylation of basic proteins (Wüthrich and Steck, 1981).

Recent studies *in vivo* have compared phosphorylation and methylation of basic proteins during development (Des Jardins and Morell, 1983). The phosphorylation of MBP increases with maturation in proportion to the total amount of basic protein available. This suggests that the phosphate groups on basic protein are in equilibrium with extramyelin phosphate pools throughout the life of the animal and that even the basic protein molecules assembled into myelin early in development are still accessible for phosphorylation in the mature animal. Conversely, the rate of methylation slows with development and appears to be proportional to the rate of synthesis of MBP. This suggests that methylation occurs only as MBP is being synthesized and that MBP molecules previously assembled into myelin are no longer available for methylation.

The carbohydrate composition of myelin-associated glycoprotein (MAG) has been characterized (Quarles, 1980) and appears to fit into the complex mannose group of glycoproteins. Harford *et al.* (1977) have shown a requirement for dolichol phosphate intermediates in the addition of mannose to the protein. MAG can be readily labeled *in vivo* with radioactive fucose, mannose, and *N*-acetylglucosamine (Quarles *et al.*, 1973*a*; Matthieu *et al.*, 1975*a*) and can also be sulfated (Matthieu *et al.*, 1975*b*). As discussed in Section 4.4, a shift to a lower-molecular-weight form is seen during development, probably involving the peptide backbone rather than the carbohydrate moiety (McIntyre *et al.*, 1978), but whether this is due to a change in the translation product or to posttranslational processing is not known.

The kinetics of posttranslational modification of basic proteins or of specific myelin glycoproteins such as MAG have not been investigated *in vivo* or in slices. Processing of total [³H]fucose-labeled glycoproteins in CNS myelin has been examined in slices (Benjamins *et al.*, 1978). These studies showed a delay between addition of [³H]fucose to protein and the appearance of newly synthesized glycoproteins in myelin. An extra-myelin pool was present that continued to provide glycoproteins to myelin at a normal rate for 30 min after inhibition of protein synthesis.

PLP was characterized a number of years ago as containing fatty acid (Stoffyn and Folch-Pi, 1971). The protein contains 2 moles fatty acid/mole protein, probably covalently bound to serine or threonine. In the isolated rat protein, palmitic, stearic, and oleic acid account for 60, 30, and 10%, respectively, of the total fatty acids (Folch-Pi and Stoffyn, 1972). Acylation of PLP with [³H]palmitic acid has been demonstrated both *in vivo* (Agrawal *et al.*, 1982*b*) and in slices (Townsend *et al.*, 1982). The distribution of labeled fatty acids is similar to the composition, with palmitic the predominant fatty acid. The subcellular site at which acylation occurs has not yet been identified. In slices, cycloheximide did not prevent the acylation, indicating that the fatty acids were added after translation (Townsend *et al.*, 1982). The time–course of addition of fatty acid to PLP in myelin was linear, in contrast to the delay seen for entry of the peptide backbone of PLP into myelin. These results suggest that in the slices, acylation of PLP is occurring late in processing, either by exchange or by *de novo* addition possibly within myelin itself. When isolated myelin was incubated directly with [³H]palmitic acid, PLP was not acylated, but various conditions that might be conducive to acylation were not investigated. The acylation continues for at least 2 hr after protein synthesis is inhibited, suggesting that a large pool of PLP is available for *de novo* acylation or exchange of fatty acids. Neither monensin nor colchicine had any effect on the acylation of PLP appearing in myelin (Townsend and Benjamins, 1983; Bizzozero *et al.*,1982), consistent with the other evidence that the acylation observed *in vitro* is occurring late in processing, that is, post-Golgi or possibly within myelin itself.

6.4. Myelin Subfractions and Precursor Membranes

Several reviews have discussed in detail the results of recent studies on characterization and metabolism of myelin subfractions and of extra myelin membranes that might serve as precursors to myelin (Benjamins and Smith, 1977; Quarles, 1980a; Danks and Matthieu, 1979; Braun *et al.*, 1980; Waehneldt and Linington, 1980; Norton, 1983). The objective of these studies has been to determine the sequence of events that occur between synthesis of myelin components and their assembly into compact myelin. Particular emphasis has been placed on the basic proteins, PLP, and galactolipids in these fractions, since they are highly specific for oligodendroglia and myelin is enriched in them. These studies can be placed in three categories depending on the strategy used for subcellular fractionation: (1) isolation of myelin-associated membranes from a crude myelin fraction by osmotic shock; (2) fractionation of an isolated myelin fraction into subfractions, by either continuous or discontinuous gradients; and (3) fractionation of homogenates to survey all subcellular fractions. All these approaches have the inherent problems of any subcellular fractionation method with identity and "purity" of a given membrane fraction. However, these studies have led to the development of several hypotheses about the mechanism of myelin assembly that can now be tested by a variety of experimental approaches.

The formation of the myelin membrane may be either a one-step discontinuous process or a multistep continuous process. If it is discontinuous, then at some site in the oligodendroglia there would be a sharp transition in membrane composition, involving enrichment of myelin proteins and lipids. However, differences in kinetics of entry of various proteins and lipids and the ability of some components to enter myelin even when other components are blocked from entry suggest that a continuous multistep assembly of myelin occurs. In keeping with findings in other cells regarding membrane assembly (Rothman and Lenard, 1977; Morré *et al.*, 1979; Wickner, 1979; Waksman *et al.*, 1980; Sabatini *et al.*, 1982), one current hypothesis is that many of the myelin constituents are synthesized in the endoplasmic reticulum as membrane components, then transported via vesicles to the myelin membrane. As noted above, some myelin components may pass through the Golgi before budding off into vesicles destined for myelin. Other components may first be inserted into plasma membrane any place in the cell, then move by membrane flow to the site of myelin assembly. Still other components may be transported into myelin via cytoplasmic lipoproteins or synthesized within the membrane itself. Once the components enter myelin, they are thought to move by lateral diffusion through the membrane. Further compaction of lamellae occurs as myelination progresses. Cytoplasmic loop regions are thought to be sites for active insertion and exchange of the myelin components within the lamellae. Thus, investigators have designed methods of membrane isolation that might give them fractions corresponding to (1) the proposed sites for transport or processing of myelin components within the cell body and (2) various stages in compaction of myelin itself.

6.4.1. Isolation of Myelin-Associated Membranes

Exposure of myelin to a hypotonic solution results in the release of membranes that can be separated from myelin by low-speed centrifugation, with myelin in the pellet and other membranes in the supernatant (Banik and Davison, 1969; Agrawal *et al.*, 1970; Norton, 1971). Membranes in this fraction contain myelin constituents and have metabolic properties that suggest that they could be a precursor to myelin (Agrawal *et al.*, 1974). Subsequent examination shows that the fraction contains endoplasmic reticulum (Norton, 1971; Waehneldt and Mandel, 1972), axonal membranes (McIlwain, 1974; DeVries *et al.*, 1972; Haley *et al*, 1981), and some Golgi membranes (Benjamins *et al.*, 1982). A number of investigations have suggested that the fraction contains glial plasma membrane, cytoplasmic loop regions of myelin, or precursor membranes of myelin. While some properties of the fraction are consistent with each of these possibilities, no direct evidence about the subcellular origin of membranes in this fraction is available. It appears to be a heterogeneous mixture of membranes from various places. A modification of the original method gives a fraction designated SN4 that is largely free of endoplasmic reticulum and highly enriched in myelin components (Waehneldt and Mandel, 1972). Morell *et al.* (1972) used continuous CsCl gradients to separate myelin from a similar membrane fraction. The enrichment of myelin proteins and lipids, and their higher turnover in these fractions compared to that in myelin, suggest a relationship to myelin; however, another possibility is that the fractions represent extramyelin membranes from the cell body that turn over independently of myelin and are never transported to myelin for assembly.

6.4.2. Fractionation of Isolated Myelin

Two different approaches have been used in these studies. In the earliest report, myelin centrifuged on a density gradient gave two fractions, designated "heavy myelin" and "light myelin," that differed in their protein : lipid ratios (Autilio *et al.*, 1964). Subsequently, a number of investigators have placed osmotically shocked myelin on discontinuous or continuous gradients so that a series of membranes are obtained (Adams and Fox, 1969; Eng and Noble, 1968; Bourre *et al.*, 1977, 1980; Matthieu *et al.*, 1973; Benjamins *et al.*, 1973; Zimmerman *et al.*, 1975; Shapira *et al.*, 1981; Fujimoto *et al.*, 1976). In a second approach, myelin is fractionated without osmotic shock, such that entrapped axoplasm or other constituents contribute to the properties of the membranes (McMillan *et al.*, 1972).

The hypothesis that prompts many of these studies is that myelin undergoes a transition to a more lipid-rich membrane as it is formed from glial plasma membrane and that myelin membranes differing in density might represent different stages in maturation of the myelin sheath. As discussed by a number of investigators and reviewed recently by Quarles (1978) and Norton (1981), we do not know to what extent the various fractions reflect the size and developmental stage of myelinated axons in a given region vs. transitional forms between oligodendroglial plasma membrane and compact myelin.

While a number of studies have characterized the composition of these fractions, relatively few have looked at their metabolic properties. The metabolic properties of proteins in the myelin subfractions generally support the idea that the denser fractions contain precursor membranes to the myelin membranes in the lighter fractions, as suggested by studies on composition. The highest specific radioactivity of total protein occurs in the denser fractions (Fujimoto et al., 1976; Hofteig and Druse, 1976). When the metabolism of individual proteins in the fractions was examined, the specific radioactivities of the basic proteins and PLPs were highest in the denser fractions, consistent with a precursor role, while the specific radioactivity of the Wolfgram protein was relatively constant throughout the gradient (Benjamins et al., 1976). A double-isotope method that gives results independent of the preexisting protein pools has suggested that some proteins may enter a particular myelin subfraction by transfer from a denser subfraction. Following time-staggered injection of a ^{14}C- and then a ^{3}H-labeled amino acid, the lowest ^{3}H/^{14}C ratio of a given protein should be in the subfraction furthest in time from the site of synthesis. Thus, an orderly progression of isotope ratios for a given protein from denser to less dense fractions would support a precursor–product relationship, while similar ratios in each fraction would indicate simultaneous entry from the site of synthesis. When this method was applied to the myelin subfractions, the results showed that PLP appeared first in the denser subfractions, those composed predominantly of vesicular single-membrane structures, then in a lighter fraction, composed of typical myelin lamellae (Benjamins et al., 1976). These results suppported the observation suggested by the specific radioactivity data that the lower subfractions contain pools of PLP that might serve as precursors to the less dense subfractions. For basic protein, the time between synthesis and entry into each subfraction is similar, since basic protein appeared simultaneously in all the fractions. Thus, the lower fractions are more enriched in newly synthesized basic proteins than the upper ones, but the basic protein either enters all the membranes simultaneously or moves rapidly from the membranes in the lower fractions to those in the upper fractions.

6.4.3. Fractionation of Brain Homogenates

The studies described in Sections 6.4.1 and 6.4.2 utilized either crude or purified myelin fractions as starting material for preparation of myelin subfractions and related membranes. Several methods have been developed for fractionation of brain homogenates, most based on the method of Eichberg *et al.* (1964). Recently, several methods have been described for preparation of Golgi-enriched fractions from brain homogenates (Deshmukh *et al.*, 1978; Siegrist *et al.*, 1979; Benjamins *et al.*, 1982). In the latter two studies, distribution of enzymes involved in synthesis of cerebroside and sulfatide was examined. However, only one study to date has systematically examined the metabolism of myelin proteins in a large series of extramyelin and myelin-related membranes (Pereyra and Braun, 1983; Pereyra *et al.*, 1983). In these studies a series of subcellular fractions were prepared by a combination of differential centrifugation and separation on discontinuous sucrose gradients. Several groups of membranes containing myelin proteins were obtained, one group containing multilamellar myelin and myelinated axons; another group containing axons, large vesicles, and membrane fragments, but fewer myelin lamellae; a third group derived from a microsomal fraction; and a fourth group enriched in Golgi membranes. Using staggered injection of ^{3}H- and ^{14}C-labeled amino acids, the investigators analyzed the ^{3}H/^{14}C ratios in basic protein and PLP in various fractions to assess their relationships (Pereyra *et al.*, 1983). They pointed out that turnover of the proteins in each fraction must be considered to interpret the data. Their results point out the complexity of determining the intracellular route of the myelin proteins. Their conclusions generally support the concept that the myelin proteins are transported through several endomembrane compartments for assembly into myelin.

7. CONCLUSIONS AND FUTURE DIRECTIONS

The *in vivo* studies on protein metabolism of oligondendroglia have confirmed morphological observations that myelin is formed rapidly during development and is then maintained by the oligodendroglia throughout the life of the cells. The rate of synthesis and total amount of each of the proteins increase dramatically during the most rapid period of myelination. Subsequently, the rate of synthesis falls, and the accumulated proteins show little turnover once they have entered the myelin sheath. When basic protein and PLP are compared, several observations indicate that the metabolism of these two proteins is regulated independently. Basic protein appears in brain before PLP; it enters myelin very rapidly after synthesis and exhibits detectable turnover once inserted into myelin. PLP appears somewhat later, undergoes extensive intracellular processing before entering myelin, and shows virtually no turnover once inserted into myelin. For short periods, each protein can enter myelin even though the other protein is partially blocked from entry.

Most of our information from *in vivo* studies has so far come from examination of newly synthesized proteins isolated with myelin. As discussed in Section 6, attempts to study the myelin proteins in subcellular fractions other than myelin have a number of limitations. However, the combined use of well-defined subcellular fractions and specific identification of a given protein by a combination of immunological and electrophoretic methods will allow examination of the extra myelin pools of these proteins. To avoid the contributions of other cell types to subcellular fractions, isolation of oligodendroglia followed by subcellular fractionation is the method of choice. With the availability of methods for isolation of oligodendroglia from whole brain of small animals, specifically rats and mice, radioactive amino acids can be injected, oligodendroglia isolated, and subcellular fractions prepared. The major difficulties with this approach are (1) the danger of degradation or loss of protein during isolation, (2) the large amount of tissue and radioactivity that might be required to obtain subcellular fractions in adequate quantity and with sufficient radioactivity to detect labeling of individual proteins, and (3) the question of whether the oligodendroglia isolated are representative of the population *in vivo*.

Another area that can be exploited more fully is the identification and use of agents that can disrupt synthesis or processing of specific proteins. A drawback here is the difficulty in using these agents *in vivo*. In these kinds of studies, the *in vitro* slice system may continue to provide a useful tool for examining the sequence of intracellular processing for a given protein.

Studies on posttranslational modification of the myelin proteins have gone through an initial descriptive phase. The methodology is now available to investigate where in the cell these modifications are occurring and what effects the modifications have on the function and further processing of a given protein. For example, studies on the effects of tunicamycin on the P_0 glycoprotein in PNS show that the carbohydrate portion may not be needed for insertion of P_0 into myelin. Does the same hold for myelin-associated glycoprotein in CNS myelin?

Finally, the question of how the oligodendroglia metabolize the myelin proteins in cases where myelination is impaired or where demyelination is occurring needs further exploration. Sites of synthesis, posttranslational modification, assembly into myelin, and long-term turnover of the proteins can now be investigated in detail in the several models of perturbed oligodendroglial function currently being studied.

8. REFERENCES

Abramsky, O., Lisak, R.P., Pleasure, D., Gilden, D.H., and Silberberg D. H., 1978, Immunologic characterization of oligodendroglia, *Neurosci. Lett.* **9**:311–316.

Adams, D. H., and Fox, M. E., 1969, The homogeneity and protein composition of rat brain myelin, *Brain Res.* **14**:647–661.

Adams, D. H. and Osborne, J., 1973, A developmental study of the relationship between the protein components of rat CNS myelin, *Neurobiology* **3**:91–112.

Agrawal, H. C., and Hartman, B. K., 1980, Proteolipid protein and other proteins of myelin, in: *Proteins of the Nervous System,* 2nd ed. (R. A. Bradshaw and D. M. Schneider, eds.), pp. 145–169, Raven Press, New York.

Agrawal, H. C., Banik, N. L., Bone, A. H., Davison, A. N., Mitchell, R. F., and Spohn, M., 1970, The identity of a myelin-like fraction isolated from developing brain, *Biochem. J.* **120**:635–642.

Agrawal, H. C., Trotter, J. L., Burton, R. M., and Mitchell, R. F., 1974, Evidence for a precursor role of a myelin subfraction, *Biochem. J.* **140**:99–109.

Agrawal, H. C., O'Connell, K., Randle, C. L., and Agrawal, D., 1982a, Phosphorylation *in vivo* of four basic proteins of rat brain myelin, *Biochem. J.* **201**:39–47.

Agrawal, H. C., Randle, C. L., and Agrawal, D., 1982b, *In vivo* acylation of rat brain myelin proteolipid protein, *J. Biol. Chem.* **257**:4588–4592.

Autilio, L. A., Norton, W. T., and Terry, R. D., 1964, The preparation and some properties of purified myelin from the central nervous system, *J. Neurochem.* **11**:17–26.

Autilio-Gambetti, L., Gambetti, P., and Shafer, B., 1975, Glial and neuronal contribution to proteins and glycoproteins recovered in myelin fractions, *Brain Res.* **84**:336–340.

Banik, N. L., and Davison, A. N., 1969, Enzyme activity and composition of myelin and sub-cellular fractions in the developing rat brain, *Biochem. J.* **115**:1051–1062.

Banik, N. L., and Smith, M. E., 1977, Protein determinants of myelination in different regions of developing rat central nervous system, *Biochem. J.* **162**:247–255.

Banik, N. L., Davison, A. N., Ramsey, R. B., and Scott, T., 1974, Protein composition in devel-oping human brain myelin, *Dev. Psychobiol.* **7**:539–546.

Barbarese, E., Braun, P. E., and Carson, J. H., 1977, Identification of prelarge and presmall basic proteins in mouse myelin and their structural relationship to large and small basic proteins, *Proc. Natl. Acad. Sci. U.S.A.* **74**:3360–3364.

Barbarese, E., Carson, J. H., and Braun, P. E., 1978, Accumulation of the four myelin basic proteins in mouse brain during development, *J. Neurochem.* **31**:779–782.

Benjamins, J. A., and Morell, P., 1978, Proteins of myelin and their metabolism, *Neurochem. Res.* **3**:137–174.

Benjamins, J. A., and Smith, M. E., 1977, Metabolism of myelin, in *Myelin* (P. Morell, ed.) pp. 233–270, Plenum Press, New York.

Benjamins, J. A., Herschkowitz, N., Robinson, J., and McKhann, G. M., 1971, The effects of inhibitors of protein synthesis on incorporation of lipids into myelin, *J. Neurochem.* **18**: 729–728.

Benjamins, J. A., Miller, K., and McKhann, G. M., 1973, Myelin subfractions in developing rat brain: Characterization and sulfatide metabolism, *J. Neurochem.* **20**:1589–1603.

Benjamins, J. A., Jones, M., and Morell, P., 1975, Appearance of newly synthesized proteins in myelin of young rats, *J. Neurochem.* **24**:1117–1122.

Benjamins, J. A., Gray, M., and Morell, P., 1976, Metabolic relationships between myelin subfractions: Entry of proteins, *J. Neurochem.* **27**:571–575.

Benjamins, J. A., Iwata, R., and Hazlett, J., 1978, Kinetics of entry of proteins into the myelin membrane, *J. Neurochem.* **31**: 1077–085.

Benjamins, J. A., Hadden, T., and Skoff, R. P., 1982, Cerebroside sulfotransferase in Golgi-enriched fractions from rat brain, *J. Neurochem.* **38**:233–241.

Berthold, C. H., 1978, Morphology of normal peripheral axons, in: *Physiology and Pathobiology of Axons* (S. G. Waxman, ed.), pp. 3–63, Raven Press, New York.

Bizzozero, O. A., Pasquini, J. M., and Soto, E. F., 1982, Differential effect of colchicine upon the entry of proteins into myelin and myelin-related membranes, *Neurochem. Res.* 7:1415–1425.

Bourne, J. M., Pollet, S., Daudu, O., Le Saux, F., and Baumann, N., 1977, Myelin consists of a continuum of particles of different density with varying lipid composition: Major differences are found between normal mice and quaking mutants, *Biochimie* 59:819–824.

Bourre, J. M., Jacque, C., Delassalle, A., Nguyen-Legros, J., Dumont, O., Lachapelle, F., Raoul, M., Alvarez, C., and Baumann, N., 1980, Density profile and basic protein measurements in the myelin range of particulate material from normal developing mouse brain and from neurological mutants (jimpy; quaking; trembler; shiverer and its mld allele) obtained by zonal centrifugation, *J. Neurochem.* 35:458–464.

Braun, P. E., and Brostoff, S. W., 1977, Proteins of myelin, in: *Myelin* (R. Morell, ed.) pp. 201–231, Plenum Press, New York.

Brostoff, S. W. and Eylar, E. H., 1972, Localization of methylated arginine in the A_1 protein from myelin, *Proc. Natl. Acad. Sci. U.S.A.* 68:765–769.

Cammer, W., and Norton, W. T., 1976, Disc gel electrophoresis of myelin proteins: New observations on development of the intermediate proteins (DM-20), *Brain Res.* 109:643–648.

Campagnoni, A. T., and Hunkeler, M. J., 1980, Synthesis of the myelin proteolipid protein in developing mouse brain, *J. Neurobiol.* 11:355–364.

Campagnoni, A. T., Campagnoni, C. W., Dutton, G. R., and Cohen, J., 1976, A regional study of developing rat brain: The accumulation and distribution of proteolipid protein, *J. Neurobiol.* 7:313–324.

Campagnoni, A. T., Carey, G. D., and Yu, Y. T., 1980. *In vitro* synthesis of the myelin basic proteins: Subcellular site of synthesis, *J. Neurochem.* 36:677–66.

Campagnoni, C. W., Carey, G. D., and Campagnoni, A. T., 1978, Synthesis of myelin basic proteins in the developing mouse brain, *Arch. Biochem. Biophys.* 190:118–125.

Carnegie, P. R., and Moore, W. J., 1980, Myelin basic protein, in: *Proteins of the Nervous System, 2nd ed.* (R. A. Bradshaw and D. M. Schneider, eds.), pp. 119–143, Raven Press, New York.

Carnegie, P. R., Kemp, B. E., Dunkley, P. R., and Murray, A. W., 1973, Phosphorylation of myelin basic protein by an adenosine 3′-5′-cyclic monophosphate-dependent protein kinase, *Biochem. J.* 135:569–572.

Carson, J. S., Nielson, S., and Barbarese, E., 1983, Developmental regulation of myelin basic protein expression in mouse brain, *Dev. Biol.* 96:485–492.

Clausen, J., 1969, Gray–white matter differences, in: *Handbook of Neurochemistry,* Vol. 1 (A. Lajtha, ed.) pp. 273–300, Plenum Press, New York.

Cohen, S. R., and Guarnieri, M., 1976, Immunochemical measurement of myelin basic protein in developing rat brain: An index of myelin synthesis, *Dev. Biol.* 49:294–299.

Colman, D. R., Kreibich, G., Frey, A. B., and Sabatini, D. D., 1982, Synthesis and incorporation of myelin polypeptides into CNS myelin, *J. Cell Biol.* 95:598–608.

Danks, D. M., and Matthieu, J. M., 1979, Hypotheses regarding myelination derived from comparisons of myelin subfractions, *Life Sci.* 24:1425–1440.

Day, E. D., 1981, Myelin basic protein, in: *Contemporary Topics in Molecular Immunology,* Vol. 8 (F. P. Inman and W. J. Mandy, eds.), pp. 1–39, Plenum Press, New York.

Deibler, G. E., and Martenson, R. E., 1973, Chromatographic fractionation of myelin basic proteins: Partial characterization and methylarginine content of the multiple forms, *J. Biol. Chem.* 248:2392–2396.

Deshmukh, D. S., Bear, W. D., and Soifer, D., 1978, Isolation and characterization of an enriched Golgi fraction from rat brain, *Biochim. Biophys. Acta* **542**:284–295.

Des Jardins, K. C., and Morell, P., 1983, Metabolism of phosphate and methyl groups of myelin basic proteins from rat central nervous system, *J. Cell Biol.* **97**:438–446.

Detering, N. K., and Wells, M. A., 1976, The non-synchronous synthesis of myelin components during early stages of myelination in the rat optic nerve, *J. Neurochem.* **26**:253–257.

DeVries, G. H., Norton, W. T., and Raine, C. S., 1972, Axons: Isolation from mammalian CNS, *Science* **175**:1370–1371.

D'Monte, B., Mela, P., and Marks, N., 1971, Metabolic instability of myelin protein and proteolipid fractions, *Eur. J. Biochem.* **23**:355–365.

Droz, B., and Koenig, H. L., 1970, Localization of protein metabolism in neurons, in: *Protein Metabolism of the Nervous System* (A. Lajtha, ed.), pp. 93–108, Plenum Press, New York.

Drummond, R. J., and Dean, G., 1980, Comparison of 2′,3′-cyclic nucleotide 3′-phosphodiesterase and the major component of Wolfgram protein Wl, *J. Neurochem.* **35**:1155–1165.

Druse, M. J., Brady, R. O., and Quarles, R. H., 1974, Metabolism of a myelin-associated glycoprotein in developing rat brain, *Brain Res.* **76**:423.

Eichberg, J., Whittaker, V. P., and Dawson, R. M. C., 1964, Distribution of lipids in subcellular particles of guinea pig brain, *Biochem. J.* **92**:91–100.

Einstein, E. R., Dalal, K. B., and Csejtey, J., 1970, Biochemical maturation of the central nervous system. I. Proteins and proteolytic enzyme changes, *Brain Res.* **18**:35–49.

Endo, T., and Hidaka, H., 1980, Calmodulin dependent phosphorylation of myelin isolated from rabbit brain, *Biochem. Biophys. Res. Commun.* **97**:553–558.

Eng. L. F., and Noble, E. P., 1968, The maturation of rat brain myelin, *Lipids* **3**:1577161.

Fischer, C. A., and Morell, P., 1974, Turnover of proteins in myelin and myelin-like material of mouse brain, *Brain Res.* **74**:51–65.

Fishman, M. A., Agrawal, H. C., Alexander, A., and Golterman, J., 1975, Biochemical maturation of human central nervous system myelin, *J. Neurochem.* **24**:689–694.

Folch-Pi, J., and Stoffyn, P. J., 1972, Proteolipids from membrane systems, *Ann. N. Y., Acad. Sci.* **195**:86–107.

Fujimoto, K., Roots, B. I., Burton, R. M., and Agrawal, H. C., 1976, Morphological and biochemical characterization of light and heavy myelin isolated from developing rat brain, *Biochim. Biophys. Acta* **426**:659–668.

Giorgi, P. P., and DuBois, H., 1981, Labeling by axonal transport of myelin-associated proteins in the rabbit visual pathway, *Biochem. J.* **196**:537–545.

Giorgi, P. P., Karlsson, J. O., Sjöstrand, J., and Field, E. J., 1973, Axonal flow and myelin protein in the optic pathway, *Nature (London)New Biol.* **244**:121124.

Glasgow, M. S., Quarles, R. H., and Grollman, S., 1972, Metabolism of fucoglycoproteins in the developing rat brain, *Brain Res.* **42**:129–137.

Greenfield, S., Weise, M. J., Gantt, G., Hogan, E. L., and Brostoff, S. W., 1982, Basic proteins of rodent peripheral nerve myelin: Identification of the 21.5K, 18.5K, 17K, 14K, and P2 proteins, *J. Neurochem.* **39**:1279–1282.

Haley, J. E., and Ledeen, R. W., 1979, Incorporation of axonally transported substances into myelin lipids, *J. Neurochem.* **32**:735–742.

Haley, J. E., Samuels F. G., and Ledeen, R. W., 1981, Study of myelin purity in relation to axonal contaminants, *Cell. Mol. Neurobiol.* **1**:175–187.

Hall, C., and Lim, L., 1981, Developmental changes in the composition of polyadenylated RNA isolated from free and membrane-bound polyribosomes of the rat forebrain, analyzed by translation *in vitro*, *Biochem. J.* **196**:327–336.

Hall, C., Mahadevan, L., Whatley, S., Ling, T.-S. and Lim, L., 1982, The polyadenylated RNA directing the synthesis of the rat myelin basic proteins is present in both free and membrane-bound forebrain polyribosomes, *Biochem. J.* **202:**407–417.

Harford, J. B., Waechter, C. J., and Earl, F. L., 1977, Effect of exogenous dolichyl monophosphate on a developmental change in mannosylphosphoryl-dolichol biosynthesis, *Biochem. Biophys. Res. Commun.* **76:**1036–1043.

Hartman, B. K., Agrawal, H. C., Agrawal, D., and Kalmbach, S., 1982, Development and maturation of central nervous myelin: Comparison of immunohistochemical localization of proteolipid protein and basic protein in myelin and oligodendrocytes, *Proc. Natl. Acad. Sci. U.S.A.,* **79:**4217–4220.

Hofteig, J.H., and Druse, M. J., 1976, Metabolism of three subfractions of myelin in developing rats, *Life Sci.* **18:**543–552.

Jacobson, S., 1963, Sequence of myelinization in the brain of the albino rat. A. Cerebral cortex, thalamus and related structures, *J. Comp. Neurol.* **121:**5–29.

Johnson, D., Quarles, R. H., and Brady, R. O., 1980, A radioimmunoassay for the myelin-associated glycoprotein, *Fed. Proc. Fed. Am. Soc. Exp. Biol.* **39:**1831.

Konat, G., and Clausen, ., 1980, Suppressive effect of triethyllead on entry of proteins into the CNS myelin sheath *in vitro, J. Neurochem.* **35:**382–387.

Lajtha, A., Toth, J., Fujimoto, K., and Agrawal, H. C., 1977, Turnover of myelin proteins in mouse brain *in vivo, Biochem. J.* **164:**323–329.

Lane, J. D., and Fagg, G. E., 1980, Protein and glycoprotein composition of myelin subfractions from the developing rat optic nerve and tract, *J. Neurochem.* **34:**163–171.

Lerner, P., Campagnoni, A. T., and Sampugna, J., 1974, Proteolipids in the developing brains of normal and mutant mice, *J. Neurochem.* **22:**163–170.

Lim, L., White, J. O., Hall, C., Berthold, W., and Davison, A. N., 1974, Isolation of microsomal poly(A) RNA from rat brain directing the synthesis of the encephalitogenic protein in *Xenopus* oocytes, *Biochim. Biophys. Acta* **318:**313–325.

Macklin, W. B., and Lees, M. B., 1982, Solid-phase immunoassays for quantitation of antibody to bovine white matter proteolipid apoprotein, *J. Neurochem.* **38:**348–355.

Magno-Sumbilla, C., and Campagnoni, A. T., 1977, Factors affecting the electrophoretic analysis of myelin proteins: Application to changes occurring during brain development, *Brain Res.* **126:**131–148.

Margolis, R. U., 1967, Acid mucopolysaccharides and glycoproteins of bovine whole brain, white matter and myelin, *Biochim. Biophys. Acta* **141:**91–102.

Matthees, J., and Campagnoni, A. T., 1980, Cell-free synthesis of the myelin basic proteins in a wheat germ system programmed with brain messenger RNA, *J. Neurochem.* **4:**867–872.

Matthieu, J. M., Quarles, R. H., Poduslo, J. F., Brady, R. O., and Webster, H. De F., 1973, Variation of proteins, enzyme markers and gangliosides in myelin subfractions, *Biochim. Biophys. Acta* **329:**305–317.

Matthieu, J. M., Brady, R. O., and Quarles, R. H., 1975a, Change in myelin-associated glycoprotein in rat brain during development: Metabolic aspects, *Brain Res.* **86:**55–65.

Matthieu, J. M., Quarles, R. H., Poduslo, J. F., and Brady, R. O., 1975b, [35s] Sulfate incorporation into myelin glycoproteins. Central nervous system, *Biochim. Biophys. Acta* **392:**159–166.

Matthieu, J. M., Webster, H. D., DeVries, G. H., Corthay, S., and Koellreutter, B., 1978, Glial versus neuronal origin of myelin proteins and glycoproteins studied by combined intraocular and intracranial labeling, *J. Neurochem.* **31:**93–102.

Matus, A. DePatris, S., and Raff, M. D., 1973, Mobility of concanavalin-A receptors in myelin and synaptic membranes, *Nature (London) New Biol.* **244:**278–280.

McIlwain, D. L., 1974, Localization of the acetylcholinesterase-containing membranes in purified myelin fractions, *Brain Res.* **69**:182–184.

McIntyre, L. J., Quarles, R. H., and Brady, R. O., 1978. The effect of trypsin on myelin-associated glycoprotein, *Trans. Am. Soc. Neurochem.* **9**:106.

McIntyre, L. J., Quarles, R. H., and Brady, R. O., 1979, Lectin-binding proteins in central-nervous-system myelin: Detection of glycoproteins of purified myelin on polyacrylamide gels by ^{3}H concanavalin A binding, *Biochem. J.* **183**:205–212.

McMillan, P. N., Williams, N. I., Kaufman, B., and Day, E. D., 1972, The isolation and biochemical characterization of three subfractions of myelin from central nervous tissue of the adult rat, *J. Neurochem.* **19**:1839–1848.

Miyamoto, E., and Kakiuchi, S., 1974, *In vitro* and *in vivo* phosphorylation of myelin basic protein by exogenous and endogenous adenosine 3′,5′-monphosphate-dependent protein kinases in brain, *J. Biol. Chem.* **249**:2769–2777.

Morell, P., Greenfield, S., Costantino-Ceccarini, E., and Wisniewski, H., 1972, Changes in the protein composition of mouse brain myelin during development, *J. Neurochem.* **19**:2545–254.

Morré, D. J., Kartenbeck, J., and Franke, W. W., 1979, Membrane flow and interconversions among endomembranes, *Biochim. Biophys. Acta* **559**:71–152.

Muller, H. W., Clapshaw, P. A., and Seifert, W., 1981, Characterization of 2′:3′-cyclic nucleotide 3′-phosphodiesterase: Limited proteolytic digestion, plant lectin affinity chromatography and immunological identification, *J. Neurochem.* **36**:2004–2013.

Norton, W. T., 1971, Recent developments in the investigation of purified myelin, in: *Chemistry and Brain Development,* Vol. 13 (R. Paoletti and A. N. Davison, eds), pp. 327–337, Plenum Press, New York.

Norton, W. T., 1981, Formation, structure, and biochemistry of myelin, in: *Basic Neurochemistry,* 3rd ed. (G. J. Siegel, R. W., Albers, B. W. Agranoff, and R. Katzman, eds.), pp. 63–92, Little Brown, Boston.

Norton, W T., 1983, Recent advances in the neurobiology of oligodendroglia, in: *Advances in Cellular Neurobiology,* Vol. 4 (S. Fedoroff and L. Hertz, eds.), pp. 3–55, Academic Press, New York.

Norton, W. T., and Poduslo, S. E., 1973, Myelination in rat brain: Changes in myelin composition during brain maturation, *J. Neurochem.* **21**: 759–773.

Nussbaum, J. L., and Mandel, P., 1973, Brain proteolipids in neurological mutant mice, *Brain Res.* **61**:295–310.

Pellkofer, R., and Jatzkewitz, H., 1976, Alteration of myelin biosynthesis in slices of rabbit spinal cord by antiserum to myelin basic protein and by puromycin, *J. Neurochem.* **27**:351–364.

Pereyra, P. M., and Braun, P. E., 1983, studies on subcellular fractions which are involved in myelin membrane assembly: Isolation from developing mouse brain and characterization by enzyme markers, electron microscopy, and electrophoresis, *J. Neurochem.* **41**: 957–973.

Pereyra, P. M., Braun, P. E., Greenfield, S., and Hogan, E. L., 1983, Studies on subcellular fractions which are involved in myelin assembly: Labeling of myelin proteins by a double radioisotope approach indicates developmental relationships, *J. Neurochem.* **41**:974–988.

Petrali, E. H., Thiessen, B. J., and Sulakhe, V., 1980, Magnesium-ion dependent, calcium-ion stimulated, endogenous protein kinase-catalyzed phosphorylation of basic proteins in myelin fraction of rat brain white matter, *Int. J. Biochem.* **11**:21–36.

Poduslo, J. F., 1981, Developmental regulation of the carbohydrate composition of glycoproteins associated with central nervous system myelin, *J. Neurochem.* **36**:1924–1931.

Poduslo, J. F., and Rodbard, D., 1980, Molecular weight estimation using sodium dodecyl sulfate-pore gradient electrophoresis, *Anal. Biochem.* **101**:394–406.

Poduslo, J. F., Harman, J. L., and McFarlin, D. E., 1980, Lectin receptors in central nervous system myelin, *J. Neurochem.* **34:** 1733–1744.

Poduslo, S. E., McFarland, H. F., and McKhann, G. M., 1977, Antiserums to neurons and to oligodendroglia from mammalian brain, *Science* **197:**270–272.

Quarles, R. H., 1980a, The biochemical and morphological heterogeneity of myelin and myelin-related membranes, in: *Biochemistry of Brain* (S. Kumar, ed.), pp. 81–102, Pergamon Press, Oxford.

Quarles, R. H., 1980b, Glycoproteins from central and peripheral myelin, in: *Myelin: Chemistry and Biology* (G. A. Hashim, ed.) pp. 55–77, Alan R. Liss, New York.

Quarles, R. H., Everly, J. L., and Brady, R. O., 1973a. Evidence for the close association of a glycoprotein with myelin in rat brain, *J. Neurochem.* **21:**1177–1191.

Quarles, R. H., Everly, J. L., and Brady, R. O., 1973b, Myelin-associated glycoprotein: A developmental change, *Brain Res.* **58:**506–509.

Quarles, R. H., McIntyre, L. J., and Pasnak, C. F., 1979, Lectin-binding proteins in central-nervous-system myelin: Binding of glycoproteins in purified myelin to immobiled lectins, *Biochem. J.* **183:**213–226.

Ramsey, J. C., and Steele, W. J., 1977, Quantitative isolation and properties of nearly homogeneous populations of undergraded free and bound polysomes from rat brain, *J. Neurochem.* **28:**517–527.

Rapaport, R. N., Benjamins, J. A., and Skoff, R. P., 1982, Effects of monensin on assembly of P_0 protein into peripheral nerve myelin, *J. Neurochem.* **39:**1101–1110.

Rothman, J. E., and Lenard, J., 1977, Membrane asymmetry, *Science* **195:**743–753.

Sabatini, D. D., Kreibich, G., Morimoto, T., and Adesnik, M., 1982, Mechanisms for the incorporation of proteins into membranes and organelles, *J. Cell Biol.* **91:**637–646.

Sabri, M. I., Bone, A. H., and Davison, A. N., 1974, Turnover of myelin and other structural proteins in the developing rat brain. *Biochem. J.* **142:**499–507.

Shapira, R., Wilhelmi, M. R., and Kibler, R. F., 1981, Turnover of myelin proteins of rat brain, determined in fractions separated by sedimentation in a continuous sucrose gradient, *J. Neurochem.* **36:**1427–1432.

Siegrist, H. P., Burkart, T., Wiesmann, U. N., Herschkowitz, N. N., and Spycher, M. A., 1979, Ceramide-galctosyl transferase and cerebroside-sulfotransferase localisation in Golgi membranes isolated by a discontinuous sucrose gradient of mouse brain microsomes *J. Neurochem.* **33:**497–504.

Singh, H., and Jungalwala, F. B., 1979, The turnover of myelin proteins in adult rat brain, *Int. J. Neurosci.* **9:**123–131.

Smith, C. B., Davidsen, L., Deibler, G., Patlak, C., Pettigrew, K.,and Sokoloff, L., 1980, A method for determination of local rates of protein synthesis in brain, *Trans Am. Soc. Neurochem.* **11:**94.

Smith, M. E., 1972, The turnover of myelin proteins, *Neurobiology* **2:**35–40.

Smith, M. E., 1973, A regional survey of myelin development: Some compositional and metabolic aspects, *J. Lipid Res.* **14:** 541–511.

Smith, M. E., 1983, Peripheral nervous system myelin: Properties and metabolism, in: *Handbook of Neurochemistry,* Vol. 3, (A. Lajtha, ed.), pp. 201–223, Plenum Press, New York.

Smith, M. E., and Hasinoff, C. M., 1971, Biosynthesis of myelin proteins *in vitro, J. Neurochem.* **18:**739–747.

Sprinkle, T. J., Zaruea, M. E., and McKhann, G. M., 1978a, Activity of 2′,3′-cyclic-nucleotide 3′-phosphodiesterase in regions of rat brain during development: Quantitative relationship to myelin basic protein, *J. Neurochem.* **30:**309–314.

Sprinkle, T. J., Zaruba, M. E., and McKhann, G. M., 1978*b*, Radioactive measurement of 2′-3′-cyclic nucleotide 3′-phosphodiesterase activity in central and peripheral nervous system and in extraneural tissue, *Anal, Biochem.* **88:**449–456.

Sprinkle, T. J., Wells, M. R., Garver, F. A., and Smith, D. B., 1980, Studies on the Wolfgram high molecular weight CNS myelin proteins: Relationship to 2′,3′-cyclic nucleotide 3′-phosphodiesterase, *J. Neurochem.* **35:**1200–1208.

Steck, A. J., and Appel, S. H., 1974, Phosphorylation of myelin basic protein, *J. Biol. Chem.* **249:**5416–5420.

Sternberger, N. H., Itoyama, Y., Kies, M. W., and Webster, H., 1978*a*, Myelin basic protein demonstrated immunocytochemically in oligodendroglia prior to myelin sheath formation, *Proc. Natl. Acad. Sci. U.S.A.* **5:**2521–2524.

Sternberger, N. H., Itoyama, Y., Kies, M. W., and Webster, H., 1978*b*, Immunocytochemical method to identify basic protein in myelin-forming oligodendrocytes of newborn rat C.N.S. *J. Neurocytol.* **7:**251–263.

Sternberger, N. H., Quarles, R. H., Itoyama, Y., and Webster, H. D., 1979, Myelin-associated glycoprotein demonstrated immunocytochemically in myelin and myelin-forming cells of developing rat, *Proc. Natl. Acad. Sci. U.S.A.* **76:**1510–1514.

Stoffyn, P., and Folch-Pi, J., 1971, On the type of linkage binding fatty acids present in brain white matter proteolipid apoprotein, *Biochem. Biophys. Res. Commun.* **44:**157–161.

Tennekoon, G. I., Cohen, S. R., Price, D. L., and McKhann, G. M., 1977, Myelinogenesis in optic nerve: A morphological, autoradiographic, and biochemical analysis, *J. Cell Biol.* **72:**604–616.

Townsend, L. E., and Benjamins, J. A., 1979, Protein synthesis by free and membrane bound polysomes from brainstem., *Trans. Am. Soc. Neurochem.* **11:**157.

Townsend, L. E., and Benjamins, J. A., 1983, The effects of monensin on post-translational processing of myelin proteins, *J. Neurochem.* **40:**1333–1339.

Townsend, L. E., and Benjamins, J. A., 1984, Effects of colchicine and monensin on myelin galactolipids, *J. Neurochem.* (in press).

Townsend, L. E., Agrawal, D., Benjamins, J. A., and Agrawal, H. C., 1982, Acylation of myelin proteolipid protein *in vitro, J. Biol. Chem.* **257:**9745–9750.

Traugott, U., Snyder, D. S., Norton, W. T., and Raine, C. S., 1978, Characterization of anti-oligodendrocyte serum, *Ann. Neurol.* **4:**431–439.

Trotter, J. L., Lieberman, L., Margolis, F. L., and Agrawal, H. C., 1981, Radioimmunoassay for central nervous system myelin-specific proteolipid protein, *J. Neurochem.* **36:**68–74.

Waehneldt, T. V., and Linington, C., 1980, Organization and assembly of the myelin membrane in: *Neurological Mutations Affecting Myelination* (N. Baumann, eds.), Inserm symposium No. 14, pp. 389–412, Elsevier, North-Holland, Amsterdam.

Waehneldt, T. V., and Mandel, 1972, Isolation of rat brain myelin, monitored by polyacrylamide gel electrophoresis of dodecyl sulfate-extracted proteins, *Brain Res.* **40:**419–432.

Waksman, A., Hubert, P., Cremel, G., Rendon, A., and Burrun, C., 1980, Translocation of proteins through biological membranes: A critical review, *Biochim. Biophys. Acta* **604:**249–296.

Wickner, W., 1979, The assembly of proteins into biological membranes: The membrane trigger hypothesis, *Annu. Rev. Biochem.* **48:**23–45.

Wolfgram, F., 1966, A new proteolipid fraction of the nervous system. I. Isolation and amino acid analyses, *J. Neurochem.* **13:**461–470.

Wolman, M., and Hestrin-Lerner, S., 1960, A histochemical contribution to the study of the molecular morphology of the myelin sheath, *J. Neurochem.* **5:**114–120.

Wüthrich, C., and Steck, A. J., 1981, A permeability change of myelin membrane vesicles towards cations is induced by MgATP but not by phosphorylation of myelin basic proteins, *Biochim. Biophys. Acta* **640**:195–206.

Yu, Y. T., and Campagnoni, A. T., 1982, *In vitro* synthesis of the four myelin basic proteins: Evidence for the lack of a metabolic relationship, *J. Neurochem.* **39**:1559–1568.

Zimmerman, A. W., Quarles, R. H., Webster, H. De F., Matthieu, J. M., and Brady, R. O., 1975, Characterization and protein analysis of myelin subfractions in rat brain: Developmental and regional comparison, *J. Neurochem.* **25**:749–757.

CHAPTER 4

PATTERNS OF OLIGODENDROCYTE FUNCTION SEEN BY IMMUNOCYTOCHEMISTRY

NANCY H. STERNBERGER

1. INTRODUCTION

The classification of cells into types and the functions assigned to each cell type have, in the past, been dependent primarily upon morphological criteria. The functions usually associated with oligodendrocytes are: (1) myelin formation by interfascicular oligodendrocytes and (2) nutrition of neurons by satellite oligodendrocytes in the gray matter, the satellite cells being presumed not to participate in myelination (for a review, see Raine, 1981). More recently, immunocytochemistry has become a useful tool for confirming and extending (or contradicting) conclusions based on morphological observations. In addition, immunocytochemical studies have led to the discovery of new functions associated with oligodendrocytes and have shown that oligodendrocytes can no longer be considered as being solely myelin-producing cells.

NANCY H. STERNBERGER ● *Center for Brain Research, University of Rochester Medical Center, Rochester, New York 14642*

While, in general, there is agreement among immunocytochemical results obtained from different groups of investigators using different antisera, discrepancies do exist. Some potential sources for different results are: (1) animal species used, (2) age of animal, (3) type of fixative and time of fixation, (4) method of preparing tissue sections, (5) use of cultures vs. tissue, (6) immunocytochemical technique used, and (7) tissue or structure penetrability. It is encouraging that despite all these variations, uniform results are usually obtained. A more important problem is the need for careful immunochemical evaluation of antisera (see Jones and Hartman, 1978). It is becoming increasingly evident that standard immunodiffusion techniques often do not detect cross-reactions of antisera that can be easily seen by immunocytochemistry. Use of the electroblot technique of Towbin *et al.* (1979) to characterize the reaction of antisera against whole-tissue homogenates as well as purified fractions or proteins will help greatly to define specificity of antisera. At this writing, electroblot analyses of the antisera discussed in this review have not been published.

Diversity of immunocytochemical results may also arise from molecular heterogeneity of the protein being localized. The complexity of neural antigens has recently been recognized by monoclonal antibodies. An example occurs in the localization of the neurofilament triplet proteins. Although neurofilaments are present in the perikarya of most neurons, a majority of the antisera prepared to neurofilaments react only with dendrites and axons. Monoclonal antibodies to neurofilaments have been produced that stain perikarya and, more important, can recognize different subpopulations of neurons in different brain regions (Goldstein *et al.*, 1982, 1983). Although molecular heterogeneity cannot be expected to be hiding behind every antigenic bush, some differences in localization seen with conventional antisera may arise from nonrecognition or poor recognition of diverse antigenic forms.

2. CELL-TYPE-SPECIFIC ANTISERA

Cell-type-specific antisera that react with a restricted population of cells have not yet been produced and used as extensively as antisera to purified components of the nervous system, but are potentially very useful for tracing the appearance, development, and pathology of specific cell types. Production of cell-specific antisera that can be used in the identification of oligodendrocytes has been facilitated by the recent development of isolation and purification techniques (McCarthy and de Vellis, 1980; Snyder *et al.*, 1980; Szuchet *et al.*, 1980). Poduslo *et al.* (1977) reported an antiserum that exhibited surface fluorescence when incubated with isolated oligodendrocytes from lamb (the antigen), calf, or human brain. Reaction could be abolished by absorbing the antiserum with isolated oligodendrocytes, but not with myelin. A series of antisera produced to bovine oligodendrocytes (Abramsky *et al.*, 1978, 1979; Lisak *et al.*, 1980) also reacted with the surface of isolated oligodendrocytes. In bovine and human brain sections, perineuronal (satellite) and interfascicular oligodendrocyte cell surfaces are stained. Cell-surface fluorescence disappeared when the antiserum was incubated with oligodendrocytes or white matter, but purified myelin did not affect reactivity. In one of these studies (Abramsky *et al.*, 1979), low levels of anti-myelin basic protein (MBP) antibodies were found in most of the rabbits injected with oligodendrocytes, and several rabbits had significant levels of antigalactocerebroside (GalCer) antibody. These antisera do not bind to Schwann-cell surfaces, but it has recently been reported that some binding to astrocytes and fibroblasts in culture does occur (Lisak *et al.*, 1980). Guinea pig antisera to oligodendrocytes (Lisak *et al.*, 1980) exhibited surface binding to oligodendrocytes in dissociated rat corpus callosum and cerebellar cultures. In primary and secondary sciatic-nerve and dorsal-root-ganglion cultures, immunofluorescent reaction was seen on Schwann cell surfaces. The common oligodendrocyte–Schwann cell antigen does not seem to be MBP, since anti-MBP antibodies cannot be demonstrated by radioimmunoassay (RIA) in the guinea pig serum (Abramsky *et al.*, 1979). Lisak and co-workers felt that the surface antigen was highly unlikely to be sulfatide or GalCer, since Schwann cells in culture stop making these myelin lipids (Mirsky *et al.*, 1980). Traugott *et al.* (1978) have reported an antioligodendrocyte serum that reacts with the plasma membrane of bovine oligodendrocytes in suspension. In tissue sections (human and bovine), cytoplasmic staining of oligodendroglial cell bodies and processes was observed (Figure 1). Absorption of the antiserum with bovine MBP or myelin did not affect the staining reaction. Absorption with oligodendrocytes completely removed staining of oligodendrocytes, but did not affect Schwann-cell staining in bovine nerve roots. All the aforementioned antisera appear to react with antigens that are not species-specific and are not present in myelin (or not accessible by the staining techniques used), and some may be detecting antigens common to both the cells responsible for myelination, oligodendrocytes and Schwann cells. An antiserum to lamb oligodendrocytes (Szuchet *et al.*, 1980) reacts with the original antigen in culture on tissue sections, but does not react with rat, hamster, guinea pig, or human brain sections. An anti-mouse oligodendrocyte antiserum (Bologa-Sandru *et al.*, 1981*a*) stains bulk-isolated mouse oligodendrocytes in suspension as well as oligodendrocytes in dissociated brain-cell culture. It cross-reacts with GalCer, but also stains another component in the oligodendrocyte membrane. As yet, the antigens being detected by these antioligodendrocyte antisera have not been characterized.

Antibodies reacting with oligodendrocytes have been found in the sera and CSF of patients with multiple sclerosis (MS) (Abramsky, *et al.*, 1977; Taugott

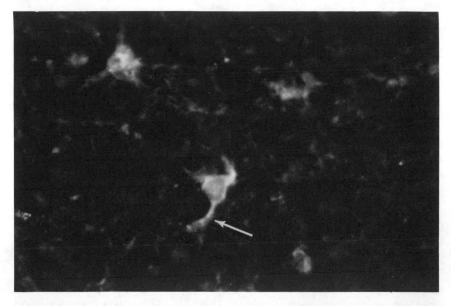

FIGURE 1. Cryostate section of bovine spinal cord. A single brightly fluorescing oligodendrocyte is seen with three cell processes, one of which partially encompasses an unstained myelinated fiber (←). Photomicrograph courtesy of U. Traugott, S. Snyder, W. T. Norton, and C. S. Raine.

et al., 1979; Kennedy and Lisak, 1979; Ma *et al.*, 1981; Traugott and Raine, 1981). However, antibody binding to oligodendrocytes was not specific for MS, since patients with other neurological diseases and normal individuals also demonstrated antioligodendrocyte antibodies (Traugott *et al.*, 1979; Kennedy and Lisak, 1979; Ma *et al.*, 1981; Traugott and Raine, 1981). Some of the binding was found to be due, not to specific antibody reaction, but to nonspecific binding of immunoglobulins to Fc receptors (Traugott *et al.*, 1979; Traugott and Raine, 1981; Ma *et al.*, 1981).

3. ANTISERA TO MYELIN–OLIGODENDROCYTE ANTIGENS: REACTION *IN SITU*

3.1. Proteolipid Protein

The most extensively studied oligodendrocyte antigens have been those involved in myelination. One of the first was proteolipid protein (PLP), which is a major component of CNS myelin, accounting for 50% of the total myelin proteins (for a review, see Agrawal and Hartman, 1980). Purification of PLP for immunological studies has been hampered by the limited solubility of PLP in aqueous solvents. However, Agrawal *et al.* (1977) have prepared an anti-serum to purified rat myelin PLP and shown that in tissue sections of adult rat, the antiserum specifically stains only myelin sheaths. In the corpus callosum of 10-day-postnatal rats, reaction was seen in the oligodendrocyte cytoplasm as well as in myelin sheaths. A more recent report (Hartman *et al.* 1982) compared the localization of PLP and MBP in developing rat brain. PLP reaction in oligodendrocyte cytoplasm had a granular, clumped appearance suggestive of packaging of this protein in the Golgi complex (Figure 2). Neither PLP nor MBP was observed in oligodendrocytes before myelination begins. Positive-reacting oligodendrocytes were always associated with axons that already had a ring of myelin staining, and the authors concluded that the signal for production of these proteins occurred after ensheathment of the axon. This is in contrast to the results of other groups showing that MBP (Sternberger *et al.*, 1978*b*; Roussel *et al.*, 1981), the myelin-associated glycoprotein (MAG) (Sternberger *et al.*, 1979*a*), Wolfgram (W1) protein (Roussel *et al.*, 1981), carbonic anhydrase (Ghandour *et al.*, 1980*c*), and 2′,3′-cyclic nucleotide 3′-phosphohydrolase (CNP) (Nishizawa *et al.*, 1981) appear in oligodendrocytes prior to myelination. During development of a particular tract, oligodendrocytes were positive for MBP before PLP, indicating a shift in priority of synthesis for these proteins. Staining for PLP decreased with development and was absent in adult oligodendrocytes (Figure 3). Varicosities or swellings in the

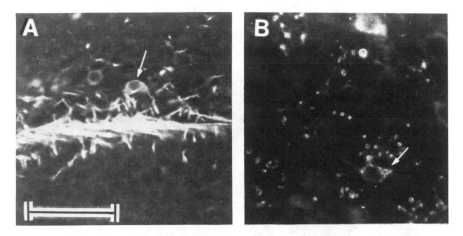

FIGURE 2. Comparison of the immunocytochemical localization of MBP (A) and PLP (B) in oligodendrocytes. Specific MBP immunofluorescence appears homogeneous in the cytoplasm, whereas PLP exhibits, a granular appearance (brain of 10-day-old rat). (←) Oligodendrocytes. Scale bar: 50μm. Photomicrograph courtesy of B. K. Hartman, H. C. Agrawal, D. Agrawal, and S. Kalmbach.

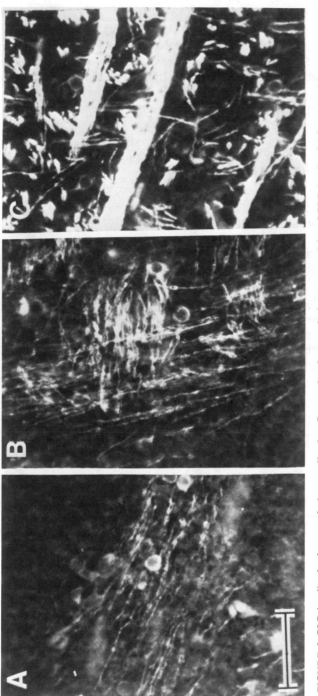

FIGURE 3. PLP in oligodendrocytes during myelination. Progressive decrease in immunoreactivity of PLP in oligodendrocytes with a concomitant increase in the intensity of fluorescence in myelinated fibers. (A–C, Changes in PLP fluorescence at 1, 3, and 10 days after birth in rat medulla. Scale bar: 50 μm. Photomicrograph courtesy of B. K. Hartman and co-workers.)

sheath were observed in early phases of myelin formation. An interesting observation was that in adjacent sections, fine myelinated fibers were more easily visualized with anti-PLP and large fibers that reacted well with anti-MBP did not show significant reactivity for PLP. It was concluded that the relative concentrations of MBP and PLP may vary as a function of myelin-sheath size.

3.2. Wolfgram Proteins

On sodium dodecyl sulfate (SDS)–polyacrylamide gels of isolated myelin, the Wolfgram proteins (Wolfgram, 1966) appear as three bands, a high-molecular-weight band of approximately 55,000 daltons and a lower-molecular-weight doublet in the range of 42,000–50,000 daltons (for a review, see Norton, 1981). Antisera have been prepared (Nussbaum *et al.*, 1977) to the rat brain doublet proteins [called W1 by Nussbaum *et al.* (1977) and more recently referred to as W1 and W2] and to the high-molecular-weight form that comigrates with tubulin [referred to as W2 by Nussbaum *et al.* (1977)].* The antiserum to W1 reacted with both purified W1 and W2 proteins (presumably this antiserum would then localize all three molecular forms) and was the antiserum used for immunocytochemical studies.

Initial results at the light-microscopic (LM) level (Roussel *et al.*, 1977) demonstrated that reaction of the antiserum was localized in myelinated tracts. Glial-cell staining was observed that was sometimes more intense at the periphery of the cell than in the perinuclear cytoplasm. Appearance of staining in developing rat-brain sections correlated with the time of onset of myelination. The reaction was shown to be specific for oligodendrocytes and myelinated axons. At the ultrastructural level (Rousse *et al.* 1978), it was observed that the cytoplasm of oligodendrocytes was labeled by the W1 antiserum. The labeling was more concentrated at the periphery of the cell, suggesting incorporation of these proteins into the plasma membrane of the cell, and often appeared in rosette, interpreted as polysomes. Staining of the plasma membrane was also seen. Staining of myelin was restricted to the innermost and outermost myelin lamellae and occurred at the major dense line (cytoplasmic side of the oligodendrocyte plasma membrane). Within the area of compact myelin, staining was not seen, possibly because of the severe restriction of antibody accessibility. A recent, comparative immunocytochemical study of the sequential appearance of MBP and the W1 protein was carried out in sections of developing rat corpus callosum (Roussel and Nussbaum, 1981). W1-protein-containing oligodendrocytes with many fine, branched processes could be seen as early as 2

---

*For details concerning the resolution of the Wolfgram proteins and their relationship to CNP species (Section 3.3), see Chapter 7 (Section 2.3.2c).

days after birth, when no myelin staining was observed. MBP staining in oligodendrocytes was also seen before myelination begins, as has been observed previously (See Figure 7), but appeared later than the W1 protein. With further development, staining of oligodendrocytes with anti-MBP disappeared. The same observation has been made with other immunocytochemical studies of MBP (Sternberger *et al.*, 1978*a*,*b*), MAG (Sternberger *et al.*,1979*a*,*b*) and PLP (Hartman *et al.*, 1979). In contrast, labeling with W1 antiserum was observed in corpus callosum from 2 days to adulthood.

3.3. 2′,3′-Cyclic Nucleotide 3′-Phosphohydrolase

CNP (EC 3.1.4.37) hydrolyzes the 3′-phosphodiester bond of 2′,3′-cyclic nucleotides to produce 2′-monophosphate nucleotides. It is found in many tissues, tumors, and cells, as well as in serum and CSF. High activity is found in the CNS with a remarkably high activity in myelin or myelin–oligodendrocytic structures, and white matter has been used for purification of CNP. The biological function of CNP is not known, but developmental changes in CNP activity suggest that it is involved in myelination. It is not clear whether 2′,3′-cyclic nucleotides are the true substrates of CNP, since these nucleotides have not been found in mammalian tissue.

Interesting recent findings by Drummond and Dean (1980) and Sprinkle *et al.* (1980) have shown that the doublet of Wolfgram myelin proteins (W1 and W2) of molecular weight 42,000–50,000 (see Section 3.2) contain CNP. Similarity of amino acid compositions between CNP and the Wolfgram proteins and reaction of antisera raised to CNP with the Wolfgram doublet proteins suggest that CNP is a major component of or identical to the Wolfgram doublet, but not of the higher 55,000-molecular-weight protein also called the Wolfgram protein.

Several antisera have been raised to CNP and used in immunocytochemical studies. Sprinkle and co-workers have used an antiserum to bovine CNP to localize the enzyme in oligodendrocytes in tissue sections of bovine optic nerve (Sprinkle *et al.*, 1981) and in oligodendrocytes isolated from fetal and newborn calf brains (Sprinkle and McDonald, 1982). Oligodendrocyte plasma membranes, rough endoplasmic reticulum, and ribosomes were stained. Periaxonal staining somewhat similar to that seen with antiserum to MAG (Sternberger *et al.*, 1979*a*) was seen. Nishizawa *et al.* (1981), using an antiserum to bovine CNP that cross-reacts with rat CNP, have found staining in 15-day-old rat associated with myelinated nerve tracts and cell bodies of glial cells within or near the tracts. These cells were identified as oligodendrocytes by their morphological appearance and the finding of stained cell processes connected with myelinated fibers. Some immature glial cells in premyelinated areas also reacted positively with the antiserum. An unexpected finding was that of

Muller *et al.* (1981), who found that antiserum to bovine CNP reacted with a cloned CNS cell line of neuronal origin (B104) and was localized in intracellular structures. The possibility that the cell line used in this study may express some glial characteristics not normally seen in neurons was not ruled out by the authors.

3.4. Myelin Basic Protein

MBP is a major structural component of CNS myelin, accounting for 30–35% of the total protein (for a review, see Kies, 1982). Since its discovery in the early 1960s, it has been extensively studied, both biochemically and immunologically. Specific localization at the LM level in the myelin sheath was first demonstrated immunocytochemically by Rauch and Raffel (1964). Later reports also demonstrated myelin-sheath staining (Lennon *et al.*, 1971; Whitaker, 1975; Eng and Bigbee, 1978), although localization in neuronal nuclei was also reported in one of these studies (Kornguth *et al.*, 1966). The absence of oligodendrocyte reaction with anti-MBP was puzzling until developmental studies showed that MBP could be detected in oligodendrocytes of young rats, but not of adult animals such as were used in most of the previous studies. Sternberger *et al.* (1978*a*) showed that cytoplasmic staining of oligodendrocyte cell bodies and processes was easily seen in the spinal cord and brainstem at birth, and such staining appeared in other brain regions later with development (Figures 4 and 5). MBP was also shown in oligodendrocyte processes that were surrounding axons and in developing myelin sheaths (Figure 6). Numbers and lengths of oligodendrocyte processes could be measured, and in one case, 10 processes 4–38 μm in length could be traced from one oligodendrocyte perikaryon to developing myelin sheaths. Anti-MBP reaction was most intense in oligodendrocytes during the early phase of myelination in any nervous tract and decreased rapidly during subsequent myelination (Sternberger *et al.*, 1978*b*). The rapid loss of staining while myelination was still occurring was unexpected and differed from the developmental pattern observed with MAG (see Figure 9) and Wolfgram proteins. Obviously, failure to detect MBP in oligodendrocytes did not indicate that the protein was not present, but only that it was no longer detectable. Staining of oligodendrocytes was dependent on age, brain region, and nerve tract studied. MBP staining in oligodendrocytes could also be demonstrated before the onset of myelination. Oligodendrocytes with a thin rim of stained cytoplasm and many fine processes (Figure 7) could be seen in premyelinating areas in which no staining around axons and no myelin sheaths could be detected. Some anatomical studies of developing neuroglia (Ramon-Molinger, 1958; Inoue *et al.*, 1973; Narang and Wisniewski, 1976; Narang, 1977) have reported the finding of cells with many branched processes that presumably are transitional forms of cells that develop classic oligoden-

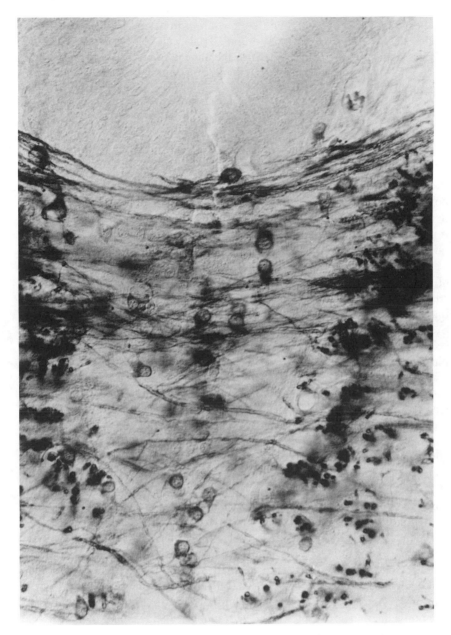

FIGURE 4. MBP staining in oligodendrocytes and developing myelin sheaths of 5-day rat pons. Vibratome section (20 μm).

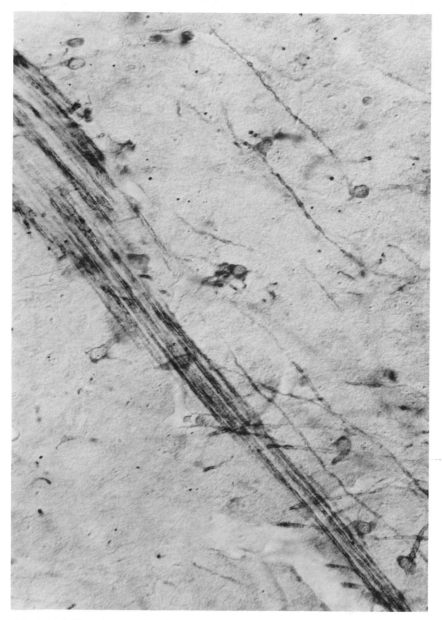

FIGURE 5. MBP staining in oligodendrocytes and developing myelin sheaths in 5-day rat brain-stem. Vibratome section (20 μm).

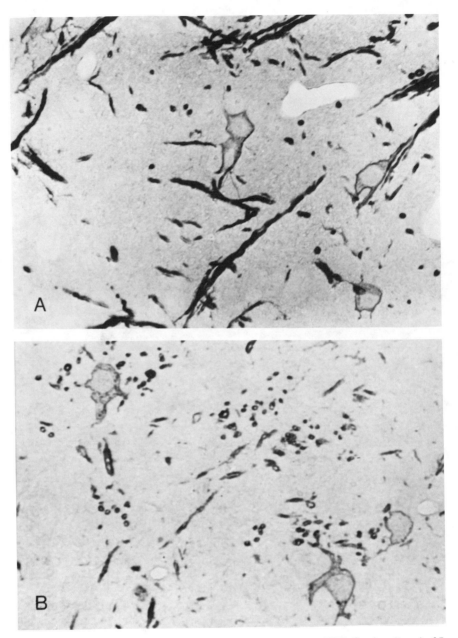

FIGURE 6. Oligodendrocyte and myelin staining with antiserum to MBP. Sections (1 μm) of 7-day rat spinal cord (A) and 7-day jimpy mouse spinal cord (B). Tissue was fixed in glutaraldehyde and osmium before dehydration and embedding in plastic. Note the fine cytoplasmic granular staining in addition to the diffuse staining in oligodendrocyte cytoplasm. Granular staining is more prominent in jimpy oligodendrocytes (B).

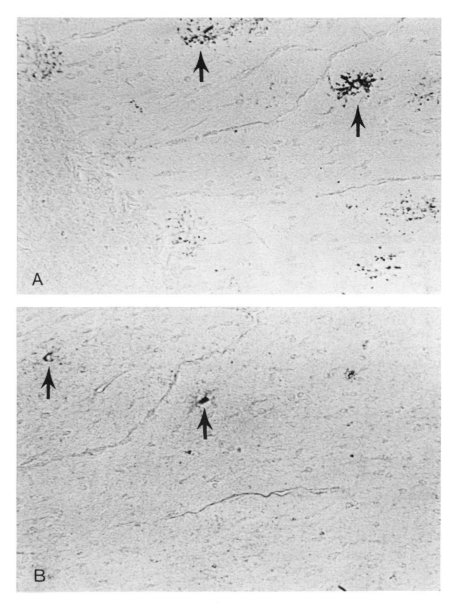

FIGURE 7. Oligodendrocytes with many processes found in developing rat brain prior to mye-lination. In adjacent paraffin sections incubated with antiserum to MBP (A) or MAG (B), stained oligodendrocytes can be seen, although many fewer cells react with MAG antiserum than with anti-MBP. Staining of the few MAG-positive cells is predominantly limited to the perikar-yon. No staining is seen in myelin or oligodendrocyte processes that have just begun to wrap around axons. (↑)Two cells that are stained by both antisera.

drocyte morphology (also see Chapter 1). In a study of human development, Borit and McIntosh (1981) have reported the finding of stained cytoplasm of cell bodies and processes in oligodendrocytes prior to the appearance of stained myelin sheaths. Roussel and Nussbaum (1981) have confirmed the appearance of MBP before myelination and the rapid disappearance of MBP staining with age. Hartman *et al.* (1979) have also found in developing chick and rat brain that the number of oligodendrocytes reacting with antiserum to MBP decreased as a particular tract became myelinated, and eventually all reactivity disappeared. However, they never observed reaction in oligodendrocytes without also seeing it in varicose-appearing myelin sheaths closely associated with the cells.

Itoyama *et al.* (1980*a*) showed that in sections of 3-month-old human infant cortex, oligodendrocytes and myelin sheaths could be stained with antiserum to MBP. In adult tissue, only myelin sheaths were stained, as had been previously shown by other investigators. An exception to lack of staining of adult human oligodendrocytes is the infrequent finding of stained oligodendrocytes in an MS shadow plaque (Itoyama *et al.*, 1980*b*), presumably indicating some remyelination in this area of the lesion. Antisera to MBP have been used in studies of experimental allergic encephalomyelitis and MS to study the pathology of myelin breakdown and distribution of MBP in myelin, astrocytes, plasma cells, macrophages, and lymphocytes in these lesions (Kies *et al.*, 1965; Johnson and Blum, 1972; Alvord *et al.*, 1976; Whitaker, 1978; Johnson *et al.*, 1971; Prineas and Graham, 1981).

More recently we have found that by use of mild fixation and modification of the staining procedure previously used for detection of MBP on vibratome sections, reaction of MBP antiserum with oligodendrocytes in adult rat brain has been obtained (del Cerro *et al.*, 1983). Stained oligodendroglia had many fine, branched processes. These results suggest that MBP in oligodendrocytes exists in a chemical or structural form that is more sensitive to tissue processing procedures than the MBP in compact myelin.

The first attempt to localize MBP at the electron-microscopic (EM) level demonstrated immunoreactivity in the major dense line (Herndon *et al.*, 1973). These investigators pointed out the problems of EM localization of myelin components that are still not completely solved today. In LM, staining for MBP occurs throughout the myelin sheath, especially when fixatives or solvents are used that disrupt the myelin sheath (Sternberger *et al.*, 1978*a*). However, when fixatives are used that retain good myelin morphology necessary for EM studies, staining usually occurs only on the outer edges of the myelin sheath and sometimes where the lamellae are disrupted. This lack of staining of compact myelin may occur if the antigenic determinants recognized by the antiserum are inaccessible within the intact sheath, as has been suggested by Lennon *et al.* (1971), or if the immunoreagents are unable to penetrate the small cytoplasmic space in the tightly compact sheath (Hirano *et al.*, 1969*a*). These problems of EM localization in myelin have been noted by other investigators in attempts at MBP localization (Eng *et al.*, 1975; Sternberger *et al.*, 1977; Roussel *et al.*, 1981; Mendell and Whitaker, 1978). Care should be taken in interpreting EM localization results of other myelin or myelin-related proteins for the same reasons. More recently, however, Omlin *et al.* (1982*b*) have shown, by using pre-embedding immunostaining techniques, that MBP is localized in the major dense line of well-preserved compact myelin. This localization supports previous biochemical evidence.

More successful have been the EM localization studies of MBP in oligodendrocytes, although different results have been reported by each group of investigators. Eng and Bigbee (1978), in a study of developing rat optic nerve, found that at the EM level, MBP could be seen in the Golgi apparatus of oligodendrocyte perikarya. Staining of oligodendrocyte processes was amorphous and in greatest abundance in processes that were wrapped around axons but had not yet started to form myelin. The observation that sheaths with more than a few wrappings were unstained demonstrates the difficulty of obtaining reliable EM results. Roussel and Nussbaum (1981) found that in the developing rat corpus callosum, positive staining for MBP was diffuse and filled the entire cytoplasm of the cell. The membranes of the rough endoplasmic reticulum and Golgi apparatus were positive. Processes just beginning to wrap around axons were intensely stained, but in myelin sheaths, only the three external dense lines were stained. Recently, a preliminary report by Omlin *et al.* (1982*a*) described staining of surface membrane and cytoplasm of oligodendrocyte processes. Reaction product was also seen in microtubules, ribosomes, and profiles of agranular endoplasmic reticulum. Staining in perikarya was described as patchy and less intense, but in the same distribution.

3.5. Myelin-Associated Glycoprotein

MAG has been shown by radioactive-fucose-labeling studies to be the most prominent glycoprotein in SDS-polyacryamide gels of purified myelin (for a review, see Quarles, 1979). Biochemical studies had shown that MAG was probably closely associated with myelin or related structures. It is present in small amounts, only about 1% of the total myelin proteins.

Several antisera prepared to purified MAG (Sternberger *et al.*, 1979*a*) have been used to identify and clarify which brain structures contain this protein. Similar to our findings with antiserum to MBP, MAG could be seen in the cytoplasm of oligodendrocyte-cell bodies and processes very early in development. Cytoplasmic staining was of two kinds: (1) diffuse staining throughout and (2) dark, irregularly distributed "granules" that were especially prominent adjacent to the nucleus and could be seen in the processes and along the developing myelin sheath (Figure 8). These granular-appearing structures presumably reflect the site of synthesis in the Golgi apparatus and vesicles involved in transport to the myelin sheath. Although cytoplasmic staining was most intense in the early phase of myelination, as was seen with MBP, the peak time of staining occurred later than with anti-MBP and staining persisted in oligodendrocytes after staining with anti-MBP had disappeared. Figure 9 shows the differences in number and intensity of staining of oligodendrocytes in a 28-day-old rat with antiserum to MBP (Figure 9A) and MAG (Figure 9B). MAG staining can also be detected in adult rats in some oligodendrocytes.

Very early in development, oligodendrocytes that reacted with anti-MAG were sometimes present in nerve tracts before myelination began, but the number was less than could be detected with MBP antiserum. Staining of cell bodies but not processes was seen (see Figure 7). These results indicate that MBP can be detected prior to the appearance of MAG. If MAG plays a role in establishing initial glial–axonal contact, as has been suggested, then it would be expected that MAG should appear before other myelin proteins. It does not seem likely that the differences in time of appearance of MAG and MBP can be attributed to the fact that MBP accounts for 30% of the total myelin protein and MAG only 1%, since the MAG antiserum is more efficient in detecting oligodendrocytes than several MBP antisera used.

In contrast to MBP, MAG is not localized throughout the myelin sheath. In the initial stages of myelination, oligodendrocyte processes stain in a similar pattern with both antisera (see Figures 6 and 8). With further development, MAG staining is seen in a periaxonal location and in the outer mesaxon [see Figure 15D (Section 5.3)]. In the adult, staining is predominantly in periaxonal and paranodal regions of CNS myelin sheaths. In the PNS, an additional locus of staining is seen in Schmidt–Lanterman incisures.

3.6. Myelin Basic Protein and Myelin-Associated Glycoprotein in Satellite Oligodendrocytes

Perineuronal satellite oligodendrocytes have morphology similar to that of interfascicular oligodendrocytes, but have been presumed not to participate in myelin formation. A report by Ludwin (1979) demonstrated by EM that satellite oligodendrocytes clearly were remyelinating axons during recovery from cuprizone intoxication. We had previously reported that satellite oligodendrocytes could be demonstrated that did not react with antiserum to MBP (Sternberger *et al.*, 1978*a*). However, staining of shiverer-mutant spinal-cord sections by antiserum to MAG revealed satellite oligodendrocytes that were intensely stained (Figure 10A). Since it was possible that the capacity for producing myelin was present in these cells but not normally expressed, we reexamined normal developing rat spinal cord. Staining of satellite oligodendrocytes was

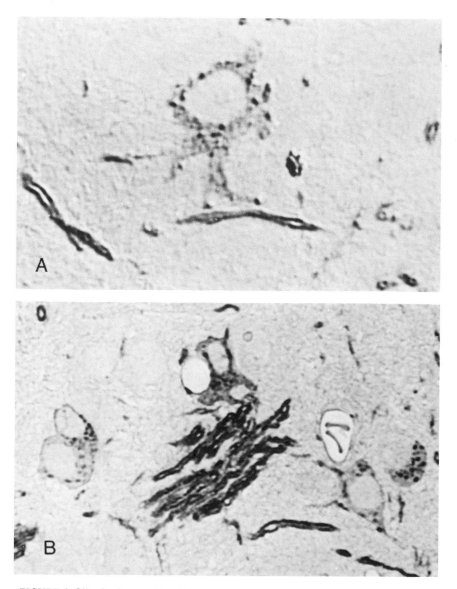

FIGURE 8. Oligodendrocytes from 7-day rat spinal cord stained with antiserum to MAG. Dark granular staining can be seen in perinuclear cytoplasm and in processes extending to developing myelin sheaths. Plastic sections (1 μm).

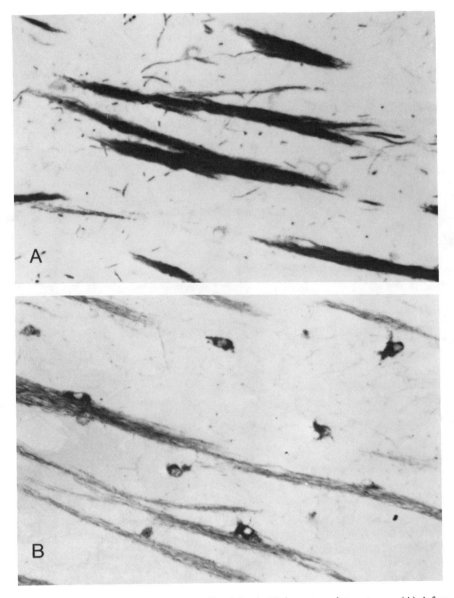

FIGURE 9. Comparison of MBP and MAG staining in 28-day rat caudate putamen. (A) A few lightly stained oligodendrocytes can be seen with antiserum to MBP. Myelin is darkly stained. (B) Many intensely stained oligodendrocytes are seen in sections incubated with anti-MAG, and myelin staining is less intense.

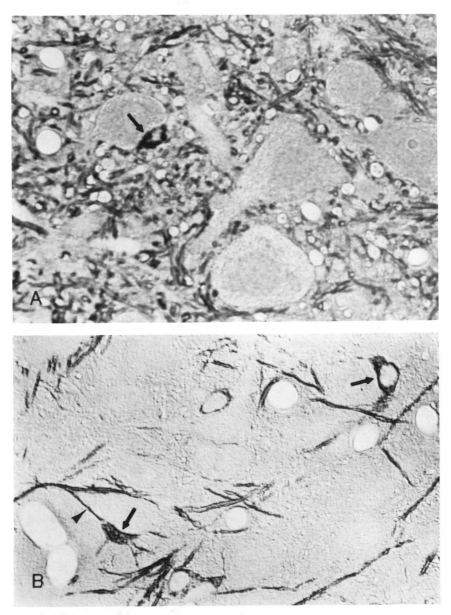

FIGURE 10. Perineuronal satellite oligodendrocytes stained with antiserum to MAG. (A) Plastic section (1 μm) of shiverer spinal cord (>90 days old). (→) Intensely stained satellite oligodendrocyte. Note also the abundant staining of oligodendrocyte processes around axons. (B) Section (1 μm) of 7-day rat spinal cord showing two stained satellite oligodendrocytes (→). Four processes can be seen extending from one oligodendrocyte perikaryon, and one of these processes is attached to a developing myelin sheath. Shiverer tissue kindly supplied by V. Friedrich and P. Massa.

seen with antisera to both MBP and MAG. Processes could be traced from oligodendrocyte-cell bodies to developing myelin sheaths (Figure 10B) confirming the role of satellite oligodendrocytes in normal myelination (Sternberger, unpublished observations). Glycerol-3-phosphate dehydrogenase (Leveille *et al.*, 1980) and unidentified antioligodendrocyte antigens (Abramsky *et al.*, 1978) have also been observed in satellite oligodendrocytes.

3.7. Limitations of Myelin–Oligodendrocyte Antigens as Oligodendrocyte "Markers"

If an antigen is to be used as an immunocytochemical "marker," that antigen must be present and detectable in oligodendrocytes throughout all stages of cell development. The results with antisera to MBP, MAG, and PLP indicate that they can be detected in oligodendrocytes only during a brief interval in the cell's life-span. In addition, it is probable that only subpopulations of oligodendrocytes are recognized during most of the interval when staining can be observed. Since absence of staining with these antisera could lead to the erroneous conclusion that (1) the cell was not an oligodendrocyte or (2) the cell did not function in myelin production, MBP, MAG, and PLP cannot be considered classic oligodendrocyte markers. They are, however, very useful for studying early myelination, if these limitations are recognized. Potentially more useful "markers" are galactocerebroside, Wolfgram protein, CNP, and other proteins reviewed below.

3.8. Galactocerebroside and Sulfatide

The myelin membrane is rich in lipids (70–85%) compared to protein (15–30%). Two galactosphingolipids, galactocerebroside [galactosylceramide (GalCer)] and sulfatide (sulfogalactosylceramide), are concentrated in the brain and have been thought to be restricted to myelin. In rat myelin, GalCer and sulfatide account for approximately 24 and 7% of the lipids present. Several early immunocytochemical studies confirmed the myelin localization of GalCer in tissue sections of developing rat (Sternberger *et al.*, 1978*a*; Eng and Bigbee, 1978) and of GalCer and sulfatide on the surface of the myelin sheath in isolated mouse myelinated axonal preparation (Dupouey *et al.*, 1979*b*). A thorough study of the localization of GalCer and sulfatide in 30-day-old mouse brains has shown that GalCer (but not sulfatide) appears to be a specific marker for oligodendrocytes and myelin (Zalc *et al.*, 1981). GalCer was found in myelinated tracts and in the interfascicular oligodendrocytes associated with those tracts. In cerebral hemisphere sections, GalCer was found in isolated cells not associated with myelin, which were thought to be cortical oligodendrocytes. Subependymal cells of a layer in contact with the corpus callosum were GalCer positive also and were identified as immature oligodendrocytes, as has been suggested by Privat and Leblond (1972). Sulfatide distribution in the brain as visualized by their antiserum was less specific for myelin and myelin-related structures. Sulfatide was localized in myelin and interfascicular oligodendrocytes. However, the GalCer positive cortical oligodendrocytes and subependymal cells were negative for sulfatide. Sulfatide staining was seen in ependymal cells, fiber processes in contact with ependymal cells, or the pia arachnoid, and Bergman glial fibers. The fiber staining resembled that seen with antiserum to the glial fibrillary acidic protein of astrocytes.

3.9. Antimyelin Antibody

An antimyelin serum has recently been reported that reacts with the cell surface of a small number of oligodendrocytes in cultures of newborn rat cerebral hemispheres (Roussel and Nussbaum, 1982). The labeled cells have multiple branched processes and have been identified as a subclass of oligodendrocytes on the basis of double-labeling studies with antiserum to MBP and to the Wolfgram proteins. Most of the cells are also MBP-positive. A number of oligodendrocytes that react with antiserum to Wolfgram proteins are not labeled by the antimyelin antibody. The nature of the antibodies in this antiserum has not been explored, but the staining pattern resembles that observed by others for GalCer.

4. ANTISERA TO MYELIN–OLIGODENDROCYTE ANTIGENS: REACTION IN CULTURE

The development of a variety of methods for growing neural cells *in vitro* has stimulated the search for specific markers to unambiguously identify cell types in culture, where morphological criteria are often not sufficient. GalCer, the major myelin glycolipid, was first, shown by Raff *et al.* (1978) to be a specific cell-surface marker for oligodendrocytes in cultures of rat optic nerve. More extensive studies in dissociated cell cultures from a variety of brain regions confirmed the exclusive localization of GalCer on oligodendrocytes and their processes (Raff *et al.*, 1979). Double-labeling experiments also indicated that all oligodendrocytes were sulfatide-positive and greater than 90% of them were labeled with antisera to the gangliosides GM_1 (also present on neurons and other cell types) and GM_3. The usefulness of GalCer as a marker for oligodendrocytes from a variety of animal species has been demonstrated in bovine (Lisak *et al.*, 1979, 1981; Pleasure *et al.*, 1981), ovine (Szuchet *et al.*,

1980), rat (Pfeiffer *et al.*, 1981; Bhat *et al.*, 1981), mouse (Bologa-Sandru *et al.*, 1981*a*; Schachner *et al.*, 1981), and cat (Gebicke-Harter *et al.*, 1981).

In an interesting study of dissociated cell cultures from neonatal rat optic nerve, corpus callosum, or cerebellum, Mirsky *et al.* (1980) demonstrated that oligodendrocytes in culture are specifically labeled by antiserum to GalCer, sulfatide, and MBP. It was possible to detect these labels for up to 10 weeks in culture even in the absence of tetanus-toxin-positive neurons, indicating that oligodendrocytes do not require a continuing signal from neurons to continue synthesizing myelin-specific proteins in culture. In contrast, Schwann cells stop making detectable amounts of these molecules after a few days *in vitro*. Oligodendrocytes in cultures of newborn optic nerve were positive for GalCer and sulfatide after 1 day in culture and for MBP only after 6–10 days in culture, indicating a temporal sequence of expression of myelin molecules. Since myelination does not begin in the rat optic nerve until 6 days after birth (Skoff *et al.*, 1976), the results of Mirsky and co-workers indicate that if a signal from axons is required for oligodendrocytes to initiate the synthesis of myelin proteins, the signal must be given many days before myelination begins. The presence of myelin-related components in oligodendrocytes before the time of myelination had previously been demonstrated in tissue sections stained for MBP and more recently in tissue sections stained with antisera to myelin-associated glycoprotein, carbonic anhydrase (CA) II, and 2′,3′-cyclic nucleotide 3′-phosphohydrolase.

A comparative study of sulfatide and GalCer appearance in embryonic rat cerebral cortex cultures (Ranscht *et al.*, 1982) has been carried out using a monoclonal antibody to GalCer and rabbit antiserum to sulfatide. After 6 days in culture, staining with the monoclonal anti-GalCer was observed in only a few oligodendrocytes (cell bodies and processes). Less than 30% of the cells were sulfatide-positive, and staining was restricted to the cell body. With further time in culture, sulfatide could also be visualized on processes as well as on cell bodies, and 95% of the GalCer-reacting cells also reacted with antisulfatide. The results with these antisera suggest that the appearance of sulfatide as an oligodendrocyte-cell-surface antigen lags behind the appearance of GalCer. Cytoplasmic expression of the antigens was not studied.

MBP antisera specifically react with myelin and some oligodendrocytes during the early phase of active myelination in tissue sections (see above). Such antisera are now being used extensively in conjunction with anti-GalCer to further define populations of oligodendrocytes in culture (Szuchet *et al.*, 1980; Bologa-Sandru *et al.*, 1981*a,b*; Lisak *et al.*, 1981; Barbarese and Pfeiffer, 1981; Pfeiffer *et al.*, 1981; Bhat *et al.*, 1981; Roussel *et al.*, 1981; Pruss *et al.*, 1981). In agreement with the observations of Mirsky *et al.* (1980), Bologa-Sandru *et al.* (1981*b*) have found in dissociated mouse brain cell cultures that during development, GalCer appears early in the membrane of oligodendrocytes and cytoplasmic MBP appears later in cells that presumably represent a more differentiated population. Two cell populations were seen: one that was GalCer positive, and one that was GalCer- and MBP-positive. The observation that more cells stain with anti-GalCer than with anti-MBP has also been pointed out by Lisak *et al.* (1981) in long-term cultures of isolated oligodendrocytes and by Barbarese and Pfeiffer (1981) in mixed primary cultures. As has been noted by many investigators, oligodendrocytes in culture have an elaborate morphology with multiple processes and complex membranous sheets and networks (Figure 11).

Antisera to several other myelin-related proteins have now been used to characterize oligodendrocytes in culture. Primary cultures of newborn rat brain hemispheres showed noticeable reaction with antiserum to MBP and Wolfgram (W1) protein after about a week in culture. In addition to the demonstration of the presence of W1 in nonmyelinating cells in culture, Roussel *et al.* (1981) have also recently shown that oligodendrocytes positive for W1 can be found in premyelinated areas of the brain in tissue sections. CA was localized in small cells scattered over the astroglial layer in cultures of embryonic mouse cerebral hemispheres (Sarlieve *et al.*, 1980). Cytoplasm and plasma membranes of putative oligodendrocytes were stained (Sarlieve *et al.*, 1981).

The studies with dissociated cell cultures and isolated oligodendrocytes have convincingly demonstrated that the expression of myelin-specific proteins and glycolipids can occur in the absence of myelin formation or continuing neuronal signals. However, evidence is accumulating (Pfeiffer *et al.*, 1981; Barbarese and Pfeiffer, 1981; Bhat *et al.*, 1981) that mechanisms that control expression of MBP are particularly disrupted in culture and that the presence of other brain-cell types enhances the ability of oligodendrocytes to express myelin-related functions.

See Chapter 7 for a further discussion of the expression of differentiated properties of oligodendroglia in culture.

5. ANTISERA TO ENZYMES THAT ARE PREDOMINANTLY OR EXCLUSIVELY IN OLIGODENDROCYTES

5.1. Cerebroside Sulfotransferase

Cerebroside sulfotransferase [(CST) EC 2.8.2.11] catalyzes the sulfation of galactocerebroside to form sulfatide. Biochemical studies (Benjamins *et al.*, 1974) of isolated cells have shown high CST activity in oligodendrocytes with very low activity in other CNS cell types. CST activity was absent from myelin.

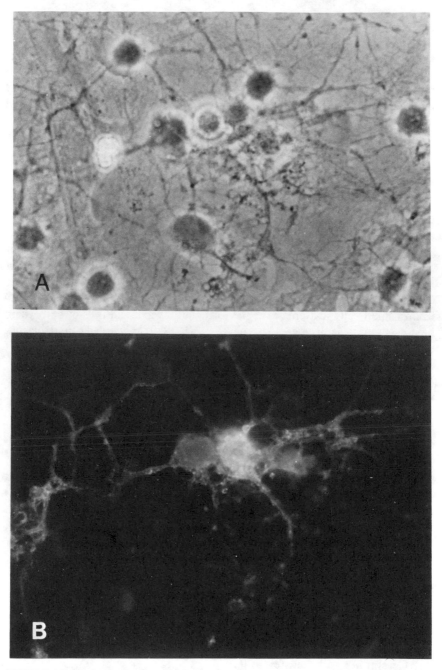

FIGURE 11. Mechanically dissociated 19- to 21-day fetal rat cerebral hemisphere culture. Approximately 30 days in culture. (A) Phase contrast. (B) Anti-MBP, showing many elaborate stained processes. Photomicrograph courtesy of E. Barbarese and S. E. Pfeiffer.

An antiserum to CST purified from rat kidney has been used to localize CST in that organ (Tennekoon *et al.*, 1981) and more recently has been used in a study of developing rat optic nerve. At 16 days, cells identified as oligodendrocytes and their processes were stained (Figure 12). Myelin, axons, and astrocytes (or their processes) were not stained, suggesting a specific oligodendrocytic localization. In view of the astrocytic and ependymal-cell localization obtained by Zalc *et al.* (1981) with their antisulfatide serum, it will be of interest to see further localization studies with CST antiserum in brain sections.

5.2. Glycerol-3-phosphate Dehydrogenase

Glycerol-3-phosphate dehydrogenase [(GPDH) L-α-glycerol-3-phosphate dehydrogenase (EC 1.1.1.8)] is an enzyme involved in glucose metabolism that catalyzes the NADH-linked generation of α-glycerol phosphate from dihydroxyacetone phosphate. Like the other oligodendrocyte antigens discussed in this section, it is widely distributed and cannot be considered a brain-specific protein. Two reports of GPDH localization in rodent cerebellum provide conflicting evidence for an exclusively oligodendrocytic localization (Leveille *et al.*, 1980) or an oligodendrocytic–Bergmann glial distribution (Fisher *et al.*, 1981). Leveille *et al.* (1980) prepared an antiserum to rat skeletal-muscle GPDH that was used to localize GPDH on 4%-formaldehyde-fixed, 100-μm-thick sections of adult rat cerebellum. At the LM level, specific reaction product was found to be confined to cells the morphological size and distribution of which were similar to those of oligodendrocytes. At the EM level, the GPDH-positive reaction product was confined to the cytoplasmic matrix of oligodendrocytic cell

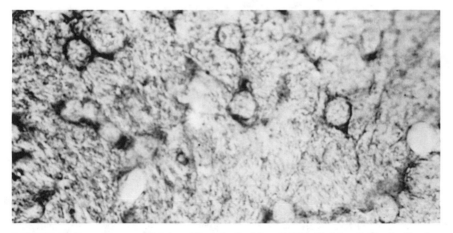

FIGURE 12. Rat optic nerve (15-day-old) stained with anti-CST. Staining is seen in oligodendrocytes. Other cell types are unstained. Photomicrograph courtesy of G. Tennekoon.

bodies and processes and absent from nuclei and organelles. GPDH-positive oligodendrocytes were found in perineuronal, interfascicular, ad perivascular positions. Direct continuity could be demonstrated between the external mesaxon of the mature myelin sheath and the cytoplasm of the oligodendrocyte (Figure 13).

The results of Fisher *et al.* (1981), using antiserum to mouse muscle GPDH on 5-μm-thick paraffin sections of Bouin's fixed 25-day-old mouse cerebellum, indicate that their antiserum reacted predominantly with cell bodies clustered within the Purkinje cell layer and with fibers that extended through the molecular layer to the pial surface. This pattern of staining is characteristic of Bergmann glia. Also seen scattered throughout the white matter and granular layer was a small number of stained cells that were identified as oligodendrocytes. Fibrous astrocytes were not stained. Neurological mutant mice were found to confirm the same localization of GPDH seen in the normal mouse. In a comparative study, cerebella from 33-day-old rats were stained with antiserum to mouse GPDH. Despite the different conditions of fixation, tissue prep-

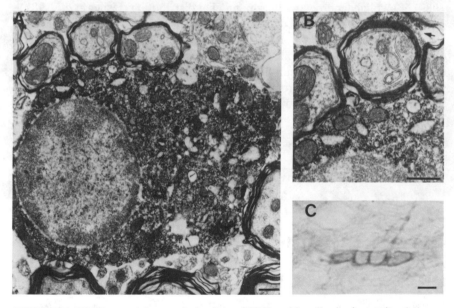

FIGURE 13. (A) Electron micrograph showing a GPDH-positive oligodendrocyte in relation to six myelinated axons. (B) Higher magnification of one of the axons to demonstrate continuity between the myelin sheath and a stained oligodendrocyte process. (C) Light micrograph showing GPDH localized to four interfascicular oligodendrocytes aligned in a row among bundles of axons in white matter. Photomicrograph courtesy of P. J. Leveille, J. F. McGinnis, D. S. Maxwell, and J. de Vellis.

aration, different animal age, and other factors, characteristic intense staining of oligodendrocytes was observed in agreement with the results of Leveille and co-workers. If the sections were viewed under dark-field illumination (this was not done by Leveille and co-workers), Bergmann glial fibers were evident. However, there can be seen an equally intense reaction surrounding some Purkinje cells and also associated with the neuron-rich granule-cell layer that differs from the diffuse glow seen in control sections. Of interest is a recent biochemical study of levels of GPDH in isolated cells of developing rat brains (Cammer *et al.*, 1982) (also see Chapter 6). Low activities of GPDH were found in bulk-isolated neurons and astrocytes of developing rats. Significant activity that increased with age was found only in isolated oligodendrocytes. It is possible that different antigenic forms of GPDH are present in these cells. Different antisera may vary in their ability to recognize these antigenic variants.

5.3. Carbonic Anhydrase

Carbonic anhydrase [(CA) carbonate hydrolase (EC 4.2.1.1)] is widely distributed in plant and animal tissues and catalyzes the interconversion of carbon dioxide and carbonic acid. In mammalian tssues, it can exist as at least two different isoenzymes, designated B (or I) and C (or II). Only the highly active isoenzyme CA C appears to be intrinsic to the CNS. CA may be involved in the regulation of ion, water, and carbon dioxide balance in the brain and play a role in CSF formation.

Two interesting questions have been raised by recent immunocytochemical studies of mammalian brain with antisera to CA C: (1) Is CA C a glial (astrocyte and oligodendrocyte) marker or exclusively an oligodendrocyte marker? (2) Is CA C a component of the myelin sheath?

Early biochemical analysis of single cells from animal and human brains demonstrated that this enzyme was in glial, rather than the neuronal cells (Giacobini, 1961, 1962). In a histochemical study by Korhonen *et al.* (1964), reaction product of CA activity was seen in areas of myelinated nerve fibers and in glial cells. Although maintenance of the brain's ionic environment is a function usually associated with astrocytes, antibodies to CA C have been shown by several groups of investigators to react predominantly or exclusively with oligodendrocytes. The finding of an enzyme involved in control of the brain's ionic environment in oligodendrocytes indicates that these cells serve other important functions besides myelin production.

Spicer *et al.*, (1979), using rabbit anti-human erythrocyte CA C, stained a population of nonneuronal cells in mouse brain. Intensely stained glial cells were tentatively identified as oligodendrocytes and were largely confined to white-matter areas. Moderate immunostaining of myelinated nerve tracts was

also seen. An LM and EM study by Roussel *et al.* (1979) demonstrated localization of CA C in developing rat brain with antiserum to CA C from rat red
cell hemolysates. At the LM level, CA C could be found at approximately a
week after birth in cell bodies and processes of oligodendrocytes. Myelinated
fibers were weakly stained. In the EM, peroxidase reaction product was seen
in the cytoplasm of oligodendrocytes. Nuclei, mitochondria, Golgi apparatus,
and rough endoplasmic reticulum were free of staining. In a series of reports,
Ghandour and co-workers (Ghandor *et al.*, 1979, 1980*a–c*; Langley *et al.*,
1980) demonstrated exclusive localization of CA in oligodendrocytes of rat cerebellum using rabbit antisera against rat red blood cell CA C. Sequential staining of adult rat cerebellar sections with antiserum to the glial fibrillary acidic
protein (GFAP), a specific marker for astrocytes (for a review, see Eng and
DeArmond, 1982), and antiserum to CA C showed that there was no overlap
in the cell populations that stained with each antiserum. During cerebellar
development in the neonatal rat, weak CA C staining of oligodendrocytes and
their processes was seen before myelin formation begins (0 and 4 days). Levels
of staining increased with development, reaching adult levels by the end of the
3rd postnatal week. Rapid accumulation of CA C was seen during oligodendrocyte maturation and at the time of myelination. Small immunofluorescent
spots were seen at the surface of myelinated fibers. EM results showed dense
deposits of peroxidase reaction product throughout the cytosol, and cytoplasmic organelles were unstained. Obliteration of intracytoplasmic membranes and oligodendrocyte plasma membranes by these dense deposits was
interpreted as support for a membrane localization of CA. The enzyme has
been localized in normal human cerebral and cerebellar tissues in cells interpreted as oligodendrocytes and in myelinated fiber tracts (Kumpulainen and
Nystrom, 1981). In contrast to the results of Ghandour and co-workers with
rat cerebellum, a vigorous reaction was observed in human cerebellar white
matter with rabbit antiserum to human erythrocyte CA C. Cerebral white
matter showed staining in areas of myelinated fibers, a few intensely stained
glial cell bodies, and a larger population of moderately stained nonneuronal
cells. Exact identification of these different types of CA C-positive cells was
not possible, although the distribution and morphology, as well as the lack of
reqction of anti-CA C with astrocytomas, suggested that they were oligodendrocytes. Kumpulainen and Korhonen (1982) recently demonstrated CA C
localization in the developing and adult mouse brain. Intense staining in the
brain was found in small oval or round cells and in granular or filamentous
patterns associated with myelinated tracts. In the spinal cord, stained cells
were located mainly in the gray matter, suggesting that at least in the spinal
cord, CA is not an adequate marker for all oligodendrocytes.

In contrast to the aforecited *in situ* studies in which CA C has been shown
or presumed to be present only in oligodendrocytes, Kimelberg *et al.* (1982)

have demonstrated immunocytochemical staining with antiserum to rat erythrocyte CA C of GFAP-positive, astrocytic monolayer cultures from rat cerebral hemispheres. Astrocytes were less intensively stained than were occasional small, round cells identified as oligodendrocytes. Treatment of the cultures with 2′,3′-dibutyryl cyclic AMP (cAMP) increased astrocytic staining with anti-CA C to the level seen in the small, round cells. Delaunoy et al. (1980) have also examined rat primary cultures for CA C staining and found that oligodendrocytes but not astrocytes reacted with anti-CA. It is interesting that immunocytochemical studies of human (Kumpulainen, 1980) and mouse (Kumpulainen and Korhonen, 1982) retina have demonstrated CA C in Müller cells. Müller cells become strongly positive for GFAP after retinal injury (Bignami and Dahl, 1979) and retinal degeneration (O'Dowd and Eng, 1979).

Although the relative distribution of CA between astrocytes and oligodendrocytes has not been resolved, it is clear that oligodendrocytes are enriched in this enzyme. The amount of CA present in astrocytes may be too low to detect consistently in immunocytochemical studies, or regional variations in the levels of CA in astrocytes in sections of developing rat cerebral cortex (Roussel et al., 1979) may be due to the recognized difficulty of distinguishing between young oligodendrocytes and astrocytes, especially at the LM level, or it may reflect regional variations in CA localization. Alternatively, CA may be present in astrocytes as an antigenically distinct molecule that is not recognized or is poorly recognized by conventional antisera to CA.

A second area of interest is the association of CA C with myelin. Biochemical studies (Yandrasitz et al., 1976; Cammer et al., 1976, 1977; Sapirstein et al., 1978) have shown that CA activity can be found in purified myelin with the greatest activity in the heaviest myelin subfractions (Cammer et al., 1977; Fagg et al., 1979). The immunocytochemical observations of myelin staining with anti-CA at the LM level range from occasional small spots, presumably associated with oligodendroglial processes at the surface of myelinated fibers (Ghandour et al., 1980a), to intense filamentous staining of myelinated tracts (Kumpulainen and Korhonen, 1982). Results from our laboratory with antiserum to CA (Figure 14) more closely resemble the patterns of myelin staining reported by Kumpulainen and Korhonen. When compared with adjacent sections stained for MBP and MAG (Figure 15), the fine pattern seen with anti-GA superficially resembles that seen with antiserum to MAG, which has a more restricted distribution (Sternberger et al., 1979a) than that of MBP, which is a component of the compact myelin sheath. Two studies at the EM level (Roussel et al., 1979; Langley et al., 1980) agree that CA is found in areas that contain cytoplasm and is not detectable in compact myelin lamellae. However, Roussel et al. (1979) reported finding CA in the internal and external loops of oligodendroglial cytoplasm in myelin. No mention was made of the presence or absence of staining in paranodal loops of cytoplasm. Langley

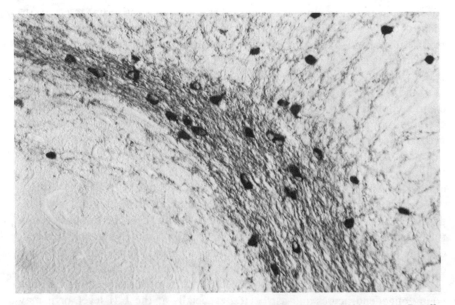

FIGURE 14. CA in oligodendrocytes and myelin of adult rat cerebellum white matter. Paraffin section. Dark reaction is seen in many cells of the white matter and some cells scattered through the granular layer. No staining is seen in the molecular layer. The staining associated with myelin appears as fine strands. Antiserum courtesy of W. van Raamsdonk and C. W. Pool.

et al. (1980) found CA only in cytoplasm of oligodendroglial processes in contact with the external portion of the myelin sheath. They concluded that CA has an exclusively oligodendroglial localization and is absent from myelin. However, lack of penetration of antibodies into the intact or slightly disrupted myelin sheath is a well-recognized problem at the EM level. The immunocytochemical evidence does suggest that CA is not distributed evenly throughout the myelin sheath like MBP, but may have a more limited localization in oligodendrocyte–myelin transition membranes.

For a further discussion of the biochemistry of those oligodendroglial enzymes, see Chapter 6.

6. CELL-COMPONENT-SPECIFIC ANTISERA

6.1. Na$^+$,K$^+$-Adenosine Triphosphatase

Another enzyme involved in biological transport is Na$^+$- and K$^+$-dependent adenosine triphosphatase [(Na$^+$,K$^+$,-ATPase) EC 3.6.1.3], a widely dis-

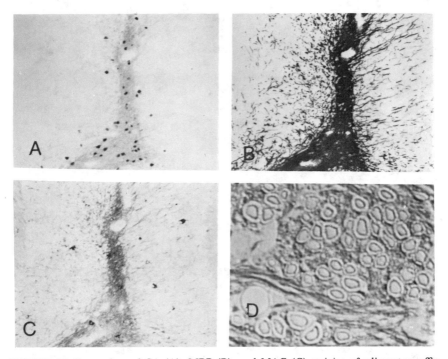

FIGURE 15. Comparison of CA (A), MBP (B), and MAG (C) staining of adjacent paraffin section of 28-day rat cerebellum. Many cells localized primarily with white matter and fine staining associated with myelinated fibers are characteristic of CA staining (A). Only a few faintly stained oligodendrocytes are present in an adjacent section incubated with anti-MBP (B). Staining of the compact myelin sheath is the predominant pattern seen. MAG antiserum reacts with oligodendrocytes in the white matter and granular layer (C). Myelin staining is more restricted compared to that seen with anti-MBP (D). Cross sections of bundles of myelinated fibers from 16-day rat pons stained with MAG antiserum. Staining is seen in the portion of the myelin sheath next to the axon and in some external mesaxons. The compact sheath is not stained.

tributed enzyme that couples ATP hydrolysis to the active transport of sodium and potassium ions during conduction of nerve impulses and transport across cellular membranes. Wood et al. (1977) used antisera to the enzyme purified from electric eel to localize Na^+,K^+-ATPase in the brain of knifefish. At the EM level, the enzyme was associated with plasma membranes of neurons, astrocytes, and oligodendrocytes (Figure 16). Membranes of oligodendrocyte processes involved in myelination were stained, and in myelin, label was seen in the outermost lamellae. At the node of Ranvier, staining appeared in the outer loop of the nodal myelin sheath. Localization of the enzyme has not been done in the mammalian brain, but a recent biochemical study (Reiss et al.,

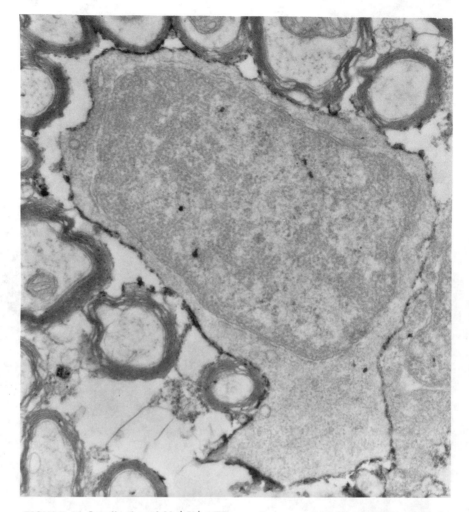

FIGURE 16. Localization of Na⁺,K⁺-ATPase antiserum on knifefish cerebellum. Reaction product is associated with the plasma membrane of an oligodendrocyte and with the outermost myelin membrane. Photomicrograph courtesy of J. D. Wood, D. H. Jean, J. N. Whitaker, B. J. McLaughlin, and R. W. Albers.

1981) provided evidence that Na^+,K^+-ATPase may be an integral component of mammalian myelin.

6.2. Cathepsin D

Cathepsin D [(CD) EC 3.4.23.5] is the major acidic endopeptidase of mammalian brain and may function in normal and pathological degradation of proteins and peptides. A study of CD localization in adult rat brain (Whitaker *et al.*, 1981) showed that the enzyme was distributed in a granular pattern, presumably lysosomal, in neurons, ependymal cells, choroid plexus epithelium, and oligodendrocytes, but not in astrocytes. In studies of the developing rat brain (Snyder and Whitaker, 1982), regional variations were observed in both the time of appearance of CD in oligodendrocytes and the intensity of staining of oligodendrocytes. Reaction with anti-CD was most intense in spinal-cord oligodendrocytes (Figure 17).

6.3. Cyclic-AMP-Dependent Protein Kinase

Cyclic-AMP-dependent protein kinase (EC 2.7.1.37) exists as two isoenzymes (I and II) that have different regulatory subunits (RI and RII) but similar catalytic subunits. The physiological effects of cAMP are mediated by activation of these specific receptor proteins. Recent immunocytochemical studies of the cAMP "second-messenger" system (Cumming *et al.*, 1981) have determined the localization of the regulatory and catalytic subunits in adult rat cerebellar cortex. In addition to the expected Purkinje-cell localization (for a

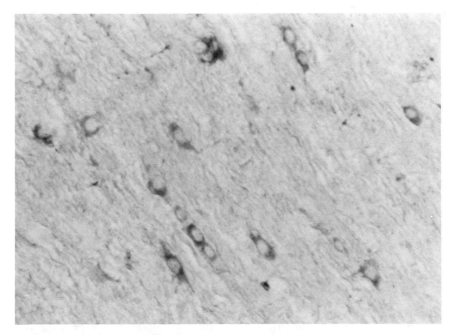

FIGURE 17. CD localization in a longitudinal section of rat spinal-cord white matter. Rows of interfascicular oligodendrocytes are stained by anti-CD. Photomicrograph courtesy of D. S. Snyder and J. N. Whitaker.

brief review, see Cumming, 1981), all subunits were also seen in glial cells Positive staining was seen for the RI subunit in nuclei and cytoplasm of glial cells in the white matter. The RII subunit was localized in glial cytoplasm, nuclei, and the nuclear membrane. Staining for the catalytic subunit (Figure 18) was restricted to nuclei of glia in a pattern characteristic of interfascicular oligodendrocytes. No staining is seen in myelin. Although the function of cAMP in oligodendrocytes is not known, presumably the cAMP system is involved in myelin formation, secretion, and transport processes.

7. IMMUNOCYTOCHEMICAL STUDIES OF OLIGODENDROCYTES IN MUTANT MICE

7.1. Jimpy

Immunocytochemical techniques have been useful for correlating biochemical studies of brain homogenates with morphological observations in nor-

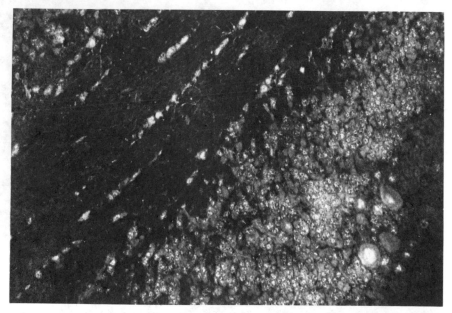

FIGURE 18. Immunofluorescent localization of cAMP-dependent protein kinase catalytic subunit in rat cerebellum. Staining is seen in the white matter and the granular and Purkinje cell layers. The nuclei of interfascicular white matter oligondendrocytes are positive for the catalytic subunit. Photomicrograph courtesy of R. Cumming, Y. Koide, M. R. Krigman, J. A. Beavo, and A. L. Steiner.

mal developing and adult brain. Application of these techniques to the study of murine mutants, particularly dysmyelinating mutants, has permitted more precise localization of antigens in brain regions, structures, and cells.

A widely studied dysmyelinating mutant is the "jimpy," first studied by Sidman and Hayes (1965) and Hirano *et al.* (1969b), who described an almost complete absence of myelin. In addition to the severe myelin deficit, the number of oligodendrocytes was drastically reduced in all brain areas studied (Farkas-Bargeton *et al.*, 1972; Privat *et al.*, 1972; Kraus-Ruppert *et al.*, 1973; Meier *et al.*, 1974; Meier and Bischoff 1975). The oligodendrocytes present were "light," immature cells as defined by Mori and LeBlond (1970). A number of biochemical studies have shown abnormalities in myelin-related components (see Hogan, 1977; Baumann, 1980). The levels of myelin basic protein (MBP) in whole brain are drastically reduced (Matthieu *et al.*, 1973; Campagnoni and Roberts, 1976; Barbarese *et al.*, 1979; Zimmerman and Cohen, 1979; Delassalle *et al.*, 1981), although synthesis occurs at a normal rate (Carson *et al.*, 1975; Delassalle *et al.*, 1981) and the concentration in the cytosol is nearly equal to control levels (Zimmerman and Cohen, 1979). Little or none of the myelin-associated glycoprotein (MAG) was found in the jimpy myelin, indicating that MAG was greatly reduced or absent from the mutant (Matthieu *et al.*, 1974).

Immunocytochemical studies of MBP and MAG in jimpy mutants (Sternberger *et al.*, 1979a) showed that MBP and MAG were found in oligodendrocyte cytoplasm and processes. Staining also surrounded axons (Figures 19 and 20). In contrast to littermate controls (Figures 19 and 20), fewer jimpy oligodendrocytes could be seen reacting with MBP and MAG antiserum. Granular staining in the cytoplasm [see Figure 6B (Section 3.4)] may reflect accumulation of MBP vesicles that are not being inserted into myelin. An unexpected finding was that staining surrounding axons was much more frequent than could be accounted for by the small number of myelin sheaths seen in phase and EM sections, although still less than that seen in control mice. This pattern of staining could also be seen in brain areas in which myelin is never found in the mutant. Staining of these axonal sheaths was intense throughout development, suggesting that they were oligodendrocyte processes or loosely wrapped myelin spirals. These results indicate that like the biochemical results for MBP and MAG, there is a deficit in the accumulation of MBP and MAG. Oligodendrocytes are present that synthesize both MBP and MAG and transport these proteins through their processes, which then surround axons. However, few of these wrapped processes ever become myelin sheaths. The inability of the mutants to consistently make compact myelin from available components is puzzling and suggests that there may be individual variations in oligodendrocyte expression or that there may be neuronal (Kristt and Butler, 1978) or astrocytic abnormalities (Skoff, 1976). The immunocyto-

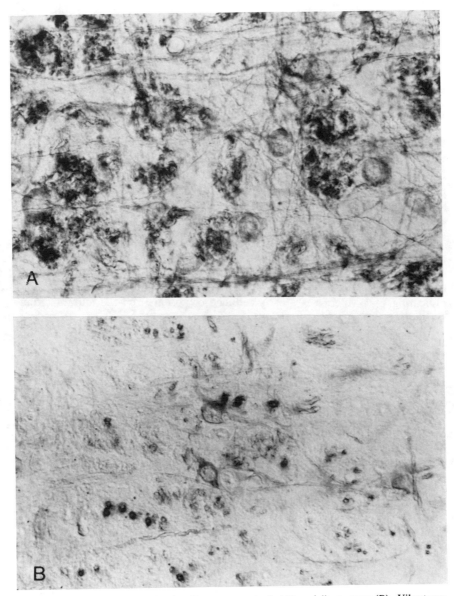

FIGURE 19. MBP staining of 8-day littermate controls (A) and jimpy pons (B). Vibratome sections (20 μm). (A) Many oligodendrocytes and developing myelin sheaths are stained. (B) Fewer oligodendrocytes are MBP-positive, but more staining is seen surrounding axons than can be accounted for by the few myelin sheaths present in the mutant.

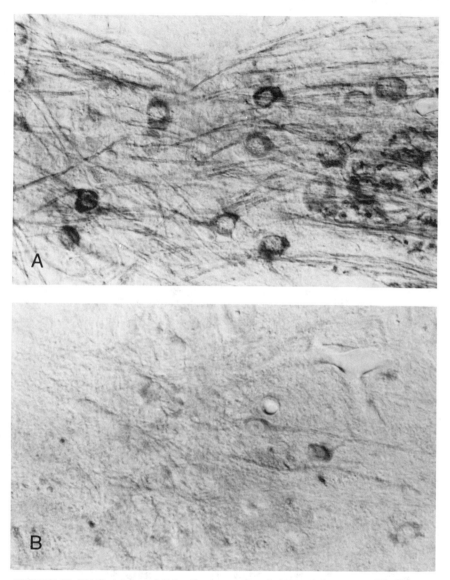

FIGURE 20. MAG staining of 8-day littermate controls (A) and jimpy pons (B). Vibratome sections (20 μm). In littermate control sections (A) many oligodendrocytes and developing myelin sheaths react with anti-MAG. In the jimpy mutant sections (B), only a few oligodendrocytes and faint staining around axons are seen.

chemical studies of Dupouey *et al.* (1980*a,b*), using antisera to MBP, showed that staining of myelin sheaths was sparse in the jimpy and intensity of staining varied according to the region. An interesting observation was that short MBP-positive segments were unequally distributed along an axon. No staining of oligodendrocytes was observed. Sandru *et al.* (1980) found that in jimpy brain cultures, the number of MBP-positive cells was only about 5% of that found in normal cultures.

Several immunocytochemical studies have shown that despite the low levels of GalCer and sulfatide detected in biochemical studies, both antigens can be localized in jimpy oligodendrocytes. Zalc *et al.* (1980) found that oligodendrocytes in the cerebellar white matter were positive for GalCer and sulfatide. Both antigens were found within the cytoplasm of cell bodies, although only surface staining was seen in control sections. No staining in myelin or oligodendrocyte processes around axons was seen. Bologa-Sandru *et al.* (1981*c*) localized GalCer in jimpy optic nerve and cerebellar sections. Staining was confined to cell-body cytoplasm, and it was estimated that approximately 30% of the oligodendrocytes were GalCer-positive. Frequently, only one of the cells in a characteristic chain of oligodendrocytes was stained. The intracytoplasmic localization was considered to be unusual, probably reflecting accumulation of GalCer, since in their experience, anti-GalCer stains only the plasma membranes of normal oligodendrocytes, in agreement with the observations of Zalc and co-workers. No staining was seen around axons. Jimpy cells in culture exhibited only plasma-membrane localization for GalCer, and staining for jimpy and normal oligodendrocytes was similar for cultures of the same age. The results of both these studies suggest that in contrast to MBP and MAG, GalCer is synthesized by oligodendrocytes but not transferred to processes around axons that could become myelin. The results would also suggest that the small amount of myelin that is present does not contain GalCer. Antiserum to another myelin component, the Wolfgram proteins, stained only a few myelinated fibers in 26-day jimpy corpus callosum or cerebellar white matter. No oligodendrocyte staining was seen (Delaunoy *et al.*, 1977).

7.2. Shiverer

Like the jimpy, the "shiverer" mutant has a severe reduction in the amount of myelin in the CNS. Jimpy myelin appears morphologically normal, but shiverer myelin is characterized by a specific structural defect; the absence of major dense lines except in occasional foci (Jacque *et al.*, 1978; Dupouey *et al.*, 1979*a*; Privat *et al.*, 1979; Bourre *et al.*, 1980; Inoue *et al.*, 1981). Absence of a major dense line is related to a specific lack of MBP detected by RIA and immunofluorescence (Jacque *et al.*, 1978; Dupouey *et al.*, 1979*a*) or by RIA of homogenates of mutant brain separated by zonal centrifugation (Bourre *et* *al.*, 1980). Myelin in the PNS is, however, morphologically normal despite the absence of basic proteins (Ganser and Kirschner, 1979). Other immunological studies (Zalc *et al.*, 1980) have shown that antiserum GalCer reacts very faintly with myelin or oligodendrocyte processes around axons, but much more intense fluorescence was seen with antisulfatide. These findings do not reflect biochemical results showing that GalCer and sulfatide are reduced compared to controls (Jacque *et al.*, 1978; Bird *et al.*, 1978; Dupouey *et al.*, 1979*a*), but the ratio is normal. Oligodendrocytes in this study were highly reactive with antisera to GalCer and sulfatide. Immunofluorescence was seen in the cytoplasm, while in controls, reaction was limited to the plasma membrane.

Reaction of antiserum to MAG was widely distributed in sections of shiverer spinal cord [see Figure 10 (Section 3.6)], suggesting that both the few abnormal myelin sheaths and the many oligodendrocyte processes (Privat *et al.*, 1979) were being stained. Intense cytoplasmic staining of many oligodendrocytes even at 90 days suggests that MAG accumulates in the mutant at normal or greater than normal amounts.

7.3. Reeler

In the "reeler" mouse cerebellum, Purkinje cells are dispersed throughout the granular layer and white matter (for reviews, see Sotelo, 1980; Ghandour *et al.*, 1981). Studies of the mutant have centered predominantly on the disturbance of neuronal connectivity. Antibodies to carbonic anhydrase have shown that the distribution of oligodendrocytes is modified beause of the abnormal cytoarchitecture, but cell density and staining are not affected (Ghandour *et al.*, 1981).

8. MONOCLONAL ANTIBODIES TO OLIGODENDROCYTES

One of the most promising approaches to obtaining cell-type-specific antibodies is the use of the hybridoma technique of Kohler and Milstein (1975, 1976). A given polyclonal antiserum to a particular cell type such as oligodendrocytes raised thus far is most likely heterogeneous with respect to the identity of the antigen (or antigens) being detected, the number and nature of antigenic sites with which the antiserum will react, and binding affinities of the various antibody molecules in that antiserum. Monoclonal antibodies raised to a complex mixture of antigens (an oligodendrocyte) are potentially able to distinguish new, highly specific, and, perhaps, minor cell components. Clearly, careful characterization of the antigen detected is just as essential for a monospecific antibody as it is for polyclonal antisera. Problems of cross-reaction with other molecules containing a common antigenic site can occur.

As yet, only a few reports of monoclonal antibodies that react with oligodendrocytes have appeared. Sommer and Schachner (1981) have studied four monoclonal antibodies (01–04) that react with the surface of live oligodendrocytes in cultures of early postnatal mouse cerebellum, optic nerve, spinal cord, or cerebrum. These antibodies were obtained from fused spleen cells of mice injected with bovine corpus callosum white matter. All GalCer-positive cells reacted with all 0 antibodies, but more cells were labeled with the 0 antibodies than with GalCer. In frozen, unfixed tissue sections of adult mouse cerebellum, all 0 antigens were detected in white-matter tracts and in vesicular structures of the neuron-rich granular layer. In fixed cerebellar cultures, oligodendrocyte surface staining is reduced or disappears (depending upon the nature of the fixative), and intracellular staining of astrocytes in a glial-fibrillary-acidic-protein-like pattern appears with three of the monoclonals. A developmental study of fetal mouse cerebellum in culture (Schachner *et al.*, 1981) showed that antigens 03 and 04 are expressed early in oligodendrocyte development. Antigens 01 and 02 are expressed on a subpopulation of oligodendrocytes that are also postive for GalCer and presumably represent more mature cells. A recent study of mouse cerebellum cultures has correlated the ultrastructural appearance of oligodendrocytes labeled with each of the 01–04 antibodies (Berg and Schachner, 1981). The nature of the 01–04 antigens has not yet been determined. Identification of the antigens being detected should greatly facilitate understanding of the somewhat complex reaction of these antibodies.

Several preliminary reports of monoclonal antibodies that react with oligodendrocytes have recently appeared (Peng *et al.*, 1981; Castiglioni and de Vellis, 1981), and it will be of interest to see further studies on the nature and specificity of these antibodies.

A monoclonal antibody to GalCer has been reported (Ranscht *et al.*, 1982) that binds specifically to the cell surface of oligodendrocytes in embryonic rat cerebral cultures (see Section 4). It is of interest that the antigen used was a preparation of synaptic plasma membranes, and this antibody was presumably produced against a minor glial contaminant in the preparation.

A monoclonal antibody to monkey MBP showing species restriction (Sires *et al.*, 1981) has been reported that reacts with a short region near the carboxy-terminal end of MBP (residues 130–137). In tissue sections, the antibody reacts with myelin from monkey cerebellum, but not with myelin from guinea pig cerebellum.

The advantages and limitations of monoclonal antibodies are just being recognized, and they may provide a new direction in the search for oligodendrocyte functions.

ACKNOWLEDGMENTS

Some of the studies reported in this review have been supported by a grant from the National Multiple Sclerosis Society and by Grant NS-17652 from the National Institutes of Health.

9. REFERENCES

Abramsky, O., Lisak, R. P., Silberberg, D. H., and Pleasure, D. E., 1977, Antibodies to oligo-dendroglia in patients with multiple sclerosis, *N. Engl. J. Med.* **297**:1207–1211.

Abramsky, O., Lisak, R. P., Pleasure, D., Gilden, D. H., and Silberger, D. H., 1978, Immuno-logic characterization of oligodendroglia, *Neurosci. Lett.* **8**:311–316.

Abramsky, O., Lisak, R. P., Silberberg, D. H., Brenner, T., and Pleasure, D., 1979, Immune response to isolated oligodendrocytes, *J. Neurol. Sci.* **43**:157–167.

Agrawal, H. C., and Hartman, B. K., 1980, Proteolipid protein and other proteins of myelin, in: *Proteins of the Nervous System,* 2nd ed. (R . A. Bradshaw and D. M., Schneider, eds.), pp. 145–169, Raven Press, New York.

Agrawal, H. C., Hartman, B. K., Shearer, W. T., Kalmbach, S., and Margolis, F. L., 1977, Purification and immunohistochemical localization of rat brain myelin proteolipid, *J. Neu-rochem.* **28**: 495–508.

Alvord, E. C., Jr., Shaw, C. M., Hruby, S., 1976, Neuro-allergic reactions in primates, in: *The Aetiology and Pathogenesis of the Demyelinating Diseases,* Proceedings of a symposium held in September 1976 (H. Shiraki, T. Yonezawa, and Y. Kuroiwa, eds.), pp. 203–216, Japan Science Press, Tokyo.

Barbarese, E., and Pfeiffer, S. E., 1981, Developmental regulation of myelin basic protein in dispersed cultures, *Proc. Natl. Acad. Sci. U.S.A.,* **78**:1953–1957.

Barbarese, E., Carson, J. H., and Braun, P. E., 1979, Subcellular distribution and structural polymorphism of myelin basic protein in normal and jimpy mouse brain, *J. Neurochem.* **32**:1437–1446.

Baumann, N. (ed.), 1980, *Neurological Mutations Affecting Myelination,* Elsevier/North-Hol-land, Amsterdam.

Benjamins, J., Guarnieri, M., Miller, K., Sonneborn, M., and McKhann, G. M., 1974, Sulfatide synthesis in isolated oligodendroglial and neuronal cells, *J. Neurochem.* **23**:751–757.

Berg, G., and Schachner, M., 1981, Immuno-electron-microscopic identification of O-antigen-bearing oligodendroglial cells *in vitro, Cell Tissue Res.* **219**:313–325.

Bhat, S., Barbarese, E., and Pfeiffer, S. E., 1981, Requirement for nonoligodendrocyte cell sig-nals for enhanced myelinogenic gene expression in long-term cultures of purified rat oligo-dendrocytes, *Proc. Natl. Acad. Sci. U.S.A.,* **78**:1283–1287.

Bignami, A., and Dahl, D., 1979, The radial glia of Müller in rat retina and their response to injury: An immunofluorescence study with antibodies to the glial fibrillary acidic (GFA) protein, *Exp. Eye Res.* **28**:63–69.

Bird, T. D., Farrell, D. F., ad Sumi, S. M., 1978, Brain lipid composition of the shiverer mouse (genetic defect in myelin development), *J. Neurochem.* **31**:387–391.

Bologa-Sandru, L., Siegrist, H. P., and Herschkowitz, N., 1981a, Immunological properties of bulk isolated mouse oligodendrocytes, *Neurosci. Lett.* **22**:131–135.

Bologa-Sandru, L., Siegrist, H. P., Z'Graggen, A., Hofmann, K., Wiesmann, U., Dahl, D., and Herschkowitz, N., 1981*b*, Expression of antigenic markers during the development of oligodendrocytes in mouse brain cultures, *Brain Res.* **210**:217–119.

Bologa-Sandru, L., Zalc, B., Herschkowitz, N. and Baumann, N., 1981*c*, Oligodendrocytes of jimpy mice express galactosylceramide: An immunofluorescence study on brain sections and dissociated brain cell cultures, *Brain Res.* **225**:425–430.

Borit, A., and McIntosh, G. C., 1981, Myelin basic protein and glial fibrillary acidic protein in human fetal brain, *Neuropathol. Appl. Neurobiol.* **7**:279–287.

Bourre, J. M., Jacque, C., Delasalle, A., Nguyen-Legros, J., Dumont, O., Lachaelle, F., Raoul, M., Alvarz, C., and Baumann, N., 1980, Density profile and basic protein measurements in the myelin range of particulate material from normal developing mouse brain and fom neurological mutants (jimpy; quaking; trembler; shiverer and its mld allele) obtained by zonal centrifugation, *J. Neurochem.* **35**:458–464.

Cammer W., Fredman, T., Rose, A. L., and Norton, W. T., 1976, Brain carbonic anhyrase: Activity in isolated myelin and the effect of hexachlorophene, *J. Neurochem.* **27**:165–171.

Cammer, W., Bieler, L., Fredman, T., and Norton, W. T., 1977, Quantitation of myelin carbonic anhydrase: Development and subfractions of rat brain myelin and comparison with myelin from other species, *Brain Res.* **138**:17–28.

Cammer, W., Snyder, D. S., Zimmerman, T. R., Jr., Faroq, M., and Norton, W. T., 1982, Glycerol phosphate dehydrogenase, glucose-6-phosphate dehydrogenase and lactate dehydrogenase: Activities in oligodendrocytes, neurons, astrocytes, and myelin isolated from developing rat brains, *J. Neurochem.* **38**:360–367.

Campagnoni, A. T., and Roberts, J. L., 1976, Isolation of myelin basic proteins from jimpy mice, *Brain Res.* **115**:351–356.

Carson, J. H., Herschkowitz, N. N., and Braun, P. E., 1975, Synthesis and degradation of myelin basic protein in normal and jimpy mouse brain, *Trans. Am. Soc. Neurochem.* **6**:207.

Castiglioni, E. T., and deVellis, J., 1981, Monoclonal antibody to a rat glial cell antigen, *Soc. Neurosci. Abstr.* **7**:698.

Cumming, R., 1981 Immunocytochemistry of second messenger systems, pp. 202–203.

Cumming, R., Koide, Y., Krigman, M. R., Beavo, J. A., and Steiner, A. L., 1981, The immunofluorescent localization of regulatory and catalytic subunits of cyclic AMP-dependent protein kinase in neuronal and glial cell types of the central nervous system, *Neuroscience* **6**:953–961.

Delassalle, A., Zalc, B., Lachapelle, F., Raoul, M., Collier, P., and Jacque, C., 1981, Regional distribution of myelin basic protein in the central nervous system of quaking, jimpy, and normal mice during development and aging, *J. Neurosci. Res.* **6**:303–313.

Delaunoy, J. P., Roussel, G., Nussbaum, J. L., and Mandel, P., 1977, Immunohistochemical studies of Wolfgram proteins in central nervous system of neurological mutant mice, *Brain Res.* **133**:29–36.

Delaunoy, J. P., Hog, F., Devilliers, G., Bansart, M., Mandel, P., and Sensenbrenner, M., 1980, Developmental changes and localization of carbonic anhydrase in cerebral hemispheres of the rat and in rat glial cell cultures, *Cell Mole. Biol.* **26**:235–240.

del Cerro, C., Sternberger, N. H., Kies, M. W., and Herndon, R. M., 1983, Immunocytochemistry of myelin basic protein in adult oligodendroglia, *Soc. Neurosci. Abstr.* **9**:451.

Drummond, R. J., and Dean, G., 1980, Comparison of 2′,3′-cyclic nucleotide 3′-phosphohyrolase and the major component of Wolfgram protein W1, *J. Neurochem.* **35**:1155–1165.

Dupouey, P., Jacque, C., Bourre, J. M., Cesseliln, F., Privat, A., and Baumann, N., Immunocytochemical studies of a myelin basic protein in Shiverer mouse devoid of major 1979*a*, *Neurosci. Lett.* **12**:113–118.

Dupouey, P., Zalo, B., Lefroit-Joly, M., and Gomes, D., 1979*b*, Localization of galactosylcer-amide and sulfatide at the surface of the myelin sheath: An immunofluorescence study in liquid medium, *Cell. Mol. Biol.* **25:**269–272.

Dupouey, P., Lucas, C., Gomes, D., and Jacque, C., 1980*a*, Immunochistochemical localization of the MBP and of the GFAP: Comparative study in normal, quaking and jimpy mice, *J. Neurosci. Res.* **5:**387–398.

Dupouey, P., Gomes, D., Raoul, M., Collier, P., and Jacque, C., 1980*b*, Abnormal myelination in the mouse: Immunohistochemical investigation on the quaking, jimpy and shiverer mutants, in: *Neurological Mutations Affecting Myelination* (N. Baumann, ed.), INSERM Symposium No. 14, pp. 327–332, Elsevier/North-Holland, Amsterdam.

Eng. L. F., and Bigbee, J. W., 1978, Immunohistochemistry of nervous system specific antigens, in: *Advances in Neurochemistry*, Vol. 3 (B. W. Agronoff and M. H. Aprison, eds.), pp. 43–98, Plenum Press, New York.

Eng, L. F., and DeArmond, S. J., 1982, Immunochemistry of the glial fibrillary acidic (GFA) protein, in: *Progress in Neuropathology* (H. M. Zimmerman, ed.), Raven Press, New York.

Eng, L. F., Burkstaller, M., Bigbee, J., Kosek, J. C., and Kies, M. W., 1975, Immunohistologic comparison of the glial fibrillary acidic protein and myelin basic protein in the myelinating brain, 5th International Meeting of the International Society of Neurochemists, Barcelona, Spain, Abstract 41.

Fagg, G. E., Lane, J. D., Neuhoff, V., and Waehneldt, T. V., 1979, Carbonic anhydrase activity in myelin fractions from rat optic nerves, *Neurosci. Lett.* **12:**219–222.

Farkas-Bargeton, E., Robain, O., and Mandel, P., 1972, Abnormal glial maturation in the white matter in jimpy mice, *Acta Neuropathol. (Berlin)* **21:**272–281.

Fisher, M., Gapp, D. A., and Kozak, L. P., 1981, Immunocytochemical localization of *sn*-glyc-erol-3-phosphate dehydrogenase in Bergmann glia and oligodendroglia in the mouse cere-bellum, *Dev. Brain Res.* **1:**341–354.

Ganser, A. L., and Kirschner, D. A., 1979, Compact myelin exists in the absence of basic protein in the shiverer mouse, *Nature (London)*, **283:**207–210.

Gebicke-Harter, P. J., Althaus, H. H., Schwartz, P., and Neuhoff, V., 1981, Oligodendrocytes from postnatal cat brain in cell culture. I. Regeneration and maintenance, *Dev. Brain Res.* **1:**497–518.

Ghandour, M. S., Langley, O. K., Vincendon, G., and Gombos, G., 1979, Double labeling immu-nohistochemical technique provides evidence of the specificity of glial cell markers, *J. His-tochem.* **27:**1634–1637.

Ghandour, M. S., Langley, O. K., Vincendon, G., Gombos, G., Filippi, D., Limozin, N., Dal-masso, C., and Laurent, G., 1980*a*, Immunochemical and immunohistochemical study of carbonic anhydrase II in adult rat cerebellum: A marker for oligodendrocytes, *Neuroscience* **5:**559–571.

Ghandour, M. S., Vincendon, G., and Gombos G., 1980*b*, Astrocyte and oligodendrocyte distri-bution in adult rate cerebellum: An immunohistological study, *J. Neurocytol.* **9:**637–646.

Ghandour, M. S., Vincendon, G., Gombos, G., Limozin, N., Filippi, D., Dalmasso, C., and Lau-rent, G., 1980*c*, Carbonic anhydrase and oligodendroglia in developing rat cerebellum: A biochemical and immunohistological study, *Dev. Biol.* **77:**73–83.

Ghandour, M. S., Derer, P., Labourdette, G., Delaunoy, J. P., and Langley, O. K., 1981, Glial cell markers in the reeler mutant mouse: A biochemical and immunohistological study, *J. Neurochem.* **36:**195–200.

Giacobini, E., 1961, Localization of carbonic anhydrase in the nervous system, *Science* **134:**1524–1525.

Giacobini, E., 1962, A cytochemical study of the localization of carbonic anhydrase in the ner-vous system, *J. Neurochem.* **9:**169–177.

Goldstein, M. E., Sternberger, L. A., and Sternberger, N. H., 1982, Developmental expression of neurotypy revealed by immunocytochemistry with monoclonal antibodies, *J. Neuroimmunol.* 3:203–217.

Goldstein, M. E., Sternberger, L. A., and Sternberger, N. H., 1983, Microheterogeneity ("neurotypy") of neurofilament proteins, *Proc. Natl. Acad. Sci. U.S.A.* **80**:3101–3105.

Hartman, B. K., Agrawal, H. C., Kalmback, S., and Shearer, W. T., 1979, A comparative study of the immunohistochemical localization of basic protein to myelin and oligodendrocytes in rat and chicken brain, *J. Comp. Neurol.* **188**:273–290.

Hartman, B. K., Agrawal, H. C., Agrawal, D., and Kalmbach, S., 1982, Development and maturation of central nevous system myelin: Comparison of immunohistochmical localization of proteolipid protein and basic protein in myelin and oligodendrocytes, *Proc. Natl. Acad. Sci. U.S.A.* **79**:4217–4220.

Herndon, R. M., Rauch, H. C., and Einstein, E. R., 1973, Immuno-electron microscopic localization of the encephalitogenic basic protein in myelin, *Immunol. Commun.* **2**:163–172.

Hirano, A., Sax, D. S., and Zimmerman, H. M., 1969a, The fine structure of the cerebella of jimpy mice and their "normal" litter mates, *J. Neuropathol. Exp. Neurol.* **28**:388–400.

Hirano, A., Becker, N. H., and Zimmerman, H. M., 1969b, Isolation of the periaxonal space of the central myelinated nerve fiber with regard to the diffusion of peroxidase, *J. Histochem. Cytochem.* **17**:512–516.

Hogan, E. L., 1977, Animal models of genetic disorders of myelin, in: *Myelin* (P. Morell, ed.), pp. 489–520, Plenum Press, New York.

Inoue, Y., Sugihara, Y., Nakagawa, S., and Shimai, K., 1973, The morphological changes of oligodendroglia during the formation of myelin sheaths: Golgi study and electron microscopy, *Okajimas Fol. Anat. Jap.* **50**:327–344.

Inoue, Y., Nakamura, R., Mikoshiba, K., and Tsukada, Y., 1981, Fine structure of the central myelin sheath in the myelin deficient mutant shiverer mouse, with special reference to the pattern of myelin formation by oligodendroglia, *Brain Res.* **219**:85–94.

Itoyama, Y., Sternberger, N. H., Kies, M. W., Cohen, S. R., Richardson, E. P., Jr., and Webster, H. de F., 1980a, Immunocytochemical method to identify myelin basic protein in oligodendroglia and myelin sheaths of the human nervous system, *Ann. Neurol.* **7**:157–166.

Itoyama, Y., Sternberger, N. H., Webster, H. de F., Quarles, R. H.,Cohen, S. R., and Richardson, E. P., Jr., 1980b, Immunocytochemical observations on the distribution of myelin-associated glycoprotein and myelin basic protein in multiple sclerosis lesions, *Ann. Neurol.* **7**:167–177.

Jacque, C., Privat, A., Dupouey, P., Bourre, J. M., Bird, T. D., and Baumann, N., 1978, Shiverer mouse: A dysmyelinating mutant with absence of major dense line and basic protein in myelin in: *2nd European Society of Neurochemistry Meeting, Proc. Europ. Soc. Neurochem.*, Vol. 1 (V. Neuhoff, ed.) p. 131, Verlag Chemie, Wiesbaden.

Johnson, A. B., and Blum, N. R., 1972, Peroxidase-labeled antigens in light and electron immunohistochemistry and their utilization in studies of experimental allergic encephalomyelitis, *Abst. Histocem. Soc.* **7**:841.

Johnson, A. B., Wisniewski, H. M., Raine, C. S., Eylar, E. H., and Terry, R. D., 1971, Specific binding of peroxidase-labeled myelin basic protein in allergic encephalomyelitis, *Proc. Natl. Acad. Sci. U.S.A.* **68**:294–2698.

Jones, E. G., and Hartman, B. K., 1978, Recent advances in neuroanatomical methodology, *Annu. Rev. Neurosci.* **1**:215–296.

Kennedy, P. G. E., and Lisak, R. P., 1979, A search for antibodies against glial cells in the serum and cerebrospinal fluid of patients with multiple sclerosis and Guillain–Barré syndrome, *J. Neurol. Sci.* **44**:125–133.

Kies, M. W., 1982, Myelin basic protein, *Scand. J. Immunol.* **15**:125–146.

Kies, M. W., Thompson, E. B., and Alvord, E. C., Jr., 1965, The relationship of myelin proteins to experimental allergic encephalomyelitis, *Ann. N. Y. Acad. Sci.* **122**:148–160.

Kimelberg, H. K., Stieg, P. E., and Mazurkiewicz, J. E., 1982, Immunocytochemical and biochemical analysis of carbonic anhydrase in primary astrocyte cultures from rat brain, *J. Neurochem.* **39**:734–742.

Kristt, D. A., and Butler, F. K., 1978, Neuronal abnormalities associated with impaired myelination during brain development: A Golgi study of neocortex in the jimpy mouse, *Neurosci. Lett.* **7**:107–113.

Kohler, G., and Milstein, C., 1975, Continuous cultures of fused cells secreting antibody of predefined specificity, *Nature (London)* **256**:495–497.

Kohler, J. G., and Milstein, C., 1976, Derivation of specific antibody producing tissue culture and tumor lines by cell fusion, *Eur. J. Immunol.* **6**:511

Korhonen, L. K., Naatanen, E., and Hyppa, M., 1964, A histochemical study of carbonic anhydrase in some parts of the mouse brain, *Acta Histochem.* **18**:336–347.

Kornguth, S. E., Anderson, J. W., and Scott, G., 1966, Temporal relationship between myelinogenesis and the appearance of basic protein in the spinal cord of the white rat, *J. Comp. Neurol.* **127**:1–18.

Kraus-Ruppert, R., Herschkowitz, N., and Furst, H., 1973, Morphological studies on neuroglial cells in the corpus callosum of the jimpy mouse, *J. Neuropathol. Exp. Neurol.* **32**:197–203.

Kumpulainen, T., 1980, Carbonic anhydrase isoenzyme C in the human retina, *Acta Ophthalmol.* **58**:397–405.

Kumpulainen, T., and Korhonen, L. K., 1982, Immunohistochemical localization of carbonic anhydrase isoenzyme C in the central and peripheral nervous system of the mouse, *J. Histochem. Cytochem.* **30**:283–292.

Kumpulainen, T., and Nystrom, S. H. M., 1981, Immunohistochemical localization of carbonic anhydrase isoenzyme C in human brain, *Brain Res.* **220**:220–225.

Langley, O. K., Ghandour, M. S., Vincendon, G., and Gombos, C., 1980, Carbonic anhydrase: An ultrastructural study in rat cerebellum, *Histochem. J.* **12**:473–483.

Lennon, V. R., Wittingham, J., Carnegie, P. R., McPherson, T. A., and MacKay, I. R., 1971, Detection of antibodies to the basic protein of human myelin by radioimmunoassay and immunofluorescence, *J. Immunol.* **107**:56–62.

Leveille, P. J., McGnnis, J. F., Maxwell, D. S., and de Vellis, J., 1980, Immunocytochemical localization of glycerol-3-phosphate dehydrogenase in rat oligodendrocytes, *Brain Res.* **196**:287–305.

Lisak, R. P., Abramsky, O., Dorfman, S. H., George, J., Manning, M. C., Pleasure, D. E., Saida, T., and Silberberg, D. H., 1979, Antibodies to galactocerebrosde bind to oligodendroglia in suspension culture, *J. Neurol. Sci.* **40**:65–73.

Lisak, R. P., Pruss, R. M., Kennedy, P. G. E., Abramsky, O., Pleasure, D. E., and Silberberg, D. H., 1981, Antisera to bovine oligodendroglia raised in guinea pigs bind to surface of rat oligodendroglia and Schwann cells, *Neurosci. Lett.* **17**:119–124.

Ludwin, S. K., 1979, The perineuronal satellite oligodendrocyte: A role in remyelination, *Acta Neuropathol.* **47**:49–53.

Ma, B. I., Joseph, B. S., Wash, M. J. Potvin, A. R., and Tourtellotte, W. W., 1981, Multiple sclerosis serum and cerebrospinal fluid immunoglobulin binding to Fc receptors of oligodendrocytes, *Ann. Neurol.* **9**:371–377.

Matthieu, J. M., Widmer, S., and Herschkowitz, N., 1973, Jimpy, an anomaly of myelin maturation: Biochemical studies of myelination phases, *Brain Res.* **55**:403–412.

Matthieu, J. M., Quarles, R. H., Webster, H. de F., Hogan, E. L., and Brady R. O., 1974, Characterization of the fraction obtained from the CNS of jimpy mice by a procedure for myelin isolation, *J. Neurochem.* **23**:517–523.

McCarthy, K. D., and de Vellis, J., 1980, Preparation of separate astroglial and oligodendroglial cell cultures from rat cerebral tissue, *J. Cell Biol.* **85**:890–902.

Meier, C., and Bischoff, A., 1975, Oligodendroglial cell development in jimpy mice and controls: An electron microscopic study in the optic nerve, *J. Neurol. Sci.* **26**:517–528.

Meier, C., Herschkowitz, N., and Bischoff, A., 1974, Morphological and biochemical observations in the jimpy spinal cord, *Acta Neuropathol.* **27**:349–362.

Mendell, J. R., and Whitaker, J. N., 1978, Immunocytochemical localization studies of myelin basic protein, *J. Cell Biol.* **76**:502–511.

Mirsky, R., Winter, J., Abney, E. R., Pruss, R. M., Gavrilovic, J., and Raff, M. C., 1980, Myelin-specific proteins and glycolipids in rat Schwann cells and oligodendrocytes in culture, *J. Cell Biol.* **84**:483–494-

Mori, S., and LeBlond, C. P., 1970, Electron microscopic identification of three classes of oligodendrocytes and a preliminary study of their proliferative activity in the corpus callosum of young rats, *J. Comp. Neurol.* **139**:1–30.

Müller, H. W., Clapshaw, P. A., and Seifert, W., 1981, Intracellular localization of 2′,3′-cyclic nucleotide 3′-phosphodiesterase in a neuronal cell line as examined by immunofluorescence and cell fractionation, *J. Neurochem.* **37**:947–955.

Narang, H. K., 1977, Electron microscopic development of neuroglia in epiretinal portion of postnatal rabbits, *J. Neurol. Sci.* **34**:391–406.

Narang, H. K., and Wisniewski, H. M., 1976, The sequence of myelination in the epiretinal portion of the optic nerve in the rabbit, *Neuropathol. Appl. Neurobiol.* **3**:15–27.

Nishizawa, Y., Kurihara, T., and Takahashi, Y., 1981, Immunohistochemical localization of 2′,3′-cyclic nucleotide 3′-phosphodiesterase in the central nervous system, *Brain Res.* **212**:219–222.

Norton, W. T., 1981, Biochemistry of myelin, in: *Demyelinating Disease: Basic and Clinical Electrophysiology* (S. G. Waxman and J. M. Ritchie, eds.) pp. 93–121, Raven Press, New York.

Nussbaum, J. L., Delaunoy, J. P., and Mandel, P., 1977, Some immunochemical characteristics of W1 and W2 Wolfgram proteins isolated from rat brain myelin, *J. Neurochem.* **28**:183–191.

O'Dowd, D. K., and Eng, L. F., 1979, Immunocytochemical localization of the glial fibrillary acidic (GFA) protein in the Müller cell of the human retina, *Neurosci. Abstr.* **5**:1456.

Omlin, F. X., Palkovits, C. G., Cohen, S. R., and Webster, H. de F., 1982a, EM immunocytochemistry of basic protein in developing glia and myelin, *Trans. Am. Soc. Neurochem.* **13**:214.

Omlin, F. X., Webster, H. de F., Palkovits, C. G., and Cohen, S. R., 1982b, Immunocytochemical localization of basic protein in major dense line regions of central and peripheral myelin, *J. Cell Biol.* **95**:242–248.

Peng, W. W., Cole, R., and de Vellis, J., 1981, A monoclonal antibody to oligodendrocytes, *Soc. Neurosci. Abstr.* **7**:698.

Pfeiffer, S. E., Barbarese, E., and Bhat, S., 1981, Noncoordinate regulation of myelinogenic parameters in primary cultures of dissociated fetal rat brain, *J. Neurosci. Res.* **6**:369–380.

Pleasure, D., Hardy, M., Johnson, G., Lisak, R., and Silberberg, D., 1981, Oligodendroglial glycerophospholipid synthesis: Incorporation of radioactive precursors into ethanolamin glycerophospholipids by calf oligodendroglia prepared by a Percoll procedure and maintained in suspension culture, *J. Neurochem.* **37**:452–460.

Poduslo, S. E., McFarland, H. F., and McKhann, G. M., 1977, Antiserums to neurons and to oligodendroglia from mammalian brain, *Science* **197**:270–272.

Prineas, J. W., and Graham, J. S., 1981, Multiple sclerosis; Capping of surface immunoglobulin G on macrophages engaged in myelin breakdown, *Ann. Neurol.* **10**:149–158.

Privat, A., and LeBlond, C. P., 1972, The subependymal layer and neighboring region in the brain of the young rat, *J. Comp. Neurol.* **146:**277–302.

Privat, A., Robain, O., and Mandel, P., 1972, Aspects ultrastructuraux du corps calleux chez la souris jimpy, *Acta Neuropathol.* **21:**282–295.

Privat, A., Jacque, C., Bourre, J. M., Dupouey, P., and Baumann, N., 1979, Absence of the major dense line in myelin of the mutant mouse "shiverer," *Neurosci. Lett.* **12:**107–112.

Pruss, R. M., Bartlett, P. F., Gavrilovic, J., Lisak, R. P., and Rattray, S., 1982, Mitogens for glial cells: A comparison of the response of cultured astrocytes, oligodendrocytes and Schwann cells, *Dev. Brain Res.* **2:**19–35.

Quarles, R. H., 1979, Glycoproteins in myelin and myelin-related membranes, in: *Complex Carbohydrates of Nervous Tissue* (R. U. Margolis and R. K. Margolis, eds.) pp. 209–233, Plenum Press, New York.

Raff, M. C., Mirsky, R., Fields, K. L., Lisak, R. P., Dorfman, S. H., Silberberg, D. H., Gregson, N. A., Leibowitz, S., and Kennedy, M. C., 1978, Galactocerebroside is a specific cell-surface antigenic marker for oligodendrocytes in culture,*Nature (London)* **274:**813–816.

Raff, M. C., Fields, K. L., Hakamori, S. I., Mirsky, R., Pruss, R. M., and Winter, J., 1979, Cell-type-specific markers for distinguishing and studying neurons and the major classes of glial cells in culture, *Brain Res.* **174:**283–308.

Raine, C. S., 1981, Neurocellular anatomy, in: *Basic Neurochemistry* (G. J. Siegel, R. W. Albers, B. W. Agranoff, and R. Katzman, eds.), pp. 21–47, Little, Brown, Boston.

Ramon-Moliner, E., 1958, A study on neuroglia: The problem of transitional forms, *J. Comp. Neurol.* **110:**157–167.

Ranscht, B., Clapshaw, P. A., Price, J., Noble, M., and Seifert, W., 1982, Development of oligodendrocytes and Schwann cells studied with a monoclonal antibody against galactocerebroside, *Proc. Natl. Acad. Sci. U.S.A* **79:**2709–2713.

Rauch, H. C., and Raffel, S., 1964, Immunofluorescent localization of encephalitogenic protein in myelin, *J. Immunol.* **92:**2452–455.

Reiss, D. S., Lees, M. B., and Sapirstein, V. S., 1981, Is Na + K ATPase a myelin-associated enzyme?, *J. Neurochem.* **36:**1418–1426.

Roussel, G., and Nussbaum, J. L., 1981, Comparative localization of Wolfgram W1 and myelin basic proteins in the rat brain during ontogenesis, *Histochem. J.* **13:**1029–1047.

Roussel, G., and Nussbaum, J. L., 1982, Surface labeling of oligodendrocytes with anti-myelin serum in cell cultures from the rat brain, *Cell Tissue Res.* **225:**581–594.

Roussel, G., Delaunoy, J. P., Nussbaum, J. L., and Mandel, P., 1977, Immunohistochemical localization of Wolfgram proteins in nervous tissue of rat brain, *Neuroscience* **2:***307–313.*

Roussel, G., Delaunoy, J. P., Mandel, P., and Nussbaum, J. L., 1978, Ultrastructural localization study of two Wolfgram proteins in rat brain tissue, *J. Neurocytol.* **7:**155–163.

Roussel, G., Delaunoy, J. P., Nussbaum, J. L., and Mandel, P., 1979, Demonstration of a specific localization of carbonic anhydrase C in the glial cells of rat CNS by an immunohistochemical method, *Brain Res.* **160:**47–55.

Roussel, G., Labourdette, G., and Nussbaum, J. L, 1981, Characterization of oligodendrocytes in primary cultures from brain hemispheres of newborn rats, *Dev. Biol.* **81:**371–378.

Sandru, L., Siegrist, H. P., Wiesmann, U. N., and Herschkowitz, N., 1980, Development of oligodendrocytes in jimpy brain cultures, in: *Neurological Mutations Affecting Myelination* (N. Baumann, ed.) INSERM Symposium No. 14, pp. 469–474, Elsevier/North-Holland, Amsterdam.

Sapirstein, V. S., Lees, M. B., and Trachtenberg, M. C., 1978, Soluble and membrane bound carbonic anhydrase from rat CNS: Regional development, *J. Neurochem.* **31:**283–287.

Sarlieve, L. L., Fabare, M., Delaunoy, J. P., Pieringer, R. A., and Rebel, G., 1980, Surface-adhering primary cultures of dissociated brain cells from embryonic mice as a tool to study myelination *in vitro,* in: *Neurological Mutations Affecting Myelination* (N. Baumann, ed.), INSERM Symposium No. 14, pp. 489–500, Elsevier/North-Holland, Amsterdam.

Sarlieve, L. L. Delaunoy, J. P., Dierich, A., Ebel, A., Fabre, M., Mandel, P., Rebel, G., Vincendon, G., Wintzerith, M., and Yusufi, A. N. K., 1981, Investigations on myelination *in vitro.* III. Ultrastructural: Brain cells from embryonic mice, *J. Neurosci. Res.* **6:**659–683.

Schachner, M, Kim, S. K., and Zehnle, R., 1981, Developmental expresson in central and peripheral nervous system of oligodendrocyte cell surface antigens (0 antigens) recognized by monoclonal antibodies, *Dev. Biol.* **83:**328–338.

Sidman, R. L., and Hayes, R., 1965, Jimpy: A mouse with inherited sudanophilic leukodystrophy, *J. Neuropathol. Exp. Neurol.* **24:**172.

Sires, L. R., Hruby, S., Alvord, E. C., Jr., Hellström, I., Hellström, K. E., Kies, M. W., Martenson, R., Diebler, C. E., Beckman, E. D., and Casnellie, J. E., 1981, Species restrictions of a monoclonal antibody reacting with residues 130 to 137 in encephalitogenic myelin basic protein, *Science* **214:**87–89.

Skoff, R. P., 1976, Myelin deficits in the jimpy mouse may be due to cellular abnormalities in astroglia, *Nature (London)* **264:**560–562.

Skoff, R. P., Price, D. L., and Stocks, A., 1976, Electron microscopic autoradiographic studies of gliogenesis in rat optic nerve. II. Time of origin, *J. Comp. Neurol.* **169:**313–333.

Snyder, D. S., and Whitaker, J. N., 1982, Immunocytochemical localization of cathepsin in rat CNS during ontogeny, *Trans. Am. Soc. Neurochem.* **13:**115.

Snyder, D. S., Raine, C. S., Farooq, M., and Norton, W. T., 1980, The bulk isolation of oligodendroglia from whole rat forebrain: A new procedure using physiologic media, *J. Neurochem.* **34:**1614–1621.

Sommer, I., and Schachner, M., 1981, Monoclonal antibodies (01 to 04) to oligodendrocyte cell surfaces: An immunocytological study in the central nervous system, *Dev. Biol.* **83:**311–327.

Sotelo, C., 1980, Mutant mice and the formtion of cerebellar circuitry, pp. 33–35.

Spicer, S. S., Stoward, P. J., and Tashian, R. E., 1979, The immunohistolocalization of carbonic anhydrase in rodent tissues, *J. Histochem. Cytochem.* **27:**820–831.

Sprinkle, T. J., and McDonald, T. F., 1982, Immunofluorescence in oligodendrocytes treated with anti-CNP antisera, *Trans. Am. Soc. Neurochem.* **13:**172.

Sprinkle, T. J., Wells, M. R., Garver, F. A., and Smith, D. B., 1980, Studies on the Wolfgram high molecular weight CNS myelin proteins: Relationship to 2′,3′-cyclic nucleotide 3′-phosphodiesterase, *J. Neurochem.* **35:**1200–1208.

Sprinkle, T. J., Baker, M. D., and McDonald, T. F., 1981, Immunocytochemical localization of CNP in adult bovine optic nerve, *Trans. Am. Soc. Neurochem.* **12:**209.

Sternberger, N., Tabira, T., Kies, M. W., and Webster, H., 1977, Immunocytochemical staining of basic protein CNS myelin, *Trans. Am. Soc. Neurochem.* **8:**157.

Sternberger, N. H., Itoyama, Y., Kies, M. W., and Webster, H., de F., 1978a, Immunocytochemical method to identify basic protein in myelin-forming oligodendrocytes of newborn rat C.N.S., *J. Neurocytol.* **7:**251–263.

Sternberger, N. H., Itoyama, Y., Kies, N. W., and Webster, H. de F., 1978b, Myelin basic protein demonstrated immunocytochemically in oligodendroglia prior to myelin sheath formation, *Proc. Natl. Acad. Sci. U. S. A.* **75:**2521–2524.

Sternberger, N. H., Quarles, R. H., Itoyama, Y., and Webster, H. de F., 1979a, Myelin-associated glycoprotein demonstrated immunocytochemically in myelin and myelin-forming cells of developing rat, *Proc. Natl. Acad. Sci. U. S. A.* **76:**1510–1514.

Sternberger, N. H., Quarles, R. H., Cohen, S. R., Winchell, K., and Webster, H. de F., 1979b Alterations in myelin basic protein and myelin-associated glycoprotein in jimpy mice, *Soc. Neurosci. Abstr.,* p. 417.

Szuchet, S., Stefannson, K., Wollmann, R. L., Dawson, G., and Arnason, B. G., 1980, Maintenance of isolated oligodendrocytes in long-term culture, *Brain Res.* **200**:151–164.

Tennekoon, G. I., Frangia, J., Aitchison, S., and Price, D. L., 1981, Cerebroside sulfotransferase: Preparation of antiboyd and localization of antigen in Kidney, *J. Cell Biol.* **91**:332–339.

Towbin, H., Staehelin, T., and Gordon, J., 1979, Electrophoretic transfer of proteins from polyacrylamide gels to nitrocellulose sheets: Procedure and some applications, *Proc. Natl. Acad. Sci. U. S.A.* **76**:4350–4354.

Traugott, U., and Raine, C. S., 1981, Antioligodendrocyte antibodies in cerebrospinal fluid of multiple sclerosis and other neurologic diseases, *Neurology* **31**:695–700.

Traugott, U., Snyder, D. S., Norton, W. T., and Raine, C. S., 1978, Characterization of antioligodendrocyte serum, *Ann. Neurol.* **4**:431–439.

Traugott, U., Snyder, D. S., and Raine, C. S., 1979, Oligodendrocyte staining by multiple sclerosis serum is nonspecific, *Ann. Neurol.* **6**:13–20.

Whitaker, J. N., 1975, The antigenicity of mylin encephalitogenic protein: Production of antibodies to encephalitogenic protein with deoxyribonucleic acid–encephalitogenic protein complexes, *J. Immunol.* **114**:823–828.

Whitaker, J. N., 1978, The distribution of myelin basic protein in central nervous system lesions of multiple sclerosis and acute experimental allergic encephalomyelitis, *Ann. Neurol.* **3**:291–298.

Whitaker, J. N., Terry, L. C., and Whetsell, W. O., Jr., 1981, Immunocytochemical localization of cathepsin D in rat neural tissue, *Brain Res.* **216**:109–124.

Wolfgram, F., 1966, A new proteolipid fraction of the nervous system. I. Isolation and amino acid analyses *J. Neurochem.* **35**:461–470.

Wood, J. G., Jean, D. H., Whitaker, J. N., McLaughlin, B. J., and Albers, R. W., 1977, Immunocytochemical localization of the sodium, potassium activated ATPase in knifefish brain, *J. Neurocytol.* **6**:571–581.

Yandrasitz, J. R., Ernst, S. A., and Salganicoff, L., 1976, The subcellular distribution of carbonic anhydrase in homogenates of perfused rat brain, *J. Neurochem.* **17**:707–715.

Zalc, B., Monge, M., and Baumann, N., 1980 Immunohistochemical localization of galactosylceramide and sulfogalactosylceramide in the cerebellum of the quaking, shiverer and jimpy mice, in: *Neurological Mutations Affecting Myelination,* (N. Baumann, ed.), INSERM Symposium No. 14, pp. 263–268, Elsevier/North-Holland, Amsterdam.

Zalc, B., Monge, M., Dupouey, P., Hauw, J. J., and Baumann, N. A., 1981, Immunohistochemical localation of glactosyl and sulfogalactosyl ceramide in the brain of the 30-day-old mouse, *Brain Res.* **211**:341–354.

Zimmerman, T. R., Jr., and Cohen, S. R., 1979, The distribution of myelin basic protein in subcellular fractions of developing jimpy mouse brain, *J. Neurochem.* **32**:817–821.

CHAPTER 5

IN VITRO STUDIES OF OLIGODENDROGLIAL LIPID METABOLISM

DAVID PLEASURE, SEUNG U. KIM, and DONALD H. SILBERBERG

1. INTRODUCTION

The only known function of oligodendroglia at present is to myelinate axons in the CNS. Myelin is a lipid-rich oligodendroglial plasma-membrane derivative containing galactolipids, cholesterol, and phospholipids in a molar ratio of about 1:2:2. *In vivo* studies have established the normal sequences of oligo-dendroglial maturation and myelination and have identified diseases in which initial CNS myelination is not carried to completion, such as phenylketonuria (PKU) and Krabbe's disease, or in which normally myelinated CNS becomes demyelinated, such as multiple sclerosis (MS). Identification of the special metabolic characteristics of oligodendroglia that facilitate and regulate myelin synthesis and myelin maintenance will lead to a better understanding of the pathogenesis of dysmyelinative and demyelinative diseases.

DAVID PLEASURE and DONALD H.SILBERBERG • Children's Hospital of Philadelphia and Departments of Neurology and Pediatrics, University of Pennsylvania, Philadelphia, Pennsylvania 19104   SEUNG U. KIM • Division of Neurology, University of British Columbia, Vancouver, B. C. V6T 1W5, Canada

Tissue-culture techniques have proved useful for studies of oligodendroglial metabolism. The cultured cells can be serially observed in the living state and readily processed for electron microscopy (EM). Concentrations of substrates, cofactors, and hormones can be held at desired levels, and radioactive substrates can be introduced without hindrance by blood–neural barriers or fear of transformation by nonneural tissues.

Myelination *in vitro* was first reported in avian PNS by Peterson and Murray (1955) and in mammalian CNS by Hild (1957). Culture methods used by Bornstein and Murray (1958) were employed for the first EM demonstration of myelination *in vitro* (Ross *et al.*, 1962), to explore the pathogenesis of demyelination in experimental allergic encephalomyelitis (EAE) (Bornstein and Appel, 1961; Kies *et al.*, 1973; Lehrer *et al.*, 1978; Grundke-Iqbal *et al.*, 1981) and of hypomyelination in PKU (Silberberg, 1967) and in mutant mouse strains (Billings-Gagliardi *et al.*, 1980; Bologa-Sandru *et al.*, 1981*b*), to follow synthesis of myelin constituents by use of radioactive precursors (Silberberg *et al.*, 1972; Pleasure and Kim, 1976a; Lehrer *et al.*, 1978; Satomi and Kishimoto, 1981), and to isolate and analyze myelin synthesized *in vitro* (Bradbury and Lumsden, 1979). Dissociated, reaggregate, and reconstituted CNS cultures also form myelin (Yavin and Yavin, 1977; Sheppard *et al.*, 1978; Matthieu *et al.*, 1979; Trapp *et al.*, 1979; Sarlieve *et al.*, 1980; Wood and Bunge, 1980; Seil and Blank, 1981; Okada, 1982; Wood *et al.*, 1983), though not to the same extent as the organotypic CNS explants (Trapp *et al.*, 1979).

In addition to CNS cultures in which net myelin synthesis takes place, a number of other *in vitro* systems are of value for the study of oligodendroglial metabolism. Brain slices have been incubated with radioactive precursors to follow the kinetics of synthesis of myelin lipids (Smith, 1964, 1969, 1973; Maker and Hauser, 1967; Benjamins and Iwata, 1979). Though useful only for short-term experiments, the slices provide larger quantities of tissue for analysis than do CNS cultures. Methods have been devised for purification of oligodendroglia from mammalian cerebrum and for their maintenance in suspension or monolayer culture (Fewster *et al.*, 1967; Fewster and Mead, 1968; Raine *et al.*, 1971; Poduslo and Norton, 1972; Trapp *et al.*, 1975; Chao and Rumsby, 1977; Poduslo *et al.*, 1978; Pleasure *et al.*, 1977, 1979, 1981; McCarthy and de Vellis, 1980; D. S. Snyder *et al.*, 1980; Szuchet *et al.*, 1980; Farooq *et al.*, 1981; Lisak *et al.*, 1981; Gebicke-Harter *et al.*, 1981; Norton *et al.*, 1982; Bhat and Pfeiffer, 1982), and these methods permit analysis of oligodendroglial composition and metabolism free of contributions by other neural-cell types. Gliomas that express galactolipids characteristic of myelin (Dawson *et al.*, 1977; Dawson and Kernes, 1978, 1979; Steck and Perruisseau, 1980; Neskovic *et al.*, 1981) and oligodendrocyte–glioma hybrids that synthesize myelin basic protein, galactocerebroside, and sulfogalactocerebroside

(McMorris *et al.*, 1981) are now available and provide the opportunity to follow metabolic pathways typical of oligodendroglia in continuous cell lines.

In this chapter, data concerning the regulation of oligodendroglial lipid metabolism obtained by tissue-culture methods will be reviewed.

2. GALACTOLIPIDS

Biochemical assay and immunohistological localization of galactolipids synthesized by oligodendroglia and characteristic of myelin [e.g., galactocerebroside (GalCer), GalCer sulfate (sulfatide), monogalactosyl diglyceride] have proved useful in following the course of myelination of CNS *in vitro* and in the unequivocal identification of oligodendrocytes in the cultured tissue (Raff *et al.*, 1978*b*; Fields, 1979; Mirsky *et al.*, 1980; Lisak *et al.*, 1981; Schachner *et al.*, 1981). These galactolipids become detectable by gas chromatographic or liquid chromatographic methods in organotypic CNS cultures prepared from newborn rats or mice and maintained for 9 days or more *in vitro* (Latovitzki and Silberberg, 1973; Satomi and Kishimoto, 1981). The "myelin-marker" galactolipids are also detectable in dissociated cultures prepared from late fetal rat brain and maintained for 10 days or more *in vitro* (Singh and Pfeiffer, 1983). A sialyltransferase catalyzing the synthesis of GM_4 (sialosyl galactosylceramide), a ganglioside characteristic of myelin and oligodendroglia (Yu and Iqbal, 1979), is measurable in dissociated cultures of 15- or 16-day postfertilization mouse cerebrum that have been maintained for 11 days or more (Shanker and Pieringer, 1983).

Indirect immunofluorescence or immunoperoxidase methods show that oligodendroglia purified from calf, ovine, and rat brain express plasma-membrane-surface GalCer (Abramsky *et al.*, 1979; Szuchet *et al.*, 1980; Kennedy *et al.*, 1980; Lisak *et al.*, 1981; Hirayama *et al.*, 1983). No other CNS cell types bind anti-GalCer antibodies (Raff *et al.*, 1978*b*, 1979; Fields, 1979; Mirsky *et al.*, 1980).

GalCer-positive oligodendroglia often contain cytoplasmic myelin basic protein (MBP), as shown by immunochemical methods applied to fixed cells (Mirsky *et al.*, 1980; Lisak *et al.*, 1981). Appearance of cytoplasmic MBP in oligodendroglia in culture has been reported to be later than that of proteolipid protein (PLP) or GalCer (Barbarese and Pfeiffer, 1981; Bologa-Sandru *et al.*, 1981*a*; Herschkowitz *et al.*, 1982; Macklin and Pfeiffer, 1983), whereas *in vivo* immunohistological studies suggest that MBP appears within oligodendroglia prior to detectable PLP (Hartman *et al.*, 1982). It is possible that this discrepancy reflects only a difference in titers of the antisera used in the various laboratories for detection of these "myelin-marker" constituents. The proportion of GalCer-positive cells that also become positive for MBP is markedly reduced in cultures of CNS prepared from the jimpy mouse mutant, suggesting an oligodendroglial maturational arrest in this disease (Bologa-Sandru *et al.*, 1981*b*). The processes extended by cultured oligodendroglia express plasma-membrane-surface GalCer, as does the cell body, and indirect immunofluorescence with antiGalCer antibodies is helpful in visualizing the sheets of membrane synthesized by such cultured cells, which are difficult to appreciate by phase-contrast light microscopy alone (Szuchet *et al.*, 1980: Lisak *et al.*, 1981; Hirayama *et al.*, 1983). Indirect immunofluorescence with antisera direct against sulfoGalCer or GM_3 ganglioside (ceramide-glucose-galactose-N-acetylneuraminic acid) indicates that these galactolipids are also present on the surface of cultured rat oligodendroglia, but not detectable on the surfaces of other cultured rat CNS cells (Raff *et al.*, 1979). The apparent specificity of G_{M3} is surprising, since this is a ubiquitous ganglioside in both nervous and non-nervous tissue.

Chemical analysis indicates that GalCer and sulfo-GalCer are the major glycolipids of oligodendroglia isolated from calf and ovine brains. The ratio of sulfo-GalCer to GalCer in the isolated oligodendroglia is similar to that in myelin (Poduslo and Norton, 1972; Poduslo, 1975; Farooq *et al.*, 1981). The ratio of total galactolipid to total lipid in oligodendroglia, and in oligodendroglial plasma membrane prepared by sucrose-gradient ultracentrifugation, is about half that in CNS myelin (Poduslo and Norton, 1972; Poduslo, 1975; Abe and Norton, 1979; Farooq *et al.*, 1981). Minor oligodendroglial galactolipids include the galactosyl diglycerides and their sulfate esters, esterified GalCer (Kishimoto *et al.*, 1968; Abe and Norton, 1979), and gangliosides (Poduslo and Norton, 1972; Yu and Iqbal, 1979; Szuchet *et al.*, 1980; Mack *et al.*, 1981). Human oligodendroglia, like human CNS myelin, contain GM_4 ganglioside (ceramide-galactose-N-acetylneuraminic acid) (Yu and Iqbal, 1979), and this ganglioside is diminished to undetectable levels in plaques from the brains of patients with MS (Yu *et al.*, 1974).

Oligodendroglia are enriched over whole brain, white matter, and other CNS cell types in activities of the UDP:galactosyl transferases and in GalCer sulfotransferase, and suspension- or monolayer-cultured oligodendroglia incorporate radioactive precursors into the galactolipids (Benjamins *et al.*, 1974; Deshmukh *et al.*, 1974; Poduslo and McKhann, 1977; Pleasure *et al.*, 1977; Poduslo *et al.*, 1978; Szuchet *et al.*, 1980; Mack *et al.*, 1981; also see Chapter 6). Oligodendroglia are also enriched over other CNS cells in specific activities of the lysosomal enzymes that degrade galactolipids (Abe *et al.*, 1979). The recessively inherited diseases in which these enzymes are diminished, sulfo-GalCer sulfatase deficiency in metachromatic leukodystrophy (Morell and Braun, 1972) and galactocerebrosidase deficiency in Krabbe's disease (Suzuki and Suzuki, 1970), are characterized by dysmyelination or demyelination. *In vitro,* ceramide analogues that inhibit galactocerebrosidase cause inhibition of myelination or demyelination in organotypic CNS cultures (Benjamins *et al.,* 1976).

In vitro methods now available should make it possible to answer a number of important questions about oligodendroglial galactolipid metabolism that have not yet been answered: What are the rate-limiting steps in oligodendroglial synthesis of the galactolipids? How are these modulated by contact with neurons?

3. CHOLESTEROL

Under normal circumstances, the rate-limiting step in cholesterol synthesis in oligodendroglia, as in other cell types, is the production of mevalonate by the microsomal enzyme (Maltese and Volpe, 1979a) 3-hydroxy-3-methylglutaryl-coenzyme A reductase (HMG-CoA reductase) (Pleasure and Kim, 1976a; Pleasure *et al.,* 1977, 1979). This enzyme is enriched in oligodendroglia over other CNS cell types (Pleasure *et al.,* 1977) and is present at highest specific activity in organotypic CNS tissue culture at the point when myelination is most rapid (Pleasure and Kim, 1976a,b). The rate of mitochondrial provision of carbons for lipid synthesis can be made rate-limiting for cholesterol synthesis by use of inhibitors of mitochondrial citrate export (Pleasure *et al.,* 1979), and a similar mechanism might diminish CNS cholesterol synthesis in malnutrition.

In most nonneural tissues, activity of HMG-CoA reductase is regulated chiefly by the concentration of low-density lipoprotein (LDL) in the extracellular fluid. Specific receptors for LDL are present on the plasma membranes of such cells. After binding to such receptors, LDL is internalized by the cells by a mechanism involving coated pits, reaches the Golgi–endoplasmic reticulum–lysosomal (GERL) complex and causes the repression of HMG-CoA reductase synthesis. Removal of LDL from the extracellular fluid bathing such cells causes induction of HMG-CoA reductase synthesis, and this results in a 2-fold or greater increase in cholesterol synthesis by the cells within 24 hr (Brown and Goldstein, 1980; Brown *et al.,* 1981).

The LDL-mediated regulation of cholesterol synthesis does not appear to be a significant factor in the modulation of oligodendroglial cholesterol formation. Diminution of LDL concentration in the medium causes a fall, rather than the expected rise, in cholesterol synthesis by organotypic cultures of mouse CNS (Kim and Pleasure, 1978a,b), and LDL does not appear to penetrate the blood–brain barrier *in vivo* (Roheim *et al.,* 1979).

It has been demonstrated that HMG-CoA reductase in brain, as in other tissues, is a substrate for phosphorylation by a microsomal protein kinase, resulting in enzyme inhibition, and for dephosphorylation by a cytosolic protein phosphatase, resulting in reactivation (Beg *et al.,* 1979; Arebalo *et al.,* 1980). A considerable fraction of brain HMG-CoA reductase is in the phosphorylated, inactive form, particularly before the onset of CNS myelination (Saucier and Kandutsch, 1979; Maltese and Volpe, 1979*b*). It has not yet been established whether this phosphorylation–dephosphorylation mechanism has a significant role in the modulation of oligodendroglial cholesterol synthesis (Kleinsek *et al.,* 1980; Arebalo *et al.,* 1981). Inhibition of purified HMG-CoA reductase by very low concentrations of two of its products, free CoA and NADP (Edwards *et al.,* 1980), may also have a role in regulation of its activity in CNS.

Using the mouse glioblastoma C6, Volpe (1979) and Volpe and Obert (1981) demonstrated that HMG-CoA reductase activity is rapidly diminished by agents that depolymerize microtubules or disrupt microfilaments. Cytochalasin D, the antimicrofilament agent, causes the normally long, thick C6 cellular processes to be replaced by much shorter and thinner processes, and this morphological alteration recedes the diminution in HMG-CoA reductase activity, suggesting that the change in cell shape, rather than the agent itself, is responsible for the alteration in cholesterol metabolism. It can be speculated that changes in oligodendroglial shape caused, for example, by the presence of an axonal framework for myelination might similarly have secondary effects on oligodendroglial cholesterol synthesis, but experiments to determine the effects of agents that depolymerize microtubules or disrupt microfilaments on the metabolism of cholesterol by CNS or oligodendroglial cultures have not yet been reported.

4. GLYCEROPHOSPHOLIPIDS

The lipids of oligodendroglia contain more choline glycerophospholipid (CGP) than do those of myelin, and slightly less ethanolamine glycerophospholipid (EGP). Together, these glycerophospholipids make up three quarters of the total oligodendroglial phospholipid, with lesser amounts of serine glycerophospholipid (SGP), inositol glycerophospholipid (IGP), and sphingomyelin (Fewster and Mead, 1968; Poduslo and Norton, 1972; Poduslo, 1975; Pleasure *et al.,* 1981; Farooq *et al.,* 1981). As in myelin (Horrocks, 1967), most EGP in oligodendroglia is alkenylacyl (plasmalogen) or alkylacyl rather than diacyl. However, oligodendroglial alkenylacyl EGP constitutes a smaller proportion of total EGP than in myelin, while alkylacyl EGP, the precursor for alkenylacyl EGP, makes up a greater proportion of oligodendroglial EGP than of myelin EGP (Pleasure *et al.,* 1981). When dissociated cultures prepared from newborn rat cerebrum are incubated with radiolabeled 1-alkyl-*sn*-glycerophosphoethanolamine, acylation to form alkylacyl EGP is rapid, but subsequent transformation to alkenylacyl EGP (ethanolamine plasmalogen) is slow (Witter and Debuch, 1982). Plasmalogenase, which hydrolyzes the alkenyl ether bond of alkenylacyl glycerophospholipids, is present in much higher specific activity in oligodendroglia than in other CNS cells (Dorman *et al.*, 1977).

Cultured oligodendroglia actively incorporate radioactive precursors into the glycerophospholipids. Whereas phospholipid base exchange is a major route for incorporation of bases into glycerophospholipids in disrupted oligodendroglia (Brammer and Carey, 1980), such base exchange appears to be at most a minor pathway for incorporation of ethanolamine into EGP by viable oligodendroglia (Pleasure *et al.*, 1981). As in other tissues, L-serine is an EGP precursor, presumably by decarboxylation of SGP (Pleasure *et al.*, 1981). Transformation of EGP to CGP by methylation is not a quantitatively significant route for CGP synthesis in cultured oligodendroglia, though the presence of this pathway (Hirata *et al.*, 1978; Blusztajn *et al.*, 1979; Schneider and Vance, 1979) at very low activity has not been ruled out (Pleasure *et al.*, 1981). As in nonneural tissues, radioactive precursor studies of purified, cultured oligodendroglia suggest that synthesis of alkylacyl and alkenylacyl EGP proceeds largely via dihydroxyacetone phosphate (Pleasure *et al.*, 1981).

5. SEQUENCE OF MATURATION OF OLIGODENDROGLIA *IN VITRO*

Oligodendroglial maturation in rat optic nerve and corpus callosum *in vivo* has been analyzed by transmission EM, tritiated thymidine ($[^3H]$-TdR) radioautography, and immunochemical and biochemical techniques (Skoff *et al.*, 1976a,b; Tennekoon *et al.*, 1977, 1980; Imamoto *et al.*, 1978). Four stages have been described. The oligodendroblast is first recognizable in rat optic nerve about 16 days postfertilization (5 days before birth). This cell has a cytoplasm of moderate to high density packed with clusters of ribosomes, thin Golgi cisternae, endoplasmic reticulum, and many small mitochondria and microtubules, and is capable of mitosis. The next stage, the "light oligodendrocyte," is the first postmitotic stage in oligodendroglial maturation and has a large, organelle-rich cytoplasm containing stacks of endoplasmic reticulum and bundles of microtubules. Light oligodendrocytes appear 1–2 days before the onset of myelination and remain in this form, as judged by $[^3H]$-TdR kinetics, for about 1 week. The third stage in oligodendroglial maturation, the "medium oligodendrocyte," is smaller than the light oligodendrocyte and has a more densely staining cytoplasm. Medium oligodendroglia remain in this form for about 2 weeks. The "dark oligodendrocyte" is still smaller, with clumped nuclear chromatin and dense cytoplasm that contains fewer mitochondria than previous oligodendrocytes persist indefinitely in the CNS. (See Chapter 1 for a more complete discussion of this subject.)

Galactocerebroside first appears in the tissue at the time of emergence of light oligodendroglia from oligodendroblasts, a few days before the first myelin lamellae are formed. The myelin-lipid-synthetic enzymes GalCer sulfotransferase and UDP galactose:ceramide galactosyl transferase, and other enzymes important in myelin lipid synthesis, such as sphingosine acyltransferase and the microsomal fatty acid chain elongation system, also appear at the time of the oligodendroblast–light oligodendrocyte transition. These enzymes reach peak activities 12 days later, synchronous with the period of most rapid myelin formation (Tennekoon et al., 1980).

Though morphological and radioautographic studies of glial development in culture have not been as detailed as those in vivo, the time–course of development in CNS dissociated culture of oligodendroglia with surface GalCer detectable by indirect immunofluorescence (Raff et al., 1978b; Mirsky et al., 1980; Abney et al., 1981) and of cells that, by EM, resemble mature oligodendroglia and, by [^{3}H]-TdR radioautography, are postmitotic (Rioux et al., 1980) suggests that oligodendroglial maturation in culture is similar to that in the intact animal. With cultures initiated from 3-day-old mouse brain, the number of GalCer-positive cells increases 10-fold from 7 to 14 days in vitro (Bologa-Sandru et al., 1981a). Limiting dilution analysis of dispersed cultures prepared from late fetal rat brain and maintained in vitro for 5 weeks suggested that oligodendroglial progenitor cells undergo about 11 divisions during the course of CNS maturation (Barbarese et al., 1983).

Silberberg and co-investigators (Latovitzki and Silberberg, 1975, 1977; Younkin and Silberberg, 1976; Dorfman et al., 1976; Silberberg et al., 1980) used pulses of 5-bromodeoxyuridine (BUdR), cytosine arabinoside (ARA-C), or sera from rabbits with EAE induced by immunization with whole CNS white matter to perturb oligodendroglial maturation in organotypic rat cerebellum cultures. Glial mitotic activity was visualized by [^{3}H]-TdR autoradiography, and morphological observations and assay for the myelin-lipid-synthetic enzyme UDP-galactose:ceramide galactosyl transferase were used to follow myelin formation. Results indicated that the oligodendroglia responsible for myelin synthesis at 15 days in vitro derive from the terminal mitosis of oligodendroblasts 8 or 9 days earlier. Delay of the transition from oligodendroblast to oligodendrocyte produced by BUdR or ARA-C causes delay in subsequent myelination of the culture. If the nucleotide analogue is added after terminal oligodendroblast mitosis has taken place, however, there is no delay in myelination. The EAE sera, which inhibited myelination and, by morphological criteria, blocked oligodendroglial differentiation (Raine, 1973), proved not to prevent terminal oligodendroblast mitosis, for addition of BUdR or ARA-C after removal of the EAE serum from the medium did not prevent rapid myelination of the cultures.

After selective killing of surface GalCer-positive oligodendroglia in 14-day *in vitro* dissociated cultures of newborn mouse cerebrum by use of anti-GalCer antiserum and complement, surface GalCer-positive oligodendroglia subsequently reappear (Bologa *et al.*, 1982). This observation indicates that oligodendroglial precursor cells that do not express surface GalCer exist in the 14-day *in vitro* cultures and are capable of differentiation to more mature forms. Further, cells that demonstrate both surface GalCer and interior myelin basic protein (MBP) by indirect immunofluorescent visualization reappear in such cultures at a slower rate than do GalCer-positive, MBP-negative oligodendroglia, suggesting that the MBP-negative cells are precursors from the MBP-positive ones (Bologa *et al.*, 1982).

Few cells in the oligodendroglial line past the oligodendroblast take up [^{3}H]-TdR either *in vivo* or in culture (Rioux *et al.*, 1980; Pruss *et al.*, 1982). Two exceptions to this generalization have been reported. Herndon *et al.*, (1977) found that as many as half the oligodendroglia in regions of mouse brain remyelinating after demyelination induced by the hepatitis virus JHM take up [^{3}H]-TdR. Pruss *et al.*, (1982) noted that occasional oligodendroglia harvested from long-term monolayer cultures of neonatal rat brain take up [^{3}H]-TdR when placed on a feeder layer of irradiated Swiss 3T3 cells. It remains to be established whether such cells are derived from oligodendroglial precursors latent in the tissue or are mature oligodendroglia that have regained the capacity to proliferate.

While myelination requires axons, transformation of oligodendroblasts to oligodendrocytes does not. This conclusion emerges from studies by McCarthy and de Vellis (1980). Cells were dissociated from newborn rat cerebrum and seeded in monolayer. Neurons did not survive, but GalCer- and MBP-positive oligodendroglia (Barbarese and Pfeiffer, 1981) gradually accumulated on the surface of the dense astroglial basal layer and could be harvested by vigorous shaking of the flasks. Though neurons are not necessary for the oligodendroblast–oligodendrocyte transition, it appears that neurons facilitate this transition, since GalCer-positive, MBP-positive cells emerge more rapidly in dissociated mouse brain cell cultures that contain neurons than in cultures without neurons (Bologa *et al.*, 1983).

6. COMPARISON OF THE BEHAVIOR OF OLIGODENDROGLIA AND SCHWANN CELLS *IN VITRO*

Both oligodendroglia and Schwann cells can myelinate both central and peripheral axons (Aguayo *et al.*, 1978; Weinberg and Spencer, 1979; Wood *et al.,* 1980, 1983; Okada, 1982). Behavior of these two myelin-forming cell types in culture differs in two major respects. Schwann cells cultured without axons lose "myelin-marker" features such as surface GalCer and interior P_1 and P_2 basic proteins and P_0 glycoprotein within a week *in vitro* (Mirsky *et al.,* 1980; Kennedy *et al.,* 1980; Kreider *et al.,* 1981), while oligodendroglia retain surface GalCer and interior myelin basic protein for several months in the absence of neurons (Mirsky *et al.,* 1980; Szuchet *et al.,* 1980; Lisak *et al.,* 1981). Whereas few oligodendroglia take up [^{3}H]-TdR, Schwann cells do proliferate in culture, and the rate of their division can be increased by contact with axons or axonal fragments (Wood and Bunge, 1975; Salzer and Bunge, 1980; Salzer *et al.,* 1980) or by addition of a pituitary growth factor (Brockes *et al.,* 1980) and cholera toxin (Raff *et al.,* 1978a) to the medium (Kreider *et al.,* 1982).

7. IS THERE A "CRITICAL PERIOD OF MYELINATION" *IN VITRO*?

Initial CNS myelination *in vivo* occurs during a relatively brief period. In humans, this is during the third trimester of gestation and first year of life. In rat optic nerve, myelination begins a week after birth and proceeds rapidly for several weeks (Tennekoon *et al.,* 1980). Myelination of organotypic explants prepared from mouse or rat cerebellum or spinal cord follows a similar temporal pattern. EM, assays for constituent characteristics of myelin, such as 2′,3′-cyclic nucleotide-3′-phosphohydrolase galactolipids, and cholesterol, and measurements of rates of incorporation of radioactive precursors into myelin lipids and specific activities of myelin-lipid-synthetic enzymes yield results comparable to or slightly below those in the intact animal (Fry *et al.,* 1972; Silberberg *et al.,* 1972; Latovitzki and Silberberg, 1973, 1975; Pleasure and Kim, 1976a,b; Satomi and Kishimoto, 1981). Also, the formation of immunohistologically identifiable oligodendroglia from their progenitors in dissociated cultures of embryonic rat brain occurs chronologically in parallel with that observed *in vivo* (Abney *et al.,* 1981). Thus, the "critical period of myelination" *in vitro* is similar to that *in vivo*. Furthermore, because the cultures used in these studies were prepared from late fetal or newborn mice and rats a week or more before myelination was scheduled to begin *in vivo,* triggering of the oligodendroblast–oligodendrocyte transition and of myelination in culture must be either by a mechanism resident in the cultured CNS tissue or, alternatively, the endpoint of a process beginning a week or more previously *in vivo,* for example, the initiation of terminal differentiation of oligodendroblasts.

8. MINIMAL REQUIREMENTS FOR FORMATION OF MYELIN *IN VITRO*

No artificial substitutes for axons have thus far been successful in evoking myelination (Raine, 1973). However, purified oligodendroglia cultured in monolayer in the absence of axons do form sheets of redundant plasma membrane (Szuchet *et al.,* 1980; Lisak *et al.,* 1981).

What medium constituents are required for myelination? The first investigator to achieve myelination in CNS in culture (Hild, 1957) used a medium containing embryo extract and human ascites fluid. It was soon established that neither of these components is necessary for myelination, but that serum must be present for myelination to proceed *in vitro* at a rate similar to that in the intact animal. Diminution in medium serum concentration from 15% (vol./vol.) to 10 or 5% retards myelination, as does extraction of lipids from the serum (Kim and Pleasure, 1978*a,b*), and removal of serum from the medium causes cessation of myelination (Satomi and Kishimoto, 1981).

The use of serum precludes total definition of the culture medium. Substrates, hormones, trophic factors, immunoglobulins, and other compounds that might affect myelination and oligodendroglial metabolism are present in the serum in concentrations difficult to measure. Variations in content of these unmeasured or undefined compounds are probably responsible for the ability of some sera to support myelination well while others from animals of the same age and species do not.

Clearly, identification of factors that regulate oligodendroglial metabolism and that are important in myelin synthesis and maintenance would be more straightforward if a medium free of serum but able to sustain oligodendroglial viability and myelination were devised. Progress has been made with other tissues (Barnes and Sato, 1980), and it is now possible to maintain neuroblastoma (Bottenstein and Sato, 1979), normal neurons (E. Y. Snyder and Kim, 1979; Bottenstein *et al.,* 1980), rat C6 glioma (Wolfe *et al.,* 1980), and mouse and rat Schwann cells (Manthorpe *et al.,* 1980; Dubois-Dalcq *et al.,* 1981; Sobue *et al.,* 1983) in a totally defined medium. Two reports of CNS myelination *in vitro* in a chemically defined medium have been published (Honegger *et al.,* 1979; Kleinschmidt and Bunge, 1980). In each instance, myelination was considerably delayed in onset and diminished in magnitude.

Thyroid hormones and glucocorticoids have effects on the synthesis of myelin lipids and are likely to be among the factors important for support of myelination. This topic is discussed in detail in Chapter 8 and is therefore only outlined here. Hypothyroidism induces a lag in myelination in the intact animal (Walravens and Chase, 1969; Mantzos *et al.,* 1973; Flynn *et al.,* 1977). *In vitro,* use of serum from hypothyroid rather than normal animals causes a

decreased incorporation of radiolabeled precursors into galactolipids, and sup-
plementation of the medium with triiodothyronine restores synthesis of these
lipids to control values (Bhat *et al.,* 1979, 1981).

In vivo, adrenalectomy of 14-day-old rats causes a diminution in the
extent of CNS myelination, though adrenalectomy of rats 16 days old or older
does not (Preston and McMorris, 1983). *In vitro,* addition of glucocorticoids to
the medium stimulates sulfatide synthesis by G26 glioma (Dawson and Kernes,
1978, 1979). Glucocorticoids also induce glycerol phosphate dehydrogenase
(GPDH) activity in C6 glioma (McGinnis and deVellis, 1978) and rat brain-
cell cultures (Breen and deVellis, 1974). Oligodendroglia are enriched in
GPDH (Leveille *et al.,* 1980: Cammer *et al.,* 1982; Cammer and Zimmerman,
1983), and this enzyme may be of importance as a source for glycerol phosphate for synthesis of myelin glycerophospholipids (Laatsch, 1962).

9. MAJOR SUBSTRATES FOR SYNTHESIS OF MYELIN
   LIPIDS

There is an extensive literature on the substrates utilized by brain *in vivo*
as a function of species and stage of development, but little work has been done
in vitro to establish the substrates preferred by oligodendroglia for lipid synthesis. It has long been felt that myelination in tissue culture is favored by
enrichment of the medium with D-glucose, and dissociated cultures of CNS
maintained in a medium containing very low D-glucose concentrations show
sharply diminished numbers of cells having surface galactocerebroside (Zuppinger *et al.,* 1981). Radioactive D-galactose is an efficient precursor for radio-
labeling of oligodendroglial and myelin galactolipids (Poduslo and McKhann,
1977; Mack and Szuchet, 1981; Mack *et al.,* 1981), but UDP-galactose-4'-
epimerase is present in glial cells (Neskovic *et al.,* 1981), and the quantitative
significance of galactose as a galactolipid precursor remains to be established.

The ketone bodies D-(-)-β-hydroxybutyrate and acetoacetate are major
precursors for lipid synthesis by CNS during the "critical period of myelination" *in vivo* (DeVivo *et al.,* 1973; Buckley and Williamson, 1973; Edmond,
1974: Yeh *et al.,* 1977). Experiments with isolated oligodendroglia indicated
that like liver and other active lipid-synthesizing tissues (Stern, 1971), these
cells are able to incorporate acetoacetate into lipids by a cytoplasmic pathway
dependent on the presence of acetoacetyl-CoA synthetase, an enzyme enriched
in oligodendroglia (Pleasure *et al.,* 1979).

Isolated oligodendroglia readily take up radioactively labeled fatty acids
and are able to perform fatty acid chain elongation and desaturation (Cohen
and Bernsohn, 1973; Fewster *et al.,* 1975). Inhibition of myelination by organotypic CNS cultures in media made up with delipidated serum or in the

absence of serum may reflect a requirement for such exogenous fatty acids for myelin synthesis (Kim and Pleasure, 1978b; Satomi and Kishimoto, 1981), but the relative quantitative significances of endogenous and exogenous fatty acid syntheses for myelination have not been established.

10. PRECURSOR–PRODUCT RELATIONSHIPS BETWEEN OLIGODENDROGLIAL AND MYELIN LIPIDS

Purified oligodendroglia in suspension or monolayer culture synthesize galactolipids, cholesterol, and the phospholipids (Benjamins *et al.*, 1974; Deshmukh *et al.*, 1974; Fewster *et al.*, 1975; Poduslo and McKhann, 1977; Poduslo *et al.*, 1978; Pleasure *et al.*, 1977, 1979, 1981; Szuchet *et al.*, 1980), and the oligodendroglial plasma membrane, isolated by sucrose-gradient ultracentrifugation, has resemblances to myelin in lipid composition (Poduslo, 1975). Direct demonstration of a precursor-to-intermediary-to-product relationship between a lipid in oligodendroglial endoplasmic reticulum and Golgi apparatus, the lipid in oligodendroglial plasma membrane, and the lipid in myelin has not yet been accomplished. Such a demonstration, to be definitive, would require serial determinations of specific activity of the lipid in each of these oligodendroglial compartments during continuous labeling or pulse–chase with a radioactive precursor.

Lacking direct evidence for a precursor–product relationship between lipids synthesized by oligodendroglia and those deposited in myelin, indirect and partial data relevant to this point must be considered. Since galactocerebroside and the galactoglycerolipids are restricted to myelin and myelin-forming oligodendroglia and Schwann cells, and since cultured oligodendroglia actively incorporate radioactive precursors into these lipids and contain measurable activities and enzymes required for their synthesis, it is unlikely that these lipids are derived from other sources. But since UDP-galactose:ceramide galactosyl transferase is present in CNS myelin (Costantino-Ceccarini and Suzuki, 1975), it is possible that some of the processing required for synthesis of the myelin galactolipids takes place in myelin itself, rather than in the oligodendroglial endoplasmic reticulum and Golgi apparatus (Benjamins and Iwata, 1979).

In ovo experiments indicate that the cholesterol required for myelination of chick CNS is synthesized endogenously in brain, not derived from nonneural tissues (Connor *et al.*, 1969). The demonstration that the cholesterol biosynthesis inhibitor *trans*-1,4-*bis*(2-chlorobenzylaminomethyl)cyclohexane (AY9944) retards the myelination of organotypic cultures of fetal mouse spinal cord despite the presence of abundant cholesterol in the medium (Kim, 1975) suggests that cholesterol synthesized endogenously in brain by oligodendroglia is also necessary for myelination in mammals. The rapid disappearance of desmosterol from CNS myelin *in vivo* after maturation of demosterol reductase activity (Kritchevsky *et al.*, 1965) suggests that there is a rapid interchange of sterol between myelin and oligodendroglial microsomes. Whether such interchanges (Banik and Davison, 1971) must pass through an intermediary oligodendroglial plasma membrane sterol pool has not been established.

The origins of CNS myelin glycerophospholipids are less well understood than are those of the other lipid classes in myelin. Effects of inhibitors of glycerophospholipid synthesis on myelination *in vitro* in the presence of adequate supplies of exogenous glycerophospholipid have not been reported. Such a study would be useful in establishing the significance of endogenous oligodendroglial glycerophospholipid synthesis for the formation of myelin, since the glycerophospholipids, unlike the galactolipids, are abundant in all CNS cell types. *In vivo* experiments indicating that the half-lives of the glycerophospholipid bases are shorter in microsomes and longer in myelin are compatible with a precursor–product relationship between these compartments (Miller *et al.*, 1977). Several of the enzymes required for glycerophospholipid synthesis are present in myelin as well as in other subcellular fractions in brain (Deshmukh *et al.*, 1978; Wu and Ledeen, 1980). Oligodendroglia are enriched in alkylacyl glycerophosphatidylethanolamine (Pleasure *et al.*, 1981), and it is likely that this lipid is the precursor for the major myelin glycerophospholipid, ethanolamine plasmalogen (alkenylacyl glycerophosphatidylethanolamine) (Horrocks, 1967).

11. CONCLUSIONS

It is now possible to maintain viable oligodendroglia *in vitro* in the presence or absence of other cell types for long periods. By application of radioisotopic, immunochemical, and enzyme-assay techniques, oligodendroglial metabolism of lipids characteristic of myelin can conveniently be studied. Using techniques available at present, much has been learned about the composition of oligodendroglia and about pathways for synthesis and degradation of oligodendroglial lipids. The next major challenge is to identify control mechanisms that regulate oligodendroglial metabolism and permit myelin synthesis and maintenance.

ACKNOWLEDGMENTS

The help of R. P. Lisak is appreciated. The authors' research reported herein is supported by grants from the National MS Society, Muscular Dystrophy Association, and the National Institutes of Health (HD-08536, NS-11037, and NS-08075).

12. REFERENCES

Abe, T., and Norton, W. T., 1979, The characterization of sphingolipids of oligodendroglia from calf brain, *J. Neurochem.* **32**:823–832.

Abe, T., Miyatake, T., Norton, W. T., and Suzuki, K., 1979, Activities of glycolipid hydrolases in neurons and astroglia from rat and calf brains and in oligodendroglia from calf brain, *Brain Res.* **161**:179–182.

Abney, E. R., Bartlett, P. B., and Raff, M. C., 1981, Astrocytes, ependymal cells, and oligodendrocytes develop on schedule in dissociated cell cultures of embryonic rat brain, *Dev. Biol.* **83**:301–310.

Abramsky, O., Lisak, R. P., Silberberg, D. H., Brenner, T., and Pleasure, D., 1979, Immune response to isolated oligodendrocytes, *J. Neurol. Sci.* **43**:157–167.

Aguayo, A. J., Dickson, R., Trecarten, J., Attiwell, M., Bray, G. M., and Richardson, P., 1978, Ensheathment and myelination of regenerating PNS fibres by transplanted optic nerve glia, *Neurosci. Lett.* **9**:97–104.

Arebalo, R. E., Hardgrave, J. E., Noland, B. J., and Scallen, T. J., 1980, *In vivo* regulation of rat liver 3-hydroxy-3-methylglutaryl coenzyme A reductase: Enzyme phosphorylation as an early regulatory response after intragastric administration of mevalonolactone, *Proc. Natl. Acad. Sci. U.S.A.* **77**:6429–6433.

Arebalo, R. E., Hardgrave, J. E., and Scallen, T. J., 1981, The *in vivo* reguation of rat liver 3-hydroxy–methylglutaryl coenzyme A reductase: Phosphorylation of the enzyme as an early regulatory response following cholesterol feeding, *J. Biol. Chem.* **256**:571–574.

Banik, N. L., and Davison, A. N., 1971, Exchange of sterols between myelin and other membranes of developing rat brain, *Biochem. J.* **122**:751–758.

Barbarese, E., and Pfeiffer, S. E., 191, Developmental regulation of myelin basic protein in dispersed cultures, *Proc. Natl. Acad. Sci. U.S.A.* **78**:1953–1957.

Barbarese, E., Pfeiffer, S. E., and Carson, J. H., 1983, Progenitors of oligodendrocytes: Limiting dilution analysis in fetal rat brain culture, *Dev. Biol.* **96**:84–88.

Barnes, D., and Sato, G., 1980, Methods for growth of cultured cells in serum-free medium, *Anal. Biochem.* **102**:255–270.

Beg, Z. H., Stonik, J. A., and Brewer, H. B. Jr., 1979, Characterization and regulation of reductase kinase, a protein kinase that modulates the enzyme activity of 3-hydroxy-3-methylglutaryl-coenzyme A reductase, *Proc. Natl. Acad. Sci. U.S.A.* **76**:4375–4379.

Benjamins, J.A., and Iwata, R., 1979, Kinetics of entry of galactolipids and phospholipids into myelin, *J. Neurochem.* **32**:921–926.

Benjamins, J. A., Guarnieri, M., Miller, K., Sonneborn, M., and McKhann, G. M., 1974, Sulphatide synthesis in isolated oligodendroglia and neuronal cells, *J. Neurochem.* **23**:751–757.

Benjamins, J. A., Fitch, J., and Radin, N. S., 1976, Effects of ceramide analogs on myelinating organ cultures, *Brain Res.* **102**:267–281.

Bhat, S., and Pfeiffer, S. E., 1982, Myelinogenic gene expression intrinsic to cultured oligodendrocytes, *Trans. Am. Soc. Neurochem.* **13**:154 (abstract).

Bhat, N. R., Sarlieve, L. L., Subba Rao, G., and Pieringer, R. A., 1979, Investigations on myelination *in vitro:* Regulation by thyroid hormone in cultures of dissociated brain cells from embryonic mice, *J. Biol. Chem.* **254**:9342–9344.

Bhat, N. R., Subba Rao, G., and Pieringer, R. A., 1981, Investigations on myelination *in vitro:* Regulation of sulfolipid synthesis by thryoid hormone in cultures of dissociated brain cells from embryonic mice, *J. Biol. Chem.* **256:**1167–1171.

Billings-Gagliardi, S., Adcock, L. H., Schwing, G. B., and Wolf, M. K., 1980, Hypomyelinated mutant mice. II. Myelination *in vitro, Brain Res.* **200:**135–150.

Blusztajn, J. K., Zeisel, S. H., and Wurtman, R. J., 1979, Synthesis of lecithin (phosphatidyl choline) from phosphatidylethanolamine in bovine brain, *Brain Res.* **179:**319–327.

Bologa, L., Z'Graggen, A., Rossi, E., and Herschkowitz, N., 1982, Differentiation and proliferation: Two possible mechanisms for the regeneration of oligodendrocytes in culture, *J. Neurol. Sci.* **57:**419–434.

Bologa, L., Bisconte, J. C., Joubert, R., Marangos, P. J., Derbin, C., Rioux, F., and Herschkowitz, N., 1983, Accelerated differentiation of oligodendrocytes in neuronal-rich embryonic mouse brain cell cultures, *Brain Res.* **252:**129–136.

Bologa-Sandru, L., Siegrist, H. P., Z'Graggen, A., Hofmann, K., Wiesmann, U., Dahl, D., and Herschkowitz, N., 1981*a*, Expression of antigenic markers during the development of oligodendrocytes in mouse brain cell cultures, *Brain Res.* **210:**217–229.

Bologa-Sandru, L., Zalc, B., Herschkowitz, N., and Baumann, N., 1981*b*, Oligodendrocytes of Jimpy mice express galactosylceramide: An immunofluorescence study of brain sections and dissociated brain cell cultures, *Brain Res.* **225:**425–430.

Bornstein, M. B., and Appel, S. H., 1961, The application of tissue culture to the study of experimental "allergic" encephalomyelitis. I. Patterns of demyelination, *J. Neuropathol. Exp. Neurol.* **20:**141*157.*

Bornstein, M. B., and Murray, M. R., 1958, Serial observations of growth, myelin formation, maintenance and degeneration in cultures of newborn rat and kitten cerebellum, *J. Biophys. Biochem. Cytol.* **4:**499–504.

Bottenstein, J. E., and Sato, G. H., 1979, Growth of a rat neuroblastoma cell line in serum-free supplemented medium, *Proc. Natl. Acad. Sci. U.S.A.* **76:**514–517.

Bottenstein, J. E., Skaper, S. K., Varon, S. S., and Sato, G. H., 1980, Selective survival of neurons from chick embryo sensory ganglionic dissociates utilizing serum-free supplemented medium, *Exp. Cell Res.***125:**183–190.

Bradbury, K., and Lumsden, C. E., 1979, The chemical composition of myelin in organ cultures of rat cerebellum, *J. Neurochem.* **32:**145–154.

Brammer, M. J., and Carey, S. G., 1980, Incorporation of choline and inositol into phospholipids of isolated oligodendrocyte perikaya, *J. Neurochem.* **35:**873–879.

Breen, G., and de Vellis, J., 1974, Regulation of glycerol phosphate dehydrogenase by rat cerebral cell cultures, *Dev. Biol.* **41:**255–266.

Brockes, J. P., Lemke, G. E., and Balzer, D. R., Jr., 1980, Purification and preliminary characterization of a glial growth factor from the bovine pituitary, *J. Biol. Chem.* **255:**8374–8377.

Brown, M. S., and Goldstein, J. L., 1980, Multivalent feedback regulation of HMG CoA reductase, a control mechanism coordinating isoprenoid synthesis and cell growth, *J. Lipid Res.* **21:**505–517.

Brown, M. S., Kovanen, P. T., and Goldstein, J. L., 1981, Regulation of plasma cholesterol by lipoprotein receptors, *Science* **212:**628–635.

Buckley B. M., and Williamson, D. H., 1973, Acetoacetate and brain lipogenesis: Developmental pattern of acetoacetyl-coenzyme A synthetase in the soluble fraction of rat brain, *Biochem. J.* **132:**653–656.

Crammer, W., and Zimmerman, T. R., Jr., 1983, Glycerol phosphate dehydrogenase, glucose-6-phosphate dehydrogenase, lactate dehydrogenase and carbonic anhydrase activities in oligodendrocytes and myelin: Comparisons between species and CNS regions, *Dev. Brain Res.* 6:21–26.

Crammer, W., Snyder, D. S., Zimmerman, T. R., Jr., Farooq, M., and Norton, W. T., 1982, Glycerol phosphate dehydrogenase, glucose-6-phosphate dehydrogenase, and lactate dehydrogenase: Activities in oligodendrocytes, neurons, astrocytes, and myelin isolated from developing rat brains, *J. Neurochem.* 38:i360–367.

Chao, S. W., and Rumsky, M. D., 1977, Preparation of astrocytes, neurons and oligodendrocytes from the same rat brain, *Brain Res.* 124:347–351.

Cohen, S. R., and Bensohn, J., 1973, Incorporation of 1-^{14}C labelled fatty acids into isolated neuronal soma, astroglia and oligodendroglia from calf brain, *Brain Res.* 60:521–525.

Connor, W., Johnston, R., and Lin, D., 1969, Metabolism of cholesterol in the tissues and blood of the chick embryo, *J. Lipid Res.* 10:388–394.

Costantino-Ceccarini, E., and Suzuki, K., 1975, Evidence for presence of UDP-glactose:ceramide galactsyl transferase in rat myelin, *Brain Res.* 93:358–362.

Dawson, G., and Kernes, S. M., 1978, Induction of sulfogalactosylceramide (sulfatide) synthesis by hydrocortisone (cortisol) in mouse G-26 oligodendroglioma cell strains. *J. Neurochem.* 31:1091–1094.

Dawson, G., and Kernes, S. M., 1979, Mechanism of action of hydrocortisone potentiation of sulfogalactosyl ceramide synthesis in mouse oligodendroglioma clonal cell lines, *J. Biol. Chem.* 254:163–167.

Dawson, G., Sundarra, J. N., and Pfeiffer, S. E., 1977, Synthesis of myelin glycosphingolipids [galactosylceramide and galactosyl (3-0-sulfate) ceramide (sulfatide)] by cloned cell lines derived from mouse neurotumors, *J. Biol. Chem.* 252:2777–2779.

Deshmukh, D. S., Flynn, T. J., and Pieringer, R. A., 1974, The biosynthesis and concentration of galactosyl diglyceride in glial and neuronal enriched fractions of actively myelinating rat brain, *J. Neurochem.* 22:479–485.

Deshmukh, D. S., Bear, W. D., and Brockerhoff, H., 1978, Polyphosphoinositide biosynthesis in three subfractions of rat brain myelin, *J. Neurochem.* 30:1191–1193.

DeVivo, D. C., Fishman, M. A., and Agrawal, H. C., 1973, Preferential labelling of brain cholesterol by (3-^{14}C)-D-(-)-3-hydroxybutyrate, *Lipids* 8:649–651.

Dorfman, S. H., Holtzer, H., and Silberberg, D. H., 1976, Effect of 5-bromo-2'-deoxyuridine or cytosine-beta-D-arabinofuranoside hydrochloride on myelination in newborn rat cerebellum cultures following removal of myelination inhibiting antiserum to whole cord or cerebroside, *Brain Res.* 104:283–294.

Dorman, R. V., Toews, A. D., and Horrocks, L. A., 1977, Plasmalogenase activities in neuronal perikarya, astroglia, and oligodendroglia isolated from bovine brain, *J. Lipid Res.* 18:115–117.

Dubois-Dalcq, M., Rentier, B., Baron, A., van Evercooren, N., and Burge, B. W., 1981, Structure and behavior of rat primary and secondary Schwann cells *in vitro, Exp. Cell Res.* 131:283–297.

Edmond, J., 1974, Ketone bodies as precursors of sterols and fatty acids in the developing rat, *J. Biol. Chem.* 249:72–80.

Edwards, P. A., Lemongello, D., Kane, J., Shechter, I., and Fogelman, A. M., 1980, Properties of purified rat hepatic 3-hydroxy-3-methylglutaryl coenzyme A reductase and regulation of enzyme activity, *J. Biol Chem.* 255:3715–3725.

Farooq, M., Cammer, W., Snyder, D. S., Raine, C. S., and Norton, W. T., 1981, Properties of bovine oligodendroglia isolated by a new procedure using physiologic conditions, *J. Neurochem.* 36:431–440.

Fewster, M. E., and Mead, J. F., 1968, Lipid composition of glial cells isolated from bovine white matter, *J. Neurochem.* 15:1041–1052.

Fewster, M. E., Scheibel, A. B., and Mead, J. F., 1967, The preparation of isolated glial cells from rat and bovine white matter, *Brain Res.* **6**:401–408.

Fewster, M. E., Ihrig, T., and Mead, J. R., 1975, Biosynthesis of long chain fatty acids by oligodendroglia isolated from bovine white matter, *J. Neurochem.* **25**:207–213.

Fields, K. L., 1979, Cell type-specific antigens of cells of the central and peripheral nervous system, *Cur. Top. Dev. Biol.* **13**:237–257.

Flynn, T. J., Deshmukh, D. S., and Pieringer, R. A., 1977, Effects of altered thyroid function of galactosyl diacylglycerol metabolism in myelinating rat brain, *J. Biol. Chem.* **252**:5864–5870.

Fry, J. M., Lehrer, G. M., and Bornstein, M. B., 1972, Sulfatide synthesis: Inhibition by experimental allergic encephalomyelitis serum, *Science* **175**:192–194.

Gebicke-Harter, P. J., Althaus, H. H., Schwartz, P., and Neuhoff, V., 1981, Oligodendrocytes from postnatal cat brain in cell culture. I. Regeneration and maintenance, Dev. Brain Res. **1**:497–518.

Grundke-Iqbal, I., Raine, C. S., Johnson, A. B., Brosnan, C. F., and Bornstein, M. B., 1981, Experimental allergic encephalomyelitis: Characterization of serum factors causing demyelination and swelling of myelin, *J. Neurol. Sci.* **50**:63–79.

Hartman, B. K., Agrawal, H. C., Agrawal, D., and Kalmbach, S., 1982, Development and maturation of central nervous sytem myelin: Comparison of immunohistochemical localization of proteolipid protein and basic protein in myelin and oligodendrocytes, *Proc. Natl. Acad. Sci. U.S.A.* **79**:4217–4220.

Herndon, R. M., Price. D. L., and Weiner, L. P., 1977, Regeneration of oligodendroglia during recovery from demyelinating disease, *Science* **195**:693–694.

Herschkowitz, N. Bologa, L., and Siegrist, H. P., 1982, Characterization of mouse oligodendrocytes during development, *Trans. Am. Soc. Neurochem.* **13**:173 (abstract).

Hild, W., 1957, Myelinogensis in cultures of mammalian central nervous tissue, *Z. Zellforsch.* **46**:71–95.

Hirata, F., Viveros, O. H., Diliberto, E. J., Jr., and Axelrod, J., 1978, Identification and properties of two methyl transferases in conversion of phosphatidyl ethanolamine to phosphatidyl choline, *Proc. Natl. Acad. Sci. U.S.A.* **75**:1718–1721.

Hirayama, M., Silberberg, D. H., Lisak, R. P., and Pleasure, D., 1983, Long-term culture of oligodendrocytes isolated from rat corpus callosum by Percoll density gradient—lysis by polyclonal antigalactocerebroside serum, *J. Neuropath. Exp. Neurol.* **42**:16–28.

Honegger, P., Lenoir, D., and Favrod, P., 1979, Growth and differentiation of aggregating fetal brain cells in a serum-free defined medium, *Nature (London)* **282**:305–308.

Horrocks, L. A., 1967, Composition of myelin from peripheral and central nervous systems of the squirrel monkey, *J. Lipid Res.* **8**:569–576.

Imamoto, K., Paterson, J. A., and LeBlond, C. P., 1978, Radioautographic investigation of gliogenesis in the corpus callosum of young rats. I. Sequential changes in oligodendrocytes, *J. Comp. Neurol.* **180**:115–138.

Kennedy, P. G E., Lisak, R. P., and Raff, M. C., 1980, Cell type-pecific markers for human glial and neuronal cells in culture, *Lab Invest.* **43**:342–351.

Kies, M. W., Driscoll, B. F., Seil, F. J., and Alvord, E. C., Jr., 1973, Myelination inhibition factor: Dissociation from induction of experimental allergic encephalomyelitis, *Science* **179**:689–690.

Kim, S. U., 1975, Effects of the cholesterol biosynthesis inhibitor AY9944 on organotypic cultures of mouse spinal cord: Retarded myelinogenesis and induction of cytoplasmic inclusions, *Lab. Invest.* **32**:720–728.

Kim, S. U., and Pleasure, D. E., 1978a, Tissue culture analysis of neurogensis: Myelination and synapse formation are retarded by serum deprivation, *Brain Res.* **145**:15–25.

Kim, S. U., and Pleasure, D. E., 1978*b*, Tissue culture analysis of neurogenesis. II. Lipid-free medium retards myelination in mouse spinal cord cultures, *Brain Res.* 157:206–211.

Kishimoto, Y., Wajda, M., and Radin, N. S., 1968, 6-Acyl galactosyl ceramides of pig brain: Structure and fatty acid composition, *J. Lipid Res.* 9:27–33.

Kleinschmidt, D., and Bunge, R. P., 1980, Myelination in cultures of embryonic rat spinal cord grown in a serum-free medium, *J. Cell Biol.* 87:66 (abstract).

Kleinsek, D. A., Jabalquinto, A. M., and Porter, J. W., 1980, *In vivo* and *in vitro* mechanisms regulating rat liver beta-hydroxy-beta-methylglutaryl coenzyme A reductase activity, *J. Biol. Chem.* 255:3918–3923.

Kreider, B., Messing, A., Doan, H., Kim, S. U., Lisak, R. P., and Pleasure, D., 1981, Enrichment of Schwann cell cultures from neonatal rat sciatic nerve by differential adhesion, *Brain Res.* 207:433–444.

Kreider, B. Q., Corey-Bloom, J., Lisak, R. P., Doan, H., and Pleasure, D. E., 1982, Stimulation of mitosis of cultured rat Schwann cells isolated by differential adesion, *Brain Res.* 237:238–243.

Kritchevsky, D., Tepper, S. A., DiTullio, N. W., and Holmes, W. L., 1965, Desmosterol in developing rat brain, *J. Am. Oil Chem. Soc.* 42:1024–1028.

Laatsch, R. H., 1962, Glycerol phosphate dehydrogenase activity of developing rat central nervous system, *J. Neurochem.* 9:487–492.

Latovitzki, N., and Silberberg, D. H., 1973, Quantification of galactolipids in myelinating cultures of rat cerebellum, *J. Neurochem.* 20:1771–1776.

Latovitzki, N., and Silberberg, D. H., 1975, Ceramide glycosyltransferases in cultured rat cerebellum: Changes with age, with demyelination, and with inibition of myelination by 5-bromo-2'-deoxyuridine of experimental allergic encephalomyelitis serum, *J. Neurochem.* 24:1017–1022.

Latovitzki, N., and Silberberg, D. H., 1977, UDP-galactose:ceramide galactosyl transferase and 2',3'-cyclic nucleotide 3'-phosphohydrolase activities in cultured newborn rat cerebellum: Association with myelination and concurrent susceptibility to 5-bromodeoxyuridine, *J. Neurochem.* 29:611–614.

Lehrer, G. M., Maker, H. S., Silides, D. J., Weiss, C., and Bornstein, M. B., 1978, Antiwhole white matter serum inhibits incorporation of glucose and galactose into the lipids of myelinating spinal cord cultures, *J. Neurochem.* 30:247–251.

Leveille, P. J., McGinnis, J. F., Maxwell, D. S., and de Vellis, J., 1980, Immunocytochemical localization of glycerol-3-phosphate dejydrogenase in rat oligodendrocytes, *Brain Res.* 196:287–305.

Lisak, R. P., Pleasure, D. E., Silberberg, D. H., Manning, M. C., and Saida, T., 1981, Long-term culture of bovine oligodendroglia isolated with a Percoll gradient, *Brain Res.* 223:107–122.

Mack, S. R., and Szuchet, S., 1981, Synthesis of myelin glycosphingolipids by isolated oligodendrocytes in tissue culture, *Brain Res.* 214:180–185.

Mack, S. R., Szuchet, S., and Dawson, G., 1981, Synthesis of gangliosides by cultured oligodendrocytes, *J. Neurosci. Res.* 6:361–367.

Macklin, W. B., and Pfeiffer, S. E., 1983, Myelin proteolipid time course in primary cultures of fetal rat brain, *Trans. Am. Neurochem. Soc.* 14:212.

Maker, H. S., and Hauser, G., 1967, Incorporation of glucose carbon into gangliosides and cerebrosides by slices of developing rat brain, *J. Neurochem.* 14:457–464.

Maltese, W. A., and Volpe, J. J., 1979*a*, Developmental changes in the distribution of 3-hydroxy-3-methylglutaryl coenzyme A reductase among subcellular fractions of rat brain, *J. Neurochem.* 33:107–115.

Maltese, W. A., and Volpe, J. J., 1979*b*, Activation of 3-hydroxy-3-methylglutaryl coenzyme A reductase in homogenates of developing rat brain, *Biochem. J.*182:367–370.

Manthorpe, M., Skaper, S., and Varon, S., 1980, Purification of mouse Schwann cells using neurite-induced proliferation in serum-free monolayer culture, *Brain Res.* 196:467–482.

Mantzos, J. D., Chiotaki, L., and Levis, G. M., 1973, Biosynthesis and composition of brain galactolipids in normal and hypothyroid rats, *J. Neurochem.* 21:1207–1213.

Matthieu, J. M., Honeggar, P., Favrod, P., Gautier, E., and Dolivo, M., 1979, Biochemical characterization of a myelin fraction isolated from rat brain aggregating cell cultures, *J. Neurochem.* 32:869–881.

McCarthy, K. D., and de Vellis, J., 1980, Preparation of separate astroglial and oligodendroglial cell cultures from rat cerebral tissue, *J. Cell Biol.* 85:890–902.

McGinnis, J. F., and de Vellis, J., 1978, Glucocorticoid regulation in rat brain cell cultures: Hydrocortisone increases the rate of synthesis of glycerol phosphate dehydrogenase in C6 glioma cells, *J. Biol. Chem.* 253:8483–8492.

McMorris, F. A., Miller, S. L., Pleasure, D., and Abramsky, O., 1981, Expression of biochemical properties of oligodendrocytes in oligodendrocyte X glioma cell hybrids proliferating *in vitro, Exp. Cell Res.* 133:395–404.

Miller, S. L., Benjamins, J. A., and Morell, P., 1977, Metabolism of glycerophospholipids of myelin and microsomes in rat brain: Reutilization of precursors, *J. Biol. Chem.* 252:4025–4037.

Mirsky, R., Winter, J., Abney, E. R., Pruss, R. M., Gavrilovic, J., and Raff, M. C., 1980, Myelin-specific proteins and glycolipids in rat Schwann cells and oligodendrocytes in culture, *J. Cell Biol.* 84:483–494.

Morell, P., and Braun, P., 1972, Biosynthesis and metabolic degradation of sphingolipids not containing sialic acid, *J. Lipid Res.* 13:293–310.

Neskovic, N. M., Rebel, G., Harth, S., and Mandel, P., 1981, Biosynthesis of galactocerebrosides and glucerebrosides in glial cell lines, *J. Neurochem.* 37:1363–1370.

Norton, W. T., Farooq, M., Fields, K. L., and Raine, C. S., 1982, Long-term culture of bovine oligodendroglia, *Trans. Am. Soc. Neurochem.* 13:171 (abstract).

Okada, E., 1982, Oligodendrocyte myelination of sensory ganglion neurites in long term culture, *Okajimas Folia Anat. Jpn.* 58:957–974.

Peterson, E. R., and Murray, M. R., 1955, Myelin sheath formation in cultures of avian spinal ganglia, *Am. J. Anat.* 96:319–355.

Pleasure, D., and Kim, S. U., 1976*a*, Sterol synthesis by myelinating cultures of mouse spinal cord, *Brain Res.* 103:117–126.

Pleasure, D., and Kim, S. U., 1976*b*, Enzyme markers for myelination of mouse cerebellum *in vivo* and in tissue culture, *Brain Res.* 104:193–196.

Pleasure, D., Abramsky, O., Silberberg, D., Quinn, B., Parris, J., and Saida, T., 1977, Lipid synthesis by an oligodendroglial fraction in suspension culture, *Brain Res.* 134:377–382.

Pleasure, D., Lichtman, C., Eastman, S., Lieb, M., Abramsky, O.. and Silberberg, D., 1979, Acetoacetate and D-(-)-beta-hydroxybutyrate as precursors for sterol synthesis by calf oligodendrocytes in suspension culture: Extramitochondrial pathway for acetoacetate metabolism, *J. Neurochem.* 32:1447–1450.

Pleasure, D., Hardy, M., Johnson, G., Lisak, R. P., and Silberberg, D., 1981, Oligodendroglial glycerophospholipid synthesis: Incorporation of radioactive precursors into ethanolamine glycerophospholipids by calf oligodendroglia prepared by a Percoll procedure and maintained in suspension culture, *J. Neurochem.* 36:452–460.

Poduslo, S. E., 1975, The isolation and characterization of a plasma membrane and a myelin fraction derived from oligodendroglia of calf brain, *J. Neurochem.* 24:647–654.

Poduslo, S. E., and McKhann, G. M., 1977, Synthesis of cerebrosides by intact oligodendroglia maintained in culture, *Neurosci. Lett.* **5:**159–163.

Poduslo, S. E., and Norton, W. T., 1972, Isolation and some chemical properties of oligodendroglia from calf brain, *J. Neurochem.* **19:**727–736.

Poduslo, S. E., Miller, K., and McKhann, G. M., 1978, Metabolic properties of maintained oligodendroglia purified from brain, *J. Biol. Chem.***253:**1592–1597.

Preston, S. L., and McMorris, F. A., 1983, Adrenalectomy of rats results in hypomyelination of the CNS, *J. Neurochem.,* in press.

Pruss, R. M., Bartlett, P. F., Gavrillovic, J., Lisak, R. P., and Rattray, S., 1982, Mitogens for glial cells: A comparison of the response of cultured astrocytes, oligodendrocytes and Schwann cells, *Dev. Brain Res.* **2:**19–35.

Raff, M. C., Abney, E., Brockes, J. P., and Hornby-Smith, A., 1978*a,* Schwann cell growth factors, *Cell* **15:**813–822.

Raff, M. C., Mirsky, R., Fields, K. L., Lisak, R. P., Dorfman, S. H., Silberberg, D. H., Gregson, N. A., Leibowitz, S., and Kennedy, M. C., 1978*b,* Galactocerebroside is a specific cell-surface antigenic marker for oligodendrocytes in culture, *Nature, (London)* **274:**813–816.

Raff, M. C., Fields, K. L., Hakomori, S. I., Mirsky, R., Pruss, R. M., and Winter, J., 1979, Cell-type-specific markers for distinguishing and studying neurons and the major classes of glial cells in culture, *Brain Res.* **174:**283–308.

Raine, C. S., 1973, Ultrastructural applications of cultured nervous system tissue to neuropathology, *Prog. Neuropathol.* **2:**27–68.

Raine, C. S., Poduslo, S. E., and Norton, W. T., 1971, The ultrastructure of purified preparations of neurons and glial cells, *Brain Res.* **27:**11–24.

Rioux, F., Derbi, C., Margules, S., Joubert, R., and Bisconte, J. C., 1980, Kinetics of olgodendrocyte-like cells in primary culture of mouse embryonic brain, *Dev. Biol.* **76:**87–99.

Roheim, P. S., Carey, M., Forte, T., and Vega, G. L., 1979, Apolipoproteins in human cerebrospinal Fluid, *Proc Natl. Acad. Sci. U.S.A.* **76:**4646–4649.

Ross, L. L., Bornstein, M. B., and Lehrer, G. M., 1962, Electron microscopic observations of rat and mouse cerebellum in tissue culture, *J. Cell Biol.* **14:**19–30.

Salzer, J. ., and Bange, R. P., 1980, Studies of Schwann cell proliferation. I. An analysis in tissue culture of proliferation during development, Wallerian degeneration, and direct injury, *J. Cell Biol.* **84:**739–752.

Salzer, J. ., Williams, A. K., Glaser, L., and Bunge, R. P., 1980, Studies of Schwann cell proliferation. II. Characterization of the stimulation and specificity of the response to a neurite membrane fraction, *J. Cell Biol.* **84:**753–766.

Sarlieve, L. L., Subba Rao, G., Campbell, G. Le M., and Pieringer, R. A., 1980, Investigations on myelination *in vitro:* Biochemical and morphological changes in cultures of dissociated brain cells from embryonic mice, *Brain Res. 189:79–90.*

Satomi, D., and Kishimoto, Y., 1981, Change of galactolipids and metabolism of fatty acids in organotypic culture of myelinating mouse brain, *Biochim. Biophys. Acta* **666:**446–454.

Saucier, S. E., and Kandutsch, A. A., 1979, Inactive 3-hydroxy-3-methylglutaryl-coenzyme A reductase in broken cell preparations of various mammalian tissues and cell cultures, *Biochim. Biophys. Acta* **572:**541–556.

Schachner, M., Kim, S. U., and Zehnle, R., 1981, Developmental expression in central and peripheral nervous system of oligodendrocyte cell surface antigens (O antigens) recognized by monoclonal antibodies, *Dev. Biol.* **33:**328–338.

Schneider, W. J., and Vance, D. E., 1979, Conversion of phosphatidylethanolamine to phosphatidylcholine in rat liver: Partial purification and characterization of the enzymatic activities, *J. Biol. Chem.* **254:**3886–3891.

Seil, F. J., and Blank, N. K., 1981, Myelination of central nervous system axons in tissue culture by transplanted oligodendrocytes, *Science* **212**:1407–1408.

Shanker, G., and Pieringer, R. A., 1983, Effect of thyroid hormone on the synthesis of sialosyl galactosylceramide (G_{M4}) in myelinogenic cultures of cells dissociated from embryonic mouse brain, *Dev. Brain Res.* **6**:169–174.

Sheppard, J. R., Brus, D., and Wehner, J. M., 1978, Brain reaggregate cultures: Biochemical evidence for myelin membrane synthesis, *J. Neurobiol.* **9**:309–315

Silberberg, D. H., 1967, Phenylketonuria metabolities in cerebellum culture morphology, *Arch. Neurol.* **17**:524–529.

Silberberg, D. H., Benjamins, J., Herschkowitz, N., and McKhann, G. M., 1972, Incorporation of radioactive sulphate into sulphatide during myelination in cultures of rat cerebellum, *J. Neurochem.* **19**:11–18.

Silberberg, D. H., Dorfman, S. H., Latovitzki, N., and Younkin, L. H., 1980, Oligodendrocyte differentiation in myelinating cultures, in *Tissue Culture in Neurobiology* E. Giacobini, pp. 489–500.

Singh, H. and Pfeiffer, S. E., 1983, Expression of galactolipids by mixed primary cultures from rat brain, *Trans. Am. Soc. Neurochem.* **14**:218.

Skoff, R. P., Price, D. L., and Stocks, A., 1976*a*, Electron microscopic autoradiographic studies of gliogenesis in rat optic nerve. I. Cell proliferation, *J. Comp. Neurol.* **169**:291–312.

Skoff, R. P., Price, D. L., and Stocks, A., 1976*b*, Electron microscopic autoradiographic studies of gliogenesis in rat optic nerve. II. Time of origin, *J. Comp. Neurol.* **169**:313–334.

Smith, M. E., 1964, Lipid biosynthesis in the central nervous system in experimental allergic encaphalomyelitis, *J. Neurochem.* **11**:29–37.

Smith, M. E., 1969, An *in vitro* system for the study of myelin synthesis, *J. Neurochem.* **16**:83–92.

Smith, M. E., 1973, A regional survey of myelin development: Some compositional and metabolic aspects, *J. Lipid Res.* **14**:541–551.

Snyder, D. S., Raine, C., Farooq, M., and Norton, W. T., 1980, The bulk isolation of oligodendroglia from whole rat forebrain: A new procedure using physiologic media, *J. Neurochem.* **34**:1614–1621.

Snyder, E. Y., and Kim, S. U., 1979, Hormonal requirements for neuronal: sirvival in culture; *Neurosci. Lett.* **13**:225–230.

Sobue, G., Kreider, B. Q., Asbury, A. K., and Pleasure, D., 1983, Specific and potent mitogenic effect of axolemmal fraction on Schwann cells from rat sciatic nerves in serum-containing and defined media, *Brain Res.* **280**:263–275.

Steck, A. J., and Perruisseau, G., 1980, Characterization of membrane markers of isolated oligodendrocytes and clonal lines of the nervous sytem, *J. Neurol. Sci.* **47**:135–144.

Stern, J. R., 1971, A role for acetoacetyl-CoA synthetase in acetoacetate utilization by rat liver cell fractions, *Biochem. Biophys. Res. Commun.* **44**:1001–1007.

Suzuki, K., and Suzuki, Y., 1970, Globoid cell leucodystrophy (Krabbe's disease): Deficiency of galactocerebroside beta-galactosidase, *Proc. Natl. Acad. Sci. U.S.A.* **66**:302–309.

Szuchet, S., Stefansson, K., Wollmann, R. L., Dawson, G., and Arnason, B. G. W., 1980, Maintenance of isolated oligodendrocytes in long-term culture, *Brain Res.* **200**:151–164.

Tennekoon, G. I., Cohen, S. R., Price. D. L., and McKhann, G. M., 1977, Myelinogenesis in optic nerve: A morphological, autoradiographic and biochemical analysis, *J. Cell Biol.* **72**:604–616.

Tennekoon, G. I., Kishimoto, Y., Singh, I., Nonaka, G., and Bourre, J. M., 1980, The differentiation of oligodendrocytes in the rat optic nerve, *Dev. Biol.* **79**:149–158.

Trapp, B. D., Dwyer, B., and Bernsohn, J., 1975, Light and electron microscopic examination of isolated neurons, astrocytes and oligodendrocytes, *Neurobiology* **5**:235–248.

Trapp, B. D., Honeggar, P., Richelson, E., and Webster, H. de F., 1979, Morphological differentiation of mechanically dissociated fetal rat brain in aggregating cell cultures, *Brain Res.* **160:**117–130.

Volpe, J., 1979, Microtubules and the regulation of 3-hydroxy-3-methylglutaryl coenzyme A reductase, *J. Biol. Chem.* **254:**2568–2571.

Volpe, J., and Obert, K. A., 1981, Cytoskeletal structures and 3-hydroxy-3-methylglutaryl coenzyme A reductase in C-6 glial cells: A role formicrofilaments, *J. Biol. Chem.* **256:**2016–2021.

Walravens, P., and Chase, H. P., 1969, Influence of thyroid on formation of myelin lipids, *J. Neurochem.* **16:**1477–1484.

Weinberg, E. L., and Spencer, P. S., 1979, Studies on the control of myelinogenesis. 3. Signalling of oligodendrocyte myelination by regenerating peripheral axons, *Brain Res.* **162:**273–279.

Witter, B., and Debuch, H., 1982, On the phospholipid metabolism of glial cell primary cultures: Cell characterization and their utilization of 1-alkylglycerophosphoethanolamine, *J. Neurochem.* **38:**1029–1037.

Wolfe, R. A., Sato, G. H., and McClure, D. B., 1980, Continuous culture of rat C6 glioma in serum-free medium, *J. Cell Biol.* **87:**434–441.

Wood, P. M., and Bunge, R. P., 1975, Evidence that sensory axons are mitogenic for Schwann cells, *Nature (London)* **256:**663–664.

Wood, P., Okada, E., and Bunge, R., 1980, The use of networks of dissociated rat dorsal root ganglion neurons to induce myelination by oligodendrocytes in culture, *Brain Res.* **196:**247–252.

Wood, P., Szuchet, S., Williams, A. K., Bunge, R. P., and Arnason, B. G. W., 1983, CNS myelin formation in cocultures of rat neurons and lamb oligodendrocytes, *Trans. Am. Soc. Neurochem.* **14:**212.

Wu, P. S., and Ledeen, R. W., 1980, Evidence for the presence of CDP-ethanolamine: 1,2-*diacyl-sn*-glycerol ethanolamine-phosphotransferase in rat central nervous system myelin, *J. Neurochem.* **35:**659–666.

Yavin, Z., and Yavin, E., 1977, Synaptogenesis and myelinogensis in dissociated cerebral cells from rat embryo on polylysine coated surfaces, *Exp. Brain Res.* **29:**137–147.

Yeh, Y. Y., Streuli, U. L., and Zee, P., 1977, Ketone bodies serve as important precursors of brain lipids in the developing rat, *Lipids* **12:**957–964.

Younkin, L. H., and Silberberg, D. H., 1976, Delay of oligodendrocyte differentiation by 5-bromodeoxyuridine (BUdR), *Brain Res.* **101:**600–605.

Yu, R. K., and Iqbal, K., 1979, Sialosylgalactosyl ceramide as a specific marker for human myelin and oligodendroglial perikarya: Gangliosides of human myelin, olgodendroglia and neurons, *J. Neurochem.* **32:**293–300.

Yu, R. K., Ledeen, R. W., and Eng, L. F., 1974, Ganglioside abnormalities in multiple sclerosis, *J. Neurochem.* **23:**169–174.

Zuppinger, K., Wiesmann, U., Siegrist, H. P., Shafer, T., Sandru, L., Schwarz, H. P., and Herschkowitz, N., 1981, Effect of glucose deprivation on sulfatide synthesis and oligodendrocytes in cultured brain cells of newborn mice, *Pediatr. Res.* **15:**319–325.

CHAPTER 6

OLIGODENDROCYTE-ASSOCIATED ENZYMES

WENDY CAMMER

1. INTRODUCTION

There is strong experimental evidence that the synthesis and maintenance of myelin are the primary functions of oligodendroglia in both white matter and gray matter (Kuffler and Nicholls, 1966; Bunge, 1968; Ludwin, 1978) (also see Chapter 1). The once-popular concept that glial cells also furnish direct biochemical support to neurons (e.g., Hyden and Pigon, 1960) has remained mostly speculation. With this perspective, therefore, the enzymes that deserve consideration are those that have particular significance for the known functions of oligodendroglia and those that have relatively high activities but that do not seem to be directly related to myelination. These enzymes can be placed in four categories and are so discussed in this chapter. The first category comprises enzymes of glucose metabolism that are elevated in oligodendroglia during the phase of development when myelination is most rapid (Section 2). The activity of at least one of these enzymes remains high into adult life. The second category consists of the enzymes known to be enriched in myelin (reviewed by Norton 1980; Norton and Cammer, 1984), which might be expected to have high activities in oligodendroglia (Section 3). The third category includes the

WENDY CAMMER ● The Saul R. Korey Department of Neurology, and the Department of Neuroscience, Albert Einstein College of Medicine, Bronx, New York 10461 enzymes involved in the synthesis and degradation of myelin lipids (Section 4). The discussion of these enzymes is brief, in view of the extensive coverage of lipid metabolism in Chapters 2 and 5. The fourth category includes several enzymes, not conveniently classifiable, that have particularly high activities, although not necessarily exclusive localization, in oligodendrocytes (Section 5).

Several areas of metabolism are not discussed. These include protein metabolism, which is thoroughly covered in Chapter 3, and nucleic acid metabolism, which has recently been reviewed at length (Pevzner, 1979, 1982). With a few exceptions, this chapter also does not include evidence concerning the enzymes in "glial" fractions derived from experiments in which the authors did not make a distinction between astrocytes and oligodendrocytes. Enzymes in tumor cells, cell lines, and primary cultures are discussed only briefly, to avoid repeating the material in Chapter 7 (also see Pevzner, 1982.) It is assumed, however, that "glial clumps" obtained from white matter include large numbers of oligodendrocytes; reports of enzyme activities in preparations of that type will therefore be cited, with the understanding that myelinated axons and astrocytes may also be contributing to the observed activities.

In Section 6, the findings concerning the diverse enzymes are summarized with reference to the following questions:

1. Is a given enzyme a specific "marker" for oligodendrocytes?
2. In cases in which it is not entirely obvious, what sort of function does the enzyme serve in oligodendroglia?
3. Does the enzyme activity undergo developmental changes related to myelination?
4. Where is the enzyme localized within the oligodendrocyte?

2. ENZYMES OF GLUCOSE METABOLISM

2.1. Methods and Biological Preparations

2.1.1. *Dehydrogenases and Oxidative Metabolism: Methods and Nomenclature*

Whereas the assay methods used in studies of myelin-associated enzymes and enzymes of lipid metabolism tend to be straightforward and are described explicitly in the respective references, the conclusions concerning the rates and pathways of energy metabolism in oligodendrocytes have been inferred from more indirect histochemical data and respiration rates, as well as from enzyme-assay data. Of the cytoplasmic enzymes, lactate dehydrogenase (LDH) and hexokinase have been used to represent the contribution of the Embden–Meyerhof pathway of glucose utilization, and the rates of glucose-6-phosphate dehydrogenase (G-6-PD) and transketolase have been used to indicate the rate of flux through the pentose phosphate pathway.

Cytochrome oxidase and, in some cases, succinic dehydrogenase (SDH) have been assayed by measuring oxygen-uptake rates, usually by means of straightforward manometric methods. However, the general method used to indicate mitochondrial dehydrogenase activity in many histochemical and spectrophotometric studies requires a somewhat more detailed explanation and a definition of terms. Tetrazolium, ditetrazolium, or other dyes were used frequently as electron acceptors for reactions in which NADH or succinate was oxidized, and the formation of intensely colored reduction products indicated enzymatic activity (Seligman and Rutenburg, 1951; Farber *et al.,* 1956). In early studies, the term "diaphorase" has been used for the flavoproteins that transferred electrons from NADH or succinate to the electron-transport chain, and frequently, in papers in which dye reduction was measured, the terms "diaphorase" and "dehydrogenase" were used interchangeably (e.g., Scarpelli and Pearse, 1958). In this chapter, the term dehydrogenase will include reactions called diaphorases by some earlier authors, as well as those consistently termed dehydrogenases.

Additional techniques used in studies cited below include histochemical staining for cytochrome oxidase (e.g., Burstone, 1959) and spectrophotometric or fluorometric measurement of the reduction or oxidation of pyridine nucleotides.

2.1.2. Biological Preparations Used in Measurements of Energy Metabolism: Advantages and Pitfalls

The biological preparations that have contributed insights into oligodendroglial biochemistry have included homogenates or slices taken from discrete regions of the CNS or during defined developmental stages, histochemical preparations, and cells isolated in bulk from white matter or whole brains. The use of microassay methods in regional developmental studies has provided insights despite a lack of resolution with respect to cell types and cell parts. Histochemical stains, which provide better localization, are less quantitative and can be vulnerable to artifacts when products migrate away from their sites of formation. Cells isolated in bulk are subject to damage, to loss of part of their contents during bulk isolation, and to contamination with other CNS cells and with blood cells. During the use of any of these methods, optimal concentrations of some substrates and cofactors may not always be provided. Despite these potential or actual technical difficulties, these methods have revealed some interesting and special aspects of oligodendroglial energy metabolism.

2.2. Regional and Developmental Findings Using Homogenates and Slices

2.2.1. Evidence for Pentose Phosphate Pathway Activity: Regional Studies

2.2.1a. Glucose-6-Phosphate Dehydrogenase. Some early clues regarding the pathways of glucose metabolism in oligodendrocytes were obtained when enzyme assays were performed on tissue slices or on homogenates of tissue from discrete regions of the CNS. Measurements of cytochrome oxidase in microgram samples from rat and human brains showed relatively low activities, on a dry weight basis, in subcortical white matter (Hess and Pope, 1972), implying that white matter and, by inference, oligodendrocytes, would have to rely on anaerobic glycolysis as a significant source of energy. In fact, when lipid analyses and enzyme assays were performed on histologically identified freeze–dried fragments of rabbit CNS tissue, high glucose-6-phosphate dehydrogenase (G-6-PD) activities could be correlated with high lipid concentrations (Buell *et al.,* 1958). On the basis of their finding high G-6-PD and relatively low hexokinase activities in white matter, the authors proposed that the pentose phosphate pathway was a relatively important route for utilization of glucose-6-phosphate in that region (Buell *et al.,* 1958).

2.2.1b. Transketolase. Experimental support for high pentose phosphate pathway activity was provided by regional studies of transketolase in rat, lamb, and human CNS tissue. The values for transketolase in myelinated tracts, expressed as activity per gram protein, were relatively high, and Dreyfus (1965) proposed that transketolase activity, and possibly the other enzymes of the pentose phosphate pathway, might be a function of the number of oligodendrocytes in the samples.

That conclusion, and the additional postulate that these enzymes might have particular importance for synthesis and maintenance of myelin (Dreyfus, 1965), were not so obvious as would appear today. Until quite recently, it was believed that the pentose phosphate pathway was a rather insignificant metabolic route in the CNS, accounting for as little as 1% of the glucose utilized in the brain (e.g., Balazs, 1970). After the requirement for the cofactor, NADP, became apparent, however, it was shown that early in the developmental period of rapid myelination, up to 60% of the glucose utilized by the rat brain was metabolized via the pentose phosphate pathway and that this fraction dropped below 25% soon after the maximal rate of myelination had occurred (Hotta, 1962; Winick, 1970).

2.2.2. Glycerol Phosphate Dehydrogenase in Homogenates: Developmental Studies

The developmental data on glycerol phosphate dehydrogenase (GPDH) in tissue homogenates, although they differ somewhat from those on the pentose phosphate pathway enzymes, also implied a significant association of the enzyme activity with myelin synthesis. Laatsch (1962) observed a sharp rise in GPDH activity in the forebrains of rats at about 20 days of age, concomitant with rapid myelination, and proposed that the glycerol phosphate would be used for the synthesis of myelin lipids. Unlike G-6-PD, GPDH remained high in activity during subsequent stages of development (Laatsch, 1962; de Vellis *et al.*, 1967).

2.3. Histochemical and Microchemical Studies of Dehydrogenases and Cytochrome Oxidase

2.3.1. Comparisons among Dehydrogenase Activities

Histochemical and immunohistochemical techniques have made it possible to focus on the oligodendroglial localization, as well as the development, of G-6-PD and GPDH. In addition, although studies of CNS regions had emphasized the greater oxidative activity in gray matter compared to white matter (e.g., Heller and Elliott, 1955), histochemical techniques permitted greater resolution, within the myelinated tracts, of mitochondrial dehydrogenase activities in the developing oligodendrocytes vs. those in the neurons.

The results of an early histochemical study, which showed that the SDH activity was lower in oligodendrocytes than in neurons (Potanos *et al.*, 1959), were confirmed in Friede's laboratory, where the combination of histochemistry with microanalyses provided rather quantitative assessments of the glucose-metabolizing enzymes and the mitochondrial dehydrogenases. In primate brains, oligodendroglia had higher activities of the pentose phosphate pathway enzymes than did neurons, whereas the converse was true for the enzymes of the Krebs tricarboxylic acid cycle (Friede *et al.*, 1963). Further analysis made it possible to arrange six enzymes in decreasing order of activity in the oligodendrocytes, as follows: G-6-PD, LDH, NADH dehydrogenase, malate dehydrogenase, SDH, and cytochrome oxidase (Romanul and Cohen, 1960; Friede, 1965). Adams (1965) also presented histochemical evidence of LDH in oligodendrocytes, and an immunohistochemical report that hexokinase is relatively low in oligodendrocytes (Kao-Jen and Wilson, 1980) was consistent with the earlier finding of low hexokinase activity in white matter (Buell *et al.*, 1958).

Developmental analyses provided exceptions to the relatively low oxidative enzyme activity in white matter. In the brains of the rat, human, and lamb, marked, transient increases in oligodendroglial dehydrogenase and cytochrome oxidase activities were found in regions in which rapid myelination was taking place (Meyer and Meyer, 1964; Friede, 1966).

2.3.2. Histochemical Localization of Mitochondrial Dehydrogenases within Oligodendrocytes and among Oligodendrocyte Types

The authors of several histochemical studies have commented on the subcellular localization of mitochondrial dehydrogenases within oligodendrocytes and on the different levels of oxidative enzyme activity in the types of oligodendrocytes that can be distinguished morphologically. A common observation was staining for succinic and NADH dehydrogenases far into the processes extending from oligodendrocytes as well as in the perinuclear regions of the cells (Potanos *et al.,* 1959; Friede, 1961).

In interpreting most of the reports discussed above, it is probably safe to assume, mainly from the localization in certain spinal tracts and subcortical white matter, that interfascicular oligodendrocytes were being studied. There appears to be some heterogeneity in metabolic rates among the interfascicular oligodendrocytes of various sizes and structural features (Friede, 1966). Furthermore, it has been claimed that, in the perineuronal oligodendrocytes in gray matter, changes in the rates of oxidative enzymes and anaerobic glycolysis can be correlated with stimulated vs. resting states and sleep vs. wakefulness (Friede, 1966). Several authors have also presented histochemical evidence of high dehydrogenase activities in oligodendrocytes adjacent to axons containing low oxidase activities, as well as the converse, and have postulated an interdependence between oligodendrocytes and axons in maintaining their energy supplies (Friede, 1961, 1966; Blunt *et al.,* 1967). Because of the possibility of diffusion artifacts, such histochemical data, *per se,* may not be definitive.

2.3.3. Histochemistry and Immunocytochemistry of Glycerol Phosphate Dehydrogenase

Since the developmental study of Laatsch (1962) there has been interest in the cytoplasmic form of GPDH. The induction of GPDH by cortisol appears, within the CNS, to be an oligodendrocyte-specific process (de Vellis *et al.,* 1974). Histochemical evidence of GPDH in human white-matter oligodendrocytes has been presented by Adams (1965), and immunocytochemical studies, permitting a firm distinction between cytoplasmic and mitochondrial GPDH, have demonstrated this enzyme in the cytoplasm of oligodendrocytes in the rat CNS (Leveille *et al.,* 1980) (see Chapters 4 and 8) and of both astrocytes and oligodendrocytes in the mouse (Fisher *et al.,* 1981).

2.4. Enzymes of Energy Metabolism in Glial-Cell Clumps and Isolated Oligodendrocytes

2.4.1. Studies of Cell Respiration

A pivotal goal during early attempts to isolate oligodendrocyes from white matter was to determine how rapidly these cells could respire. From respiration rates and DNA analyses as a measure of cell number in slices of human, cat, and dog brains, Heller and Elliott (1955) had concluded that most of the cells in the corpus callosum were oligodendrocytes and that oligodendroglia respired at about 5 μl O_2/hr per 10^6 cells. This rate was higher than those of neurons of the cerebellar cortex and astrocytes, but less rapid than that of neurons of the cerebral cortex. By comparison, the rate of 12.5 μl O_2/hr per 10^6 cells in a "nonneuronal" oligodendrocytelike cell population isolated from lamb brain white matter appears reasonable (Korey and Orchen, 1959), whereas the rate of 0–115 μl O_2/hr per 10^6 cells for glial cell clumps dissected from rabbit white matter covers a wide range (Hyden and Pigon, 1960; Hyden and Lange, 1965) (see Table 1). Hyden and Pigon (1960) emphasized that the neurons in the rabbit brainstem were much larger than the oligodendrocytes, such that if the rate of respiration were expressed on a per-unit-volume basis, the latter cells had the more rapid rate, by a factor of 2.

The evidence for high mitochondrial dehydrogenase activities during myelination, discussed above, should, of course, be expected to stimulate investigations into respiration rates of oligodendrocytes isolated from appropriate CNS regions during myelination. Apparently, such studies are fraught with technical problems. In addition to cell damage, the low yields make it difficult to perform the large number of respiration measurements necessary to determine the optimal, physiologically appropriate combinations of cofactors and substrates. Although there are additional studies of cell respiration in the literature, it is often impossible to distinguish whether the cells are astrocytes, oligodendrocytes, or miscellaneous cell fragments.

2.4.2. Measurements of Dehydrogenases in Isolated Cells: G-6-PD, GPDH, and LDH

Technical improvements in bulk-isolation and tissue-culture methods have permitted the preparation of oligodendrocyte populations in which enzyme activities can be measured directly. Some such values are shown in Table 1, where, for purposes of comparison among enzymes and species, relative specific activities were calculated by dividing the specific activity in each cell preparation by that in the respective starting homogenate. The enrichment of G-6-PD in oligodendrocytes from both young rat brains and bovine white matter is

TABLE 1. Rates of Respiration and Cytoplasmic Dehydrogenases in Oligodendroglia

Species	Specific activity in oligodendrocytes[a]	RSA[b]	References
Oxygen uptake (μl/10^6 cells per hr at 37°C)			
Cat, dog	5	~1	Heller and Elliott (1955)
Lamb	12	1.3	Korey and Orchen (1959)
Rabbit	0–115	≈0.9	Hydén and Pigon (1960); Hydén and Lange (1965)
Glucose-6-phosphate dehydrogenase [nmoles NAD (or NADP)/hr per mg protein]			
Rat			
10-day-old	27	1.4	Cammer *et al.* (1982)
120-day-old	15	0.8	Cammer *et al.* (1982)
Bovine	16	2.6 (2.1)	Cammer and Zimmerman (1983*a*)
Lactate dehydrogenase [nmoles NAD (or NADP)/hr per mg protein]			
Rat			
10-day-old	510	0.6	Cammer *et al.* (1982)
120-day-old	180	0.2	Cammer *et al.* (1982)
Primary culture	1147	—	McCarthy and de Vellis (1980)
Bovine	1100	0.81 (0.45)	Cammer and Zimmerman (1983 *ι*)
Cultured "glia"	423	—	Tholey *et al.* (1980)
Rat "glia"	700	0.5	Nagata *et al.* (1974)
Glycerol phosphate dehydrogenase [nmoles NAD (or NADP)/hr per mg protein]			
Rat			
10-day-old	16	0.9	Cammer *et al.* (1982)
120-day-old	67	1.4	Cammer *et al.* (1982)
Primary culture	43	—	McCarthy and de Vellis (1980)
Bovine	29	2.0 (1.4)	Cammer and Zimmerman (1983*a*)

[a] The biological preparations for which O_2-uptake data are presented are described in the text; activities of the dehydrogenases were obtained using bulk-isolated oligodendroglia.
[b] Relative specific activity (specific activity in cells/specific activity in homogenate). The homogenates referred to are: for the respiration data, white matter; for the dehydrogenase data obtained in the rat, whole forebrains; for the bovine dehydrogenases, white matter and (in parentheses) values obtained by comparing with gray matter.

consistent with the inference from regional studies (discussed in Section 2.2.1a) that the pentose phosphate pathway activity is high in cells of this type. The values for GPDH in oligodendrocytes from adult rat brains and bovine white matter, and in primary cultures, are quite similar.

There are 3- to 7-fold differences among the values for LDH in oligoden-

drocytes in Table I, and assays for this enzyme in a large number of preparations have revealed a rather high degree of scatter, suggesting leakage of the
cytoplasmic enzymes out of the cells after varying degrees of breakage and
resealing of the plasma membranes (Snyder *et al.,* 1983). Therefore, the highest values for LDH are probably the most reliable. The likelihood that bulk-
isolated cells have suffered some leakage also suggests that the oligodendrocytes may have even higher relative specific activities of G-6-PD and GPDH
than are shown in Table 1.

The observation of GPDH, G-6-PD, and, to a lesser degree, LDH at low
activities in myelin purified from rat and bovine brains suggests that those
enzymes occur in the specialized regions of the myelin sheath, such as the inner
and outer mesaxons and paranodal loops, where oligodendroglial cytoplasm is
enclosed (Cammer *et al.,* 1982; Cammer and Zimmerman, 1983*a*).

2.5. Summary of the Implications Regarding Energy Metabolism in Oligodendroglia

The findings obtained with isolated oligodendrocytes, along with the histochemical and immunohistochemical data and the inferences from regional
and developmental studies, give a consistent if somewhat preliminary view of
oligodendrocyte energy metabolism and its relationship to the demands associated with the biosynthesis and maintenance of the myelin sheath. The
demand for NADPH, to provide reducing equivalents for the biosynthesis of
myelin lipids, was recognized by earlier investigators (McDougal *et al.,* 1961;
Friede *et al.,* 1963; Dreyfus, 1965), and indeed the enrichment of G-6-PD in
oligodendrocytes was implied by the results of regional, developmental, histochemical, and cell-isolation studies.

LDH, ranked second to G-6-PD in oligodendroglial activity by Friede
(1965), proved to have significant activity in the isolated cells, with lower relative specific activity than that of G-6-PD.

GPDH, which most likely provides material for myelin phospholipid biosynthesis (Laatsch, 1962), is indeed an oligodendrocyte-enriched enzyme,
according to developmental, immunocytochemical, and cell-isolation studies.
The early developmental peak in G-6-PD in rat brain homogenates (Lehrer *et
al.,* 1970) and oligodendrocytes (Cammer *et al.,* 1982), and the developmental
rise in GPDH, which remains at high activities in homogenates and oligodendrocytes even after the rate of myelination has slowed (Laatsch, 1962; de Vellis
et al., 1967; Cammer *et al.,* 1982), has suggested that G-6-PD may be more
important for the biosynthesis, and GPDH for the maintenance, of myelin
(Cammer *et al.,* 1982).

From the sum of the studies discussed above, a view emerges of the oligodendrocyte as a cell that is dependent on the pentose phosphate pathway,

but is capable of metabolizing, and by inference producing lactate as well, and that has an increased dependence on mitochondrial enzymes during rapid myelination.

3.   MYELIN-ASSOCIATED ENZYMES IN OLIGODENDROGLIA

3.1.   Carbonic Anhydrase

3.1.1.   Regional Studies, Dissected Glial Cells, and Histochemistry

In 1944 Ashby (1944) raised the possibility that carbonic anhydrase (CA) might be situated in the oligodendrocytes. This hypothesis was based on a correlation between the higher CA activities and the greater numbers of oligodendroglia in the cerebra than in the spinal cords of seven species and the demonstration that this distribution was independent of the amount of gray matter in those regions (Ashby, 1944). Experimental evidence supporting Ashby's proposal was presented almost 20 years later (Giacobini, 1962). Single neurons and equal volumes of tissue consisting of oligodendrocyte-rich clumps were dissected from the lower brainstems of rats, and measurements were made of the rates of conversion of bicarbonate to carbon dioxide. The glial-cell clumps were 6 times more active than the neurons, in terms of reaction rate per cell, which can be converted to a 20-fold difference in terms of activity per milligram protein (Table 2). Korhonen et al. (1964) later used histochemical staining in the mouse brain to demonstrate high CA activities in areas rich in myelinated fibers and in glial cells. These authors were explicit regarding the absence of staining in neurons.

3.1.2.   Bulk-Isolated Cells and Development

Whereas partial enrichment of CA in bulk-isolated "glial" cell fractions was subsequently obtained in several other laboratories (Table 2) (Sinha and Rose, 1971; Nagata et al., 1974; Kimelberg et al., 1978), these preparations appeared to include significant proportions of astrocytes, or astrocyte fragments, and myelin vesicles. More recently, well-characterized preparations of oligodendroglial cell bodies were obtained from rat forebrains (Snyder et al., 1980), and over 3-fold enrichment of CA was demonstrated in those cells (Snyder et al., 1983). In the latter study, it was shown that cytoplasmic enzymes, including CA, probably were lost in part during the cell isolation procedure;

TABLE 2.   Carbonic Anhydrase and Adenosine Triphosphatase Activities in Oligodendrocytes

Species	Specific activity, oligodendrocytes	RSA[a]		References
		Oligos/hom.	Oligos/myelin	
Carbonic anhydrase[b]				
Rat 20 Day	2500	3.8	2.1	Snyder et al. (1983); Cammer and Zimmerman (1981)
120-Day	6500	3.5	5.9	Cammer and Zimmerman (1981)
50-Day[c]	≈500	≈2.5	—	Sinha and Rose (1971)
Adult[c]	8.4×10^{-5}	5 × neurons	—	Nagata et al. (1974)
Adult	0.3×10^{9d}	20 × neurons[d]	—	Giacobini (1962)
26-day[c]	27.3	1.4	—	Kimelberg et al. (1978)
Mg^{2+}-Adenosine triphosphatase (nmoles/min per mg protein)				
Rat 20-Day	60	0.94	2.0	Zimmerman and Cammer (1982)
60-Day	95	0.68	7.9	Zimmerman and Cammer (1982)
Adult[c]	133	1.2	—	Nagata et al. (1974)
20-Day[c]	470	4.3	—	Medzihradsky et al. (1971)
Bovine	25	1.6	2.6	Zimmerman and Cammer (1982)
Na^+,K^+-Adensoine triphosphatase (nmoles/min per mg protein)				
Rat 20-Day	10	0.08	0.3	Zimmerman and Cammer (1982)
60-Day	10	0.07	0.3	Zimmerman and Cammer (1982)
Adult[c]	58	0.58	—	Nagata et al. (1974)
26-Day[c]	267	—	—	Kimelerg et al. (1978)
20-Day[c]	362	4.4	—	Medzihradsky et al. (1971)
Bovine	40	—	0.38	Poduslo (1975)
	2	0.12	0.5	Zimmerman and Cammer (1982)

[a] (RSA) Relative specific activity.
[b] The first two values for specific activity are in ng/mg protein and the rest in different arbitrary units.
[c] It appears from the morphology that these glial-cell preparations consisted primarily of astrocytes and membrane fragments.
[d] The activities/cell were converted to activities/mg protein by using the protein/neuron and protein/oligodendrocyte values of Farooq and Norton (1978) and Snyder et al. (1980), respectively.

thus, in individual experiments in which the cells remained relatively intact, up to 5.1-fold enrichment of CA was obtained in the oligodendroglia. A developmental pattern was also observed in which the specific activity in the oligodendrocytes increased during the period of rapid myelination and remained high in the adult (Snyder *et al.,* 1983).

3.1.3. Immunocytochemical Studies

The results of immunocytochemical studies supported the view that, of the CNS cell types, other than the cells of the choroid plexus, the oligodendroglia have the highest levels of CA II (Delaunoy *et al.,* 1980; Ghandour *et al.,* 1980), which is the only isozyme in the CNS. Staining of oligodendrocytes in gray matter, as well as in white matter, was also reported more recently in the human (Kumpulainen and Nystrom, 1981). However, there is evidence for CA at low levels in astrocytes (Roussel *et al.,* 1979; Church *et al.,* 1980; Snyder *et al.,* 1983) and possibly in neurons (Snyder *et al.,* 1983) and at moderate levels in dibutyryl 3' 5'-cyclic AMP (cAMP)-treated cultured astrocytes (Kimelberg *et al.,* 1982). Biochemical, immunocytochemical, and histochemical data indicate that there are also significant levels of this enzyme in myelin (Cammer *et al.,* 1976; Yandrasitz *et al.,* 1976; Sapirstein *et al.,* 1978; Spicer *et al.,* 1979; Kumpulainen and Nystrom, 1981; Parthe, 1981), and in myelin from rodent brains and spinal cords CA occurs at consistently higher relative specific activities than do the non-myelin-associated cytoplasmic enzymes, glucose-6-phosphate dehydrogenase and glycerol phosphate dehydrogenase (Cammer and Zimmerman, 1983*a*). Therefore, unless one is using detection methods relatively low in sensitivity, CA is not an entirely specific marker for oligodendroglia (see Chapter 4).

3.1.4. Hypothetical Functions

3.1.4a. Transport of CO_2 and of Bicarbonate and Chloride Ions. Determining the functions of CA in CNS tissue, and particularly in glial cells, was a common goal in the work of Ashby and Giacobini. This question has not been settled, although the following reasonable possibilities exist: First, Giacobini (1962) proposed a role in transport of Cl^- into the tissue, assuming that the physiologically significant direction of the CA reaction was from CO_2 to carbonic acid. The carbonic acid would rapidly ionize to HCO_3^-, which could be exchanged for Cl^- from the blood. A second, alternative, function, regeneration of CO_2 from carbonic acid, would prevent acidification of the tissue by the products of aerobic metabolism, since the CO_2, but not the ionization products of carbonic acid, could readily diffuse across membranes and, ultimately, into the circulation. Since the mature oligodendrocyte is a small cell (Mori and LeBlond, 1970) with a fairly rapid metabolic rate (e.g., Hyden and Pigon, 1960), the latter hypothetical function could protect the oligodendroglia themselves; however, removal of CO_2 from the vicinity of respiring neurons could also be a significant function. This function would be continued in the myelin sheath, where CO_2, produced by axoplasmic mitochondria and transformed spontaneously to carbonic acid, could be regenerated by CA and could hence diffuse to the outisde of the myelinated fiber.

   3.1.4b. CO_2 Fixation.   An additional possibility is that the functionally significant direction of the CA reaction in oligodendrocytes is the conversion of CO_2 to carbonic acid, which ionizes spontaneously to HCO_3^-. HCO_3^- would not diffuse rapidly out of the oligodendrocyte and would be used in the biosynthesis of fatty acids and amino acids. Specifically, HCO_3^- is utilized by acetyl-CoA carboxylase and pyruvate carboxylase, both of which occur in brain, acetyl-CoA carboxylase producing malonyl-CoA, in the first step committed to fatty acid formation, and pyruvate carboxylase serving as an early step in the biosynthesis of glutamate and aspartate (Waelsch *et al.,* 1964; Lynen, 1967; Salganicoff and Koeppe, 1968; Lane *et al.,* 1974). The last of these three proposed functions is the one that would be concerned most directly with the role of the oligodendrocyte in maintaining myelin.

3.2. Na^+,K^+-Adenosine Triphosphatase, A Putative Myelin-Associated Enzyme; Mg^{2+}-Adenosine Triphosphatase; and Adenylate Cyclase

3.2.1. Na^+,K^+-Adenosine Triphosphatase

   Of these three enzymes, only Na^+- and K^+-dependent adenosine triphosphatase (Na^+,K^+-ATPase) can be detected in purified myelin (Reiss *et al.,* 1981; Zimmerman and Cammer, 1982); however, because of their general association with membrane systems, they are grouped together. The occurrence of the transport enzyme Na^+,K^+-ATPase in bulk-isolated cells has been the subject of relatively few investigations, and among the glial-cell preparations studied, most have been predominantly astrocytes (Table 2). The Na^+,K^+-ATPase activities in well-characterized oligodendrocytes from rat brains (Zimmerman and Cammer, 1982), although lower than might be expected, are comparable to the activities in certain other types of cells, such as leukocytes and erythrocytes (Stekhoven and Bonting, 1981). Although there is a 20-fold difference in the Na^+,K^+-ATPase activities obtained in bovine oligodendrocytes in two different laboratories (Table 2), a consistent finding in the oligodendrocytes prepared from both species, in both laboratories, is activity lower than that in myelin (Table 2) (Poduslo, 1975; Zimmerman and Cammer, 1982). The immunocytochemical localization of Na^+,K^+-ATPase in knifefish brain would suggest the occurrence of this enzyme in the oligodendrocyte plasma membrane (Wood *et al.*, 1977), and in a previous study it was not possible to distinguish whether the Na^+,K^+-ATPase on the surface of oligodendrocytes was low in quantity or, alternatively, very labile (Stahl and Broderson, 1976). In the latter case, the Na^+,K^+-ATPase activity in oligodendrocytes would be higher than is suggested by the existing bulk-isolation data.

3.2.2. Mg^{2+}-Adenosine Triphosphatase and Adenylate Cyclase

Oligodendroglia isolated from rat and bovine brains have relatively high activities of Mg^{2+}-dependent adenosine triphosphatase (Mg^{2+}-ATPase), accounting for over 85% of the total ATPase activity in the bulk-isolated cells (Zimmerman and Cammer, 1982) and achieving specific activities equal to or greater than those in the forebrain or white-matter homogenates (Table 2). The results of a histochemical study (Vercelli-Retta *et al.*, 1976) are consistent with the biochemical evidence for higher Mg^{2+}-ATPase than Na^+,K^+-ATPase activity in oligodendrocytes and suggest that adenylate cyclase and Mg^{2+}-ATPase have similar, rather high, activities in cells of this type. In both cases, the reaction product was found at the cell bodies and only in the proximal regions of oligodendrocyte processes.

3.3. 2',3'-Cyclic Nucleotide 3'-Phosphohydrolase

3.3.1. 2',3'-Cyclic Nucleotide 3'-Phosphohydrolase as a Myelin-Associated Enzyme

2',3'-Cyclic nucleotide 3'-phosphohydrolase (CNP) cleaves 2',3'-cyclic nucleotides to the respective 2'-nucleotides. The high activities observed in nervous-system tissue and, subsequently, in myelin-enriched subcellular fractions from rabbit, rodent, and bovine brains suggested that CNP was a myelin-associated enzyme, and the low activities in the CNS of rodents before myelination and in the brains of the hypomyelinating mutant mice, quaking and jimpy, supported this interpretation (Drummond *et al.*, 1962; Kurihara and Tsukada, 1967; Olafson *et al.*, 1969; Kurihara *et al.*, 1970). More recently, it has been found that shiverer mutant mice, which have virtually no myelin in the CNS and diminished amounts of myelin basic protein (MBP) and proteolipid protein (PLP), have normal CNP levels (Mikoshiba *et al.*, 1980). These data have raised some doubts as to whether CNP is located primarily in myelin in normal animals. Much of the CNP and residual myelin proteins of shiverer brains can be recovered together in membrane fractions denser than myelin (Mikoshiba *et al.*, 1980; Cammer and Zimmerman, 1983*b*). It seems likely, therefore, that

CNP localization in brains of shiverer mice is not the same as in normal animals.

In normal rodents, small quantities of relatively dense myelin-related membranes with very high CNP specific activities (higher than in either normal myelin or shiverer mouse membranes) can be isolated from brain. There has been speculation that these membranes are the plasma membranes of oligodendrocyte processes, and it has been proposed, accordingly, that CNP is an oligodendrocyte enzyme marker that occurs in the myelin sheath only in specialized regions (e.g., Waehneldt *et al.,* 1977). This has not been proved, and the studies of bulk-isolated cells discussed below suggest that the cell bodies of oligodendrocytes are much lower in CNP specific activity than is myelin.

3.3.2. Bulk-Isolated Cells: Alternative Explanations for Scattered CNP Values

The variability in the CNP activities among oligodendrocyte preparations isolated in different laboratories is apparent from the data in Table 3. Some data on tissue cultures and on a "glial" cell preparation are also presented for comparison. In each of the species, bovine and rat, there is a set of specific activities greater than 1.5 μmoles/min per mg protein and a set of values less than 1 μmole/min per mg protein. At present, it does not seem possible to decide whether the high or the low values are the more realistic. If it is assumed that the high values are correct for both species, it would appear that certain isolation methods cause the loss of a particular region of the plasma membrane that contains most of the CNP; this region might be situated in the relatively distal regions of the processes, since the cell bodies appear to have intact plasma membranes, even in preparations with low CNP values (Snyder *et al.,* 1980, 1983). This interpretation is consistent with the finding that the region of the oligodendrocyte with the most intense immunocytochemical staining for CNP is the site at which the processes connect with myelinated nerve fibers (Nishizawa *et al.,* 1981). Whereas one might propose that it is necessary to permit bulk-isolated cells to regenerate such regions of membrane to obtain high CNP activities, discrepancies are also found among cultures of oligodendrocytes originating from the same species (McCarthy and deVellis, 1980; Bhat *et al.,* 1981).

It seems equally likely that the low CNP values for oligodendrocytes may be the more realistic and that the preparations with high values may be contaminated with myelin vesicles. In some cases, myelin membranes are visible in preparations of bulk-isolated cells, and such material may result in the specific activities greater than 1.5 μmoles/min per mg protein. Even when bovine oligodendroglial membranes were shown to have higher CNP activities than

TABLE 3.   2′,3′-Cyclic Nucleotide 3′-Phosphohydrolase and 5′-Nucleotidase Activities in Oligodendrocytes[a]

Species	Specific activity in oligoden- drocytes	RSA		References
		Oligo/ hom.	Oligo/ myelin	
2′,3′-Cyclic nucleotide 3′-phosphohydrolase (nmoles/min per mg protein)				
Bovine	4600	—	0.30	Poduslo and Norton (1972)
Bovine	610	—	0.13	Poduslo (1975)
Bovine	1500	0.22	—	Pleasure et al. (1977)
Bovine	4700	0.7	0.3	Farooq et al. (1981)
Lamb	1950	0.18	—	Szuchet et al. (1980)
Rat				
29-Day	4640	1.2	—	Deshmukh et al. (1974)
30-Day	3167	—	—	Banik and Smith (1976)
20-Day	600	0.40	0.03	Snyder et al. (1983); Cammer and Zimmerman (1981)
120-Day	800	0.15	0.05	Snyder et al. (1983); Cammer and Zimmerman (1981)
Adult[b]	3000	—	—	Nagata et al. (1974)
Culture	500	—	—	McCarthy and de Vellis (1980)
Culture	7000	—	—	Bhat et al. (1981)
Bovine, culture	1425–4108	—	—	McMorris et al. (1981)
5′-Nucleotidase (nmoles/min per mg protein)				
Bovine	4.3	0.10	0.09	Farooq et al. (1981)
Bovine	20	—	0.25	Poduslo (1975)
Rat				Snyder et al. (1983);
20-Day	25	2.5	1.2	Cammer and Zimmerman (1981)
120-Day	16	0.40	0.19	Snyder et al. (1983); Cammer and Zimmerman (1981)

[a] Cells were obtained from bovine and lamb white matter and from rat whole forebrains, except for the preparations of Deshmukh et al. (1974) and Banik and Smith (1976), for which rat white matter was used. The homogenates in the relative specific activity (RSA) column represent the indicated starting material.
[b] It appears, from the morphology or the methodology, that this glial-cell preparation consisted primarily of astrocytes and membrane fragments.

intact oligodendrocytes, a myelin fraction was still more active than the oligodendrocyte membranes (Poduslo, 1975).

Immunocytochemical studies have shown that certain myelin proteins can be detected in rat oligodendrocytes only very early in myelination (Agrawal et al., 1977; Sternberger et al., 1978, 1979), and it has been suggested, because CNP develops early in myelin, that high CNP activities may actually occur in oligodendrocytes of the rat only before the age of 10 days (Snyder *et al.*, 1983). A fourth, alternative, explanation for higher CNP values in oligodendrocytes from bovine white matter than from whole forebrains of the rat is that oligodendrocytes from white matter may have higher activities than those from gray matter. Progress in the immunocytochemical studies should help resolve that issue and distinguish whether oligodendrocyte processes or compact myelin membranes are the primary site of CNP.

3.3.3. Immunocytochemistry: Preliminary Studies

The immunocytochemical study by Nishizawa *et al.* (1981) detected CNP in immature oligodendrocytes in both myelinated and premyelinated areas of developing rat brains, and CNP has also been localized in oligodendrocytes from bovine CNS tissue (Sprinkle *et al.*, 1981; Sprinkle and McDonald, 1982).

Whichever values for CNP in bulk-isolated cells are correct, the specific activity of CNP in isolated oligodendrocytes appears consistently to be less than one-third the specific activity in myelin, and a survey of the studies suggests that CNP should not, at least at present, be called an exclusively "myelin-specific" or "oligodendrocyte-specific" enzyme.

3.4. 5′-Nucleotidase

3.4.1. Histochemical Studies

5′-Nucleotidase cleaves nucleoside-5′-monophosphates to the free nucleosides and inorganic phosphate. Most of the early studies, as well as more recent ones, utilized histochemical methods based on the precipitation of inorganic phosphate by lead, and several decades ago it was shown, using such a method, that the development of 5′-nucleotidase in the rat brain could be correlated with myelination and that myelinated tracts had particularly high activities of this enzyme (Naidoo and Pratt, 1954; Naidoo, 1962).

Subsequent histochemical studies have localized 5′-nucleotidase in the plasma membranes of astrocytes and oligodendrocytes in the rat brain (Vercelli-Retta *et al.*, 1976; Kreutzberg *et al.*, 1978; Bernstein *et al.*, 1978). Whereas reaction product was found in compact myelin in only one of these histochemical reports (Kreutzberg *et al.*, 1978), there is agreement concerning this enzyme activity in distal regions of oligodencrocyte processes adjoining the ensheathed axons, including the outermost myelin lamellae (Vercelli-Retta *et al.*, 1976; Bernstein *et al.*, 1978; Kreutzberg *et al.*, 1978). There is some controversy over the possibility of neuronal localization. Only one investigation of rat brain noted activity in the axolemma and at synapses (Bernstein *et al.*,

1978) although histochemical staining of neurons has been obtained in the mouse (Scott, 1965; Marani, 1977).

3.4.2. Bulk-Isolated Cells and Development

Biochemical studies carried out using bulk-isolated cells have confirmed the histochemical finding of 5′-nucleotidase in glial cells (Table 3). Significant 5′-nucleotidase was observed in oligodendrocytes from bovine and rat brains. Astrocytes from the rat brains had activities that were almost as high as those in the oligodendrocytes from the adult animals, whereas the neurons had little activity (Farooq *et al.*, 1981; Snyder *et al.*, 1983). Although there is a discrepancy between the specific activities in the two reports concerning bovine oligodendrocytes, there is agreement that the specific activity in the bovine cells is less than 25% of that in bovine myelin, and the 5′-nucleotidase activity in oligodendrocytes from rat brains is also lower than the activity in rat brain myelin (Table 3).

The development of 5′-nucleotidase in oligodendrocytes appears to be consistent with the relatively late accumulation of this enzyme in myelin (Cammer and Zimmerman, 1981). That is, the highest relative specific activity in oligodendrocytes occurred in the brains of rats at the age of 20 days, which is later than the ages at which one observes the maximal immunocytochemical staining in oligodendrocytes for MBP, myelin-associated glycoprotein, and PLP (Agrawal *et al.*, 1977; Sternberger *et al.*, 1978, 1979).

Although 5′-nucleotidase has been called a plasma-membrane marker and an ectoenzyme, there is evidence of activity in other subcellular membranes (Solyom and Trams, 1972), and in G6 glioma cells, for example, the external activity accounts for only about 50% of the total activity (Stefanovic *et al.*, 1975).

3.4.3. Hypothetical Functions

The 5′-nucleotidase in oligodendrocytes may function primarily for the benefit of the neighboring neurons; alternatively, its function may be directly related to myelination. Since the product, adenosine, is more membrane-permeant than the substrate, 5′-AMP, it is generally assumed that 5′-nucleotidase is involved in the transport of nucleosides across membranes. Thus, the primary function could be to permit access of the neurons to adenosine, a probable transmitter with modulatory effects on several biochemical and physiological processes, including the formation of cAMP (Schubert *et al.*, 1979). Alternatively, 5′-nucleotidase may be required for transport of nucleosides into the oligodendrocytes, ultimately for incorporation into RNA.

3.5. Additional Enzymes Associated with Crude or Pure Myelin

3.5.1. Cholesterol Ester Hydrolase and Basic Protein Kinase

Two myelin-associated enzymes that would be of interest in oligodendrocytes are the pH 7.2 cholesterol ester hydrolase and the basic protein kinase. The values reported for the pH 7.2 cholesterol ester hydrolase in oligodendrocytes were obtained using cultured cells (Chapter 7), and, to our knowledge, no data are available concerning the presence or absence of the latter enzyme in oligodendrocytes. The particular significance of the cholesterol ester hydrolase, in this context, is that, of the known myelin-associated enzymes, it has the highest relative specific activity in myelin (Eto and Suzuki, 1973). Since MBP is phosphorylated *in vivo* (Deibler *et al.*, 1975), probably by means of a myelin-associated enzyme (Miyamoto and Kakiuchi, 1974), it would also be desirable to have some estimate as to whether the kinase activity is higher in myelin or in oligodendrocytes.

3.5.2. Peptidase Activity

In one study, microchemical enzyme assays done on small pieces of brain taken from specific loci indicated high L-alanylglycine dipeptidase activity in white matter, and this activity was attributed to glial cells, where it was postulated to have a role in protein turnover (Pope, 1960). More recently, immunocytochemical techniques were used to demonstrate the acidic endopeptidase cathepsin D in oligodendrocytes and neurons (Snyder and Whitaker, 1983).

4. BIOSYNTHESIS AND DEGRADATION OF LIPIDS BY OLIGODENDROGLIAL ENZYMES

The activities of some lipid-metabolizing enzymes in isolated oligodendrocytes are presented in Table 4. These enzymes were chosen on the basis of their apparent enrichment in oligodendroglia or expected function in the synthesis and maintenance of myelin. Of the enzymes investigated and shown in Table 4, UDP-galactose:ceramide galactosyltransferase has a rather high relative specific activity. Since α-hydroxy fatty acid (HFA)-containing ceramides are the most favorable substrate for this enzyme, the abilities of the bovine oligodendrocytes to incorporate galactose into HFA- and nonhydroxy fatty acid (NFA)-containing ceramides were compared. In this study, the rates of incorporation of HFA by both oligodendrocytes and unfractionated white matter were about 10-fold the respective rates with NFA as a substrate (Ceccarini and Snyder, personal communication). UDP-galactose:ceramide galactosyl-

TABLE 4. Enzymes of Lipid Metabolism Measured in Isolated Oligodendrocytes

Enzyme	Species[a]	Specific activity in oligodendrocytes (pmoles/min per mg protein)	RSA[b]	References
UDP-galactose:ceramide galactosyltransferase	Rat, 16-day	16	0.94	Deshmukh et al. (1974)
	Rat, 20-day	34	4.6	E. Goldmuntz and W. T. Norton (personal communication)
	Bovine WM	92	23	E. Ceccarini and D. S. Snyder (personal communication)
Galactocerebroside β-galactosidase	Rat, 17-day	24	1.1	Radin et al. (1972)
	Bovine WM	—	2.7	Abe et al. (1979)
Arylsulfatase A	Bovine WM	—	0.53	Abe et al. (1979)
Digalactosyldiglyceride synthetase	Rat, 16-day, WM	43	3.1	Deshmukh et al. (1974)
Cerebroside sulfotransferase	Bovine WM	0.53	23	Benjamins et al. (1974)
	Bovine WM,	0.21	9.1	Pleasure et al. (1977)
HMG-CoA reductase[c]	Bovine WM	5.6	3.3	Pleasure et al. (1977)
CDP-diglyceride inositol phosphotransferase	Bovine WM	1.9	—	Brammer and Carey (1980)
	Bovine WM	2–17	—	Gibson and Brammer (1981)
CTP-independent inositol phosphotransferase	Bovine WM	≈ 2	—	Gibson and Brammer (1981)
Acetoacetyl-CoA synthetase	Bovine WM	—	>20	Pleasure et al. (1979)
Acetoacetyl-CoA thiolase	Bovine WM	—	> 4	Pleasure et al. (1979)
Sialosyltransferase ($\rightarrow$ GM$_4$)	Rat, 10-day	>12.5	—	Stoffyn et al. (1981)
	Rat, 60-day	> 4	—	Stoffyn et al. (1981)
Plasmalogenase	Bovine	112×10^3	>10 × as in neurons	Dorman et al. (1977)
Triacylglycerol synthesis	Rat, 17-day	—	≈ 2 × as in neurons	Carey et al. (1980)

[a] (WM) White matter.
[b] (RSA) Relative specific activity (specific activity in cells/specific activity in homogenate).
[c] (HMG) Hydroxymethylglutaryl.

transferase is known to occur in myelin, and using the specific activity of 22 pmoles/min per mg protein in myelin from the 20-day-old rat (Costantino-Ceccarini and Suzuki, 1975), relative specific activities of 0.7–1.5 for oligodendrocytes/myelin can be calculated.

Bovine oligodendrocytes have also been shown to have the enzymes required for elongating, desaturating, and oxidizing fatty acids and for incorporating them into phospholipids and cerebrosides (Fewster *et al.,* 1975). Polyunsaturated fatty acids, as well as saturated fatty acids, can serve as substrates for these reactions in the cells from the rat and calf, *in vivo* and *in vitro,* respectively (Cohen and Bernsohn, 1978). Bovine oligodendrocytes, *in vitro,* also incorporate choline into lecithin and inositol into phosphatidylinositol (Brammer and Carey, 1980; Freeman and Carey, 1980; Gibson and Brammer, 1981), and oligodendrocytes from lamb brains, as well as bovine brains, synthesize lipids *in vitro* under appropriate conditions (Poduslo *et al.,* 1978; Szuchet *et al.,* 1980). An acid lipase of unknown function has relative specific activities in bovine oligodendrocytes of approximately 10 and 16 compared to white matter and myelin, respectively (Hirsch *et al.,* 1977). Lipid metabolism in oligodendrocytes is discussed in greater detail in Chapters 2 and 5.

5. OTHER ENZYMES IN OLIGODENDROCYTES

5.1. Nonspecific Cholinesterase

5.1.1. Regional Studies

Although enigmatic with respect to function, and not entirely confined to oligodendrocytes, nonspecific cholinesterase (NsChE) is worthy of some discussion because it was one of the first enzymes to be observed in this cell type, because it may also be a myelin-associated enzyme, and because its disappearance may be a marker for injury to oligodendrocytes. Although the high acetylcholinesterase (AChE) activity in CNS tissue could potentially be a source of artifacts in measurements of NsChE, the different substrates and sensitivities to inhibitors have permitted well-controlled experiments in which the activities of these two enzymes were distinguished from one another and from "nonspecific esterases." Friede (1966) has summarized the other terms for NsChE and has tabulated the substrates and inhibitors of AChE and NsChE.

Values for NsChE in brain homogenates from the human and five other species suggested the association of this activity with myelinated fibers. In all the species except the dog, the NsChE activity was higher in subcortical white matter than in gray matter, and in the white matter, the NsChE activity was higher than that of AChE (Ord and Thompson, 1952; Lumsden, 1957). Significant NsChE activities were also observed in astrocytomas and fibrous astrocytes, as well as in an oligodendroglioma (Cavanagh *et al.,* 1954); therefore, this enzymatic activity cannot serve as a marker with strict specificity for oligodendrocytes.

5.1.2. Histochemical Studies

The results of histochemical studies indicated that NsChE activity was localized in glial cells in the rat brain (Koelle, 1954) and the rabbit optic nerve (Hebb *et al.,* 1953) and, in addition, in the myelinated fibers of the rabbit retina (Hebb *et al.,* 1953). The outstanding activity occurring in oligodendroglia in the subcortical white matter of the cat and human became apparent in histochemical studies from Friede's laboratory, and it was also shown that after injury, the subcortical oligodendrocytes lost NsChE, whereas astrocytes increased slightly in activity (Friede, 1966; Roessmann and Friede, 1966). The potential artifacts in the histochemical studies, and the evidence for NsChE activity in astrocytes, endothelial cells, and certain neurons in various species, as well as in oligodendrocytes in both gray matter and white matter, have been reviewed by Silver (1974). More recently, this enzyme activity was found in primate neurons and rat pituitary cells (Graybiel and Ragsdale, 1982; Das *et al.,* 1982).

Histochemical evidence of NsChE in compact myelin has also been presented (Kasa and Csillik, 1966). That observation may explain in part the apparent loss of NsChE from multiple sclerosis plaques and from sites of injury to white matter (Lumsden, 1957; Roessmann and Friede, 1966). Although the natural substrate and the function of this enzyme activity remain unknown, speculation has yielded a few proposals. First, NsChE is capable of cleaving ACh at a range of concentrations. Although NsChE turns over more slowly than does AChE, the latter is inhibited at high substrate concentrations. Thus, NsChE could serve to inactivate ACh at sites where cholinergic signals would be harmful or to regenerate acetate and choline for use in lipid bosynthesis by the oligodendrocytes. An alternative function for NsChE could be the destruction of butyrylcholine, a product of fatty acid metabolism having strong nicotinic action (see Clitherow *et al.,* 1963). The possibility has also been raised that NsChE may be an endopeptidase (Das *et al.,* 1982).

5.2. Peroxisomal Enzymes

In 1976, the occurrence of endogenous diaminobenzidine staining was observed in glial cells in the brains of rats and several other species (Keefer and Christ, 1976), and, in a morphological study at higher power, microperoxisomes were localized in oligodendrocytes, as well as certain neurons, in the rat

CNS (McKenna *et al.,* 1976). Measurements of catalase in tissue dissected from 11 areas in the rat brain have shown, since then, that some of the catalase in the CNS is located outside peroxisomes and that, compared to certain other areas, the corpus callosum has intermediate activity of catalase (Brannan *et al.,* 1981). It was proposed that within the white matter, the catalase is located in oligodendrocytes, in microperoxisomes near mitochondria. The function of catalase in these cells could be either detoxification of H_2O_2 produced by mitochondria or participation in the biosynthesis, storage, or transport of cholesterol (see Reddy, 1973).

6. SUMMARY AND CONCLUSIONS

6.1. Enrichment or Marker Specificity of Oligodendroglial Enzymes

As early as the 1940s and 1950s it was proposed that carbonic anhydrase (CA), 5′-nucleotidase, and nonspecific cholinesterase (NsChE) were localized in oligodendroglia or were essential for myelination or both (Ashby, 1944; Naidoo and Pratt, 1954; Ord and Thompson, 1952). At present, none of these is known with certainty to be an oligodendrocyte-specific marker. Although each is indeed enriched in oligodendrocytes from rat brains, compared to the brain homogenates, at some time during development (see Tables 2 and 3) or shows distinctive histochemical staining in oligodendrocytes (Friede, 1966), all three have been detected at somewhat lower levels in astrocytes as well (e.g., Cavanagh, *et al.,* 1954; Roessmann and Friede, 1966; Kreutzberg *et al.,* 1978; Roussel *et al.,* 1979; Kimelberg *et al.,* 1982; Snyder *et al.,* 1983) and at yet lower levels in neuronal perikarya or axoplasm (e.g., Roessmann and Friede, 1966; Bernstein *et al.,* 1978; Snyder *et al.,* 1983). For each enzyme, the data showing astrocytic localization are quite conclusive, whereas the findings in neurons may result from contaminants, in the case of bulk-isolated cells, or from nonspecific precipitation or diffusion, in the case of the histochemical studies. Therefore, these enzymes may be specific for glial cells and myelin. There is evidence that glycerolphosphate dehydrogenase (GPDH) is an additional glial-cell-specific enzyme (Leveille *et al.,* 1980; Fisher *et al.,* 1981).

Enzymes that are also oligodendrocyte-enriched, with little information available concerning their occurrence and levels in the other cell types, include glucose-6-phosphate dehydrogenase (G-6-PD) (see Table 1) and at least six of the enzymes involved in lipid metabolism (see Table 4).

In preparations of neurons and astrocytes 2′, 3′-cyclic nucleotide 3′-phosphohydrolase (CNP) occurs only at very low levels, which probably are due to contamination by highly active myelin vesicles (Deshmukh *et al.,* 1974; Nagata *et al.,* 1974; Snyder *et al.,* 1983). Whereas the activities found for CNP in isolated oligodendroglial cell bodies vary significantly, even the highest values (for example, those in cells from bovine white matter) are always less than one third the specific activities measured in isolated myelin (Table 3). It is likely, therefore, that CNP is not in oligodendrocyte cell bodies but that it is restricted to the distal regions of oligodendrocyte processs, membranes at specialized regions of the myelin sheath, and possibly compact myelin.

Enzymes showing moderate to high activities or detectable histochemical staining in oligodendrocytes, and likely to be present at similar or higher levels in other CNS cell types, include the mitochondrial dehydrogenases and cytochrome oxidase, lactate dehydrogenase (LDH), hexokinase, catalase, adenylate cyclase, and ATPases (Tables 1, 2, and 4). On a per-cell basis, the metabolic rates appear to be in the order neurons > oligodendrocytes > astrocytes, whereas per unit volume the oligodendrocytes may be metabolically as active as the neurons (Heller and Elliott, 1955; Korey and Orchen, 1959; Hydén and Pigon, 1960; Hydén and Lange, 1965).

According to the findings reviewed above, it appears more realistic to refer to quantitative differences of an enzyme activity among the CNS cell types than to propose any enzyme as a cell-specific marker. Although several enzymes appear to be specific for glial cells and myelin within the CNS, it would not be surprising if small amounts of at least two of these, CA and GPDH, which function in many biological systems, were eventually confirmed or demonstrated to be present in neurons.

6.2. Specialized Functions of Oligodendroglial Enzymes

This discussion of function will be biased toward the view that the metabolism of oligodendrocytes in the white matter, and possibly also in the gray matter, is directed for the most part toward maintaining the myelin sheath. CA has been detected in oligodendrocytes in both white matter and gray matter (Roussel et al., 1979; Spicer et al., 1979; Ghandour et al., 1980; Kumpulainen and Nystrom, 1981; Parthe, 1981), and the hypothetical functions of this enzyme were discussed in some detail in Section 3.1.4. It is probable that the view of oligodendroglial CA serving to exchange HCO_3^- for Cl^- arose from the putative "glial"-cell localization, and this view may be correct with regard to the enzyme in astrocytes. It seems likely that the significant direction of reaction in oligodendrocytes is the hydration of CO_2, whereas in myelin, the more important reaction is dehydration of carbonic acid. That is, CA in oligodendrocytes would generate HCO_3^-, to provide a substrate for the fixation of "CO_2" into fatty acids and amino acids, while the enzyme in the myelin sheath would be generating CO_2 from carbonic acid, to permit removal, by diffusion, of that product of axoplasmic metabolism.

The 5'-nucleotidase, as well as the CA, in myelin is believed to facilitate transport, and the 5'-nucleotidase in oligodendrocytes may also be a transport enzyme. However, whereas the significant direction of adenosine transport is assumed to be from the axoplasm out of the myelin sheath, adenosine may be transported into the oligodendroglial cytoplasm to support the biosynthesis of RNA. It is possible that the CNP, like the 5'-nucleotidase, in myelin and oligodendrocyte membranes has a role in nucleotide transport, as has been suggested with regard to the CNP in the outer membrane of liver mitochondria (Dreiling *et al.*, 1981). The ATPases are probably involved in transport of the respective ions.

Compared to neurons, oligodendrocytes and the process of myelination are highly vulnerable to conditions of metabolic stress, such as cyanide toxicity (Bass, 1968) and postnatal starvation (Wiggins *et al.*, 1976). These observations imply that the requirement for energy for the synthesis and maintenance of myelin is very high. Furthermore, the susceptibility of white matter to acute thiamine deficiency, which affects transketolase activity, has been interpreted as a sign that myelination is particularly dependent on the pentose phosphate pathway (Dreyfus, 1965). Although the mechanism of white-matter damage during thiamine deficiency is no longer so clear-cut (see Blass *et al.*, 1982), the importance of the pentose phosphate pathway in normal white matter is supported by the significant respiratory rates of oligodendrocytes and the high G-6-PD activities in white matter and bulk-isolated cells (Table 1). Furthermore, the turnover of G-6-PD and GPDH also appear to be required to generate NADPH and glycerol phosphate for the synthesis of myelin lipids, and the turnover of NsChE, with regeneration of choline, may have a similar role. The finding of catalase in oligodendrocytes is relatively recent (e.g., Brannan *et al.*, 1981), and its localization in peroxisomes near mitochondria might imply a role in detoxifying the products of oxygen reduction. Finally, whereas the function of lipid-synthesizing enzymes (Table 4) seems straightforward, the role of the myelin-associated enzyme, the pH 7.2 cholesterol ester hydrolase, in myelin and oligodendroglia remains enigmatic.

6.3. Developmental Changes in the Activities of Oligodendrocyte-Associated Enzymes

For several oligodendrocyte-associated enzymes, developmental changes in specific activity are concomitant with changes in the rate or progress of myelination. It was suggested that some myelin-associated enzymes, such as 5'-nucleotidase and CNP, might occur in relatively high concentrations in the oligodendrocyte cytoplasm early in myelination and might decline, subsequently, as these enzymes are exported into myelin (Snyder *et al.*, 1983). A second group of enzymes that appear to have their highest oligodendrocyte-associated activities during myelination are those of oxidative energy metabolism, e.g., succinate dehydrogenase (SDH) (Meyer and Meyer, 1964), and the pentose phosphate pathway, e.g., G-6-PD (Cammer *et al.,* 1982). Whereas SDH and G-6-PD provide energy and cofactors during myelination, an interesting distinction is that the enzymes that are retained at high activities in the oligodendrocytes of adult animals, namely, GPDH and CA, generate putative substrates, glycerol phosphate and HCO_3^-, which are likely to be required for the maintenance of myelin. LDH is in a fourth category, with significant activity, but not enrichment, occurring early in development, and with a decline in specific activity occurring gradually with age. Since the size of the oligodendrocyte-cell body decreases during maturation (Mori and LeBlond, 1970), the developmental decline in LDH activity per unit volume may actually be minimal.

6.4. Localization of Selected Enzymes within the Mature Oligodendrocyte

The studies cited above suggested that 5'-nucleotidase and CNP were localized in the plasma membranes of the oligodendrocyte perikarya and processes, particularly at the distal regions of the latter, and that CNP, 5'-nucleotidase, and possibly Na^+,K^+-ATPase could be found in myelin. Whereas mitochondrial dehydrogenases and cytochrome oxidase occurred in oligodendrocyte processes as well as perikarya, catalase, Mg^{2+}-ATPase and adenylate cyclase appeared to be restricted to the perikarya. Evidence from histochemical, immunohistochemical, and biochemical studies suggested the occurrence of the cytoplasmic dehydrogenases GPDH, G-6-PD, LDH, and possibly NsChE in the oligodendrocyte processes and specialized regions of the myelin sheath, such as the mesaxons and paranodal loops, as well as in the perikaryal cytoplasm. Of the oligodendrocyte-enriched enzymes, the evidence currently available suggests that CA is most widely distributed into the compartments of the extended oligodendrocyte, at both cytoplasmic and membrane-bound locations, and in gray matter and white matter.

ACKNOWLEDGMENTS

The author receives support from USPHS Grants NS-03356 and NS-12890 and from National Multiple Sclerosis Society Grant 1089. I thank E. Ceccarini, D. S. Snyder, E. Goldmuntz, and W. T. Norton for permission to use their unpublished data and gratefully acknowledge the typing skill of Ms. Reneé Sasso.

7. REFERENCES

Abe, T., Miyatake, T., Norton, W. T., and Suzuki, K., 1979, Activities of glycolipid hydrolases in neurons and astroglia from rat and calf brains and in oligodendroglia from calf brain, *Brain Res.* **161**:179–182.

Adams, C. W. M., 1965, Histochemistry of the nervous system, in: *Neurochemistry* (C. W. M., Adams, ed.), pp. 253–331, Elsevier, New York.

Agrawal, H. C., Hartman, B. K., Shearer, W. T., Kalmbach, S., and Margolis, F. L., 1977, Purification and immunocytochemical localization of rat brain myelin proteolipid protein, *J. Neurochem.* **28**:495–508.

Ashby, W., 1944, A parallelism between the quantitative incidence of carbonic anhydrase and functional levels of the central nervous system, *J. Biol. Chem.* **152**:235–240.

Balazs, R., 1970, Carbohydrate metabolism, in: *Handbook of Neurochemistry,* Vol. 3 (A. Lajtha, ed.), pp. 1–36, Plenum Press, New York.

Banik, N. L., and Smith, M. E., 1976, *In vitro* protein synthesis by oligodendroglial cells, *Neurosci. Lett.* **2**:235–238.

Bass, N. H., 1968, Pathogenesis of myelin lesions in experimental cyanide encephalopathy, *Neurology* **18**:167–177.

Benjamins, J A., Guarnieri, M. Miller, K., Sonneborn, M., and McKhann, G. M., 1974, Sulfatide syntesis in isolated oligodendroglial and neuronal cells, *J. Neurochem.* **23**:751–757.

Bernstein, H. C., Weiss, J., and Luppa, H., 1978, Cytochemical investigations on the localization of 5'-nucleotidase in the rat hippocampus with special reference to synaptic regions, *Histochemistry* **55**:261–267.

Bhat, S., Barbarese, E., and Pfeiffer, S. E., 1981, Requirement for nonoligodendrocyte cell signals for enhanced myelinogenic gene expression in long-term cultures of purified rat oligodendrocytes, *Proc. Natl. Acad. Sci. U.S.A.* **78**:1283–1287.

Blass, J. P., Piacentini, S., Boldizsar, E., and Baker, A., 1982, Kinetic studies of mouse brain transketolase, *J. Neurochem.* **39**:729–733.

Blunt, M. J., Wendell-Smith, C. P., Paisley, P. B., and Baldwin, F., 1967, Oxidative enzyme activity in macroglia and axons of cat optic nerve, *J. Anat.* **101**:13–26.

Brammer, M. J., and Carey, S. G., 1980, Incorporation of choline and inositol into phospholipids of isolated bovine oligodendrocyte perikarya, *J. Neurochem.* **35**:873–879.

Brannan, T. S., Maker, H. S., and Raes, I. P., 1981, Regional distribution of catalase in the adult rat brain, *J. Neurochem.* **36**:307–309.

Buell, M. V., Lowry, O. H., Roberts, N. R., Chang, M.-L. W., and Kapphan, J. I., 1958, The quantitative histochemistry of the brain. V. Enzymes of glucose metabolism, *J. Biol. Chem.* **232**:979–993.

Bunge, R. P., 1968, Glial cells and the central myelin sheath, *Physiol. Rev.* **48**:197–251.

Burstone, M. S., 1959, New histochemical techniques for the demonstration of tissue oxidase (cytochrome oxidase), *J. Histochem. Cytochem.* **7**:112–122.

Cammer, W., and Zimmerman, T. R., Jr., 1981, Rat brain 5'-nucleotidase: Developmental changes in myelin and activities in subcellular fractions and myelin subfractions, *Dev. Brain Res.* **1**:381–389.

Cammer, W., and Zimmerman, T. R., Jr., 1983a, Glycerolphosphate dehydrogenase, glucose-6-phosphate dehydrogenase, lactate dehydrogenase and carbonic anhydrase activities in oligodendrocytes and myelin: Comparisons between species and CNS regions, *Dev. Brain Res.* **6**:21–26.

Cammer, W., and Zimmerman, T. R., Jr., 1983b, Distribution of myelin-associated enzymes and myelin proteins into membrane fractions from the brains of adult shiverer and control (+/+) mice, *Brain Res.* **265**:73–80.

Cammer, W., Fredman, T., Rose, A. L., and Norton, W. T., 1976, Brain carbonic anhydrase: Activity in isolated myelin and the effect of hexachlorophene, *J. Neurochem.* **27**:165–171.

Cammer, W., Snyder, D. S., Zimmerman, T. R., Farooq, M., and Norton, W. T., 1982, Glycerol phosphate dehydrogenase, glucose-6-phosphate dehydrogenase and lactate dehydrogenase: Activities in oligodendrocytes, neurons, astrocytes, and myelin isolated from developing rat brains, *J. Neurochem.* **38**:360–367.

Carey, E. M., Stoll, U., and Carruthers, A., 1980, High activity for triacylglycerol formation and hydrolysis in isolated oligodendroglia from myelinating rat brain, *Biochem. Soc. Trans.* **8**:368–369.

Cavanagh, J.B., Thompson, R. H. S., and Webster, G. R., 1954, The localization of pseudo-cholinesterase activity in nervous tissue, *J. Exp. Physiol.* **39**:185–197.

Church, G. A., Kimelberg, H. K., and Sapirstein, V. S., 1980, Stimulation of carbonic anhydrase activity and phosphorylation in primary astrocyte cultures by norepinephrine, *J. Neurochem.* **34**:873–879.

Clitherow, J. W., Mitchard, M., and Harper, N. J., 1963, The possible biological function of pseudo-cholinesterase, *Nature (London)* **199**:1000–1001.

Cohen, S. R., and Bernsohn, J., 1978, The *in vivo* incorporation of linolenic acid into neuronal and glial cells and myelin, *J. Neurochem.* **30**:661–669.

Costantino-Ceccarini, E., and Suzuki, K., 1975, Evidence for the presence of UDP-galactose:ceramide galactosyltransferase in rat myelin, *Brain Res.* **93**:358–362.

Das, S., Edwardson, J. A., Hughes, D., and McDermott, J. R., 1982, Butyrylcholinesterase (BuChE)-positive glial cells in the pituitary intermediate lobe: Evidence for their role in the formation of pituitary colloid and that BuChE is an endopeptidase, *J. Physiol. (London)* **327**:45P.

Deibler, G. E., Martenson, R. E., Kramer, A. J., Kies, M. W., and Miyamoto, E., 1975, The contribution of phosphorylation and loss of COOH-terminal arginine to the microheterogeneity of myelin basic protein, *J. Biol. Chem.* **250**:7931–7938.

Delaunoy, J.-P., Hog, F., De Villiers, G., Bansart, M., Mandel, P., and Sensenbrenner, M., 1980, Developmental changes and localization of carbonic anhydrase in cerebral hemispheres of the rat and in rat glial cell cultures, *Cell. Mol. Biol.* **26**:235–240.

Deshmukh, D. S., Flynn, T. J., and Pieringer, R. A., 1974, The biosynthesis and concentration of galactosyl diglyceride in glial and neuronal enriched fractions of actively myelinating rat brain, *J. Neurochem.* **22**:479–485.

De Vellis, J., Schjeide, O. A., and Clemente, C. D., 1967, Protein synthesis and enzymatic patterns in the developing brain following head X-irradiation of newborn rats, *J. Neurochem.* **14**:499–511.

De Vellis, J., McEwen, B., Cole, R., and Inglish, D., 1974, Relations between glucocorticoid nuclear binding cytosol receptor and enzyme induction in a rat glial line, *J. Steroid Biochem.* **5**:392–393.

Dorman, R. V., Toews, A. D., and Horrocks, L. A., 1977, Plasmalogenase activities in neuronal perikarya, astroglia, and oligodendroglia isolated from bovine brain, *J. Lipid Res.* **18**:115–117.

Dreiling, C. E., Schilling, R. J., and Reitz, R. C., 1981, 2′,3′-Cyclic nucleotide 3′-phosphohydrolase in rat liver mitochodrial membranes, *Biochim. Biophys. Acta* **640**:114–120.

Dreyfus, P. M., 1965, The regional distribution of transketolase in the normal and the thiamine deficient nervous system, *J. Neuropathol. Exp. Neurol.* **24**:119–129.

Drummond, G. I., Iyer, N. T., and Keith, J., 1962, Hydrolysis of ribonucleoside 2′,3′-cyclic phosphates by a diesterase from brain, *J. Biol. Chem.* **237**:3535–3539.

Eto, Y., and Suzuki, K., 1973, Cholesterol ester metabolism in rat brain: A cholesterol ester hydrolase specifically localized in the myelin sheath, *J. Biol. Chem.* **248:**1986–1991.

Farber, E., Sternberg, W. H., and Dunlap, C. E., 1956, Histochemical localization of specific oxidative enzymes, *J. Histochem. Cytochem.* **4:**254–265.

Farooq, M., and Norton, W. T., 1978, A modified procedure for isolation of astrocyte- and neuron-enriched fractions from rat brain, *J. Neurochem.* **31:**887–894.

Farooq, M., Cammer, W., Snyder, D. S., Raine, C. S., and Norton, W. T., 1981, Properties of bovine oligodendroglia isolated by a new procedure using physiologic conditions, *J. Neurochem.* **36:**431–440.

Fewster, M. E., Ihrig, T., and Mead, J. F., 1975, Biosynthesis of long chain fatty acids by oligodendroglia isolated from bovine white matter, *J. Neurochem.* **25:**207–213.

Fisher, M., Gapp, D. A., and Kozak, L. P., 1981, Immunohistochemical localization of sn-glycerol-3-phosphate dehydrogenase in Bergmann glia and oligodendroglia in the mouse cerebellum, *Dev. Brain Res.* **1:**341–354.

Freeman, N. M., and Carey, E. M., 1980, The determination of plasmalogenase activity in isolated oligodendroglia from bovine brain white matter, *Biochem. Soc. Trans.* **8:**612–613.

Friede, R. L., 1961, A histochemical study of DPN-diaphorase in human white matter with some notes on myelination, *J. Neurochem.* **8:**17–30.

Friede, R. L., 1965, Enzyme histochemistry of neuroglia, *Prog. Brain Res.* **15:**35–47.

Friede, R. L., 1966, *Topographic Brain Chemistry,* Academic Press, New York, pp. 226–236.

Friede, R. L., Fleming, L. M., and Knoller, M., 1963, A comparative mapping of enzymes involved in hexosemonophosphate shunt and citric acid cycle in the brain, *J. Neurochem.* **10:**263–277.

Ghandour, M. S., Langley, O. K., Vincendon, G., Gombos, G., Filippi, D., Limozin, N., Dalmasso, C., and Laurent, G., 1980, Immunochemical and immunohistochemical study of carbonic anhydrase II in adult rat cerebellum: A marker for oligodendrocytes, *Neuroscience* **5:**559–571.

Giacobini, E., 1962, A cytochemical study of the localization of carbonic anhydrase in the nervous system, *J. Neurochem.***9:**169–177.

Gibson, A., and Brammer, M. J., 1981, The influence of divalent cations and substrate concentration on the incorporation of myo-inositol into phospholipids of bovine oligodendrocytes, *J. Neurochem.* **36:**868–874.

Graybiel, A. M., and Ragsdale, C. W., Jr., 1982, Pseudocholinesterase staining in the primary visual pathway of the macaque monkey, *Nature (London)* **299:**439–442.

Hebb, C. O., Silver, A., Swann, A. A. B., and Walsh, E. G., 1953, A histochemical study of cholinesterases of rabbit retina and optic nerve, *Quart. J. Exp. Physiol.* **38:**185–191.

Heller, I. H., and Elliott, K. A. C., 1955, The metabolism of normal brain and human gliomas in relation to cell type and density, *Can. J. Biochem. Physiol.* **33:**395–403.

Hess, H. H., and Pope, A., 1972, Quantitative neurochemical histology, in: *Handbook of Neurochemistry,* Vol. 7 (A. Lajtha, ed.), pp. 289–327, Plenum Press, New York.

Hirsch, H. E., Wernicke, J. F., Meyers, L. W., and Parks, M. E., 1977, Acid lipase-esterase (4-methyl-umbelliferyl oleate hydrolase) of white matter localized in oligdendrocyte cell bodies, *J. Neurochem.* **29:**979–985.

Hotta, S. S., 1962, Glucose metabolism in brain tissue: The hexosemonophosphate shunt and its role in glutathione reduction, *J. Neurochem.* **9:**43–51.

Hydén, H., and Lange, P. W., 1965, The steady state and endogenous respiration of neurons and glia, *Acta Physiol. Scand.* **64:**6–14.

Hydén, H., and Pigon, A., 1960, A cytophysiological study of the functional relationship between oligodendroglial cells and nerve cells of Deiters' nucleus, *J. Neurochem.* **6:**57–72.

Kao-Jen, J., and Wilson, J. E., 1980, Localization of hexokinase in neural tissue: Electron microscopic studies of rat cerebellar cortex, *J. Neurochem.* **35**:667–678.

Kasa, P., and Csillik, B., 1966, Electron microscopic localization of cholinesterase by a copper–lead–thiocholine technique, *J. Neurochem.* **13**:1345–1349.

Keefer, D. A., and Christ, J. F., 1976, Distribution of endogenous diaminobenzidine-staining cells in the normal rat brain, *Brain Res.* **116**:312–316.

Kimelberg, H. K., Braddlecome, S., Narumi, S., and Bourke, R. S., 1978, ATPase and carbonic anhydrase activities of bulk-isolated neuron, glia, and synaptosome fractions from rat brain, *Brain Res.* **141**:305–323.

Kimelberg, H. K., Stieg, P. E., and Mazurkiewicz, J. E., 1982, Immunocytochemical and biochemical analysis of carbonic anhydrase in primary astrocyte cultures from rat brain, *J. Neurochem.* **39**:734–742.

Koelle, G. B., 1954, The histochemical localization of cholinesterases in the central nervous system of the rat, *J. Comp. Neurol.* **100**:211–228.

Korey, S. R., and Orchen, M., 1959, Relative respiration of neuronal and glial cells, *J. Neurochem.* **3**:277–285.

Korhonen, L. K., Naatanen, E., and Hyyppa, M., 1964, A histochemical study of carbonic anhydrase in some parts of the mouse brain, *Acta Histochem.* **18**:336–347.

Kreutzberg, G. W., Barron, K. D., and Schubert P., 1978, Cytochemical localization of 5′-nucleotidase in glial plasma membranes, *Brain Res.* **158**:247–257.

Kuffler, S. W., and Nicholls, J. G., 1966, The physiology of neuroglial cells, *Ergeb. Physiol.* **57**:1–90.

Kumpulainen, T., and Nystrom, S. H. M., 1981, Immunohistochemical localization of carbonic anhydrase isoenzyme C in human brain, *Brain Res.* **220**:220–225.

Kurihara, T., and Tsukada, Y., 1967, The regional and subcellular distribution of 2′,3′-cyclic nucleotide 3′-phosphohydrolase in the central nervous system, *J. Neurochem.* **14**:1167–1174.

Kurihara, T., Nussbaum, J. L., and Mandel, P., 1970, 2′-3′-Cyclic nucleotide 3′-phosphohydrolase in brains of mutant mice with deficient myelination, *J. Neurochem.* **17**:993–997.

Laatsch, R. H., 1962, Glycerol phosphate dehydrogenase activity of developing rat central nervous system, *J. Neurochem.* **9**:487–492.

Lane, M. D., Moss, J., and Polakis, S. E., 1974, Acetyl coenzyme A carboxylase, in: *Current Topics in Cell Regulation* (B. L. Horecker and E. R. Stadtman, eds.), pp. 139–195, Academic Press, New York.

Lehrer, G. M., Bornstein, M. B., Weiss, C., Furman, M., and Lichtman, C., 1970, Enzymes of carbohydrate metabolism in the rat cerebellum developing *in situ* and *in vitro, Exp. Neurol.* **27**:410–425.

Leveille, P. J., McGinnis, J. F., Maxwell, D. S., and de Vellis, J., 1980, Immunocytochemical localization of glycerol-3-phosphate dehydrogenase in rat oligodendrocytes, *Brain Res.* **196**:287–305.

Ludwin, S. K., 1978, Central nervous system demyelination and remyelination in the mouse, *Lab. Invest.* **39**:597–612.

Lumsden, C. E., 1957, The problem of correlation of quantitative methods and tissue morphology in the central nervous system (the distribution of cholinesterases), in: *Metabolism of the Nervous System* (D. Richter, ed.), pp. 91–100, Pergamon Press, New York.

Lynen, F., 1967, The role of biotin dependent carboxylations in biosynthetic reactions, *Biochem. J.* **102**:381–400.

Marani, E., 1977, The subcellular distributon of 5′-nucleotidase activity in mouse cerebellum, *Exp. Neurol.* **57**:1042–1048.

McCarthy, K. D., and de Vellis, J., 1980, Preparation of separate astroglial and oligodendroglial cell cultures from rat cerebral tissue, *J. Cell Biol.* **85**:890–902.

McDougal, D. B., Schultz, D. W., Passonneau, J. V., Clark, J. R., Reynolds, M. A., and Lowry, O. H., 1961, Quantitative studies of white matter. I. Enzymes involved in glucose-6-phosphate metabolism, *J.Gen. Physiol.* **44**:487–498.

McKenna, O., Arnold, G., and Holtzman, E., 1976, Microperoxisome distribution in the central nervous system of the rat, *Brain Res.* **117**:181–194.

McMorris, F. A., Miller, S. L., Pleasure, D., and Abramsky, O., 1981, Expression of biochemical properties of oligodendrocytes × glioma cell hybrids proliferating *in vitro, Exp. Cell Res.* **133**:395–404.

Medzihradsky, F., Nandhasri, P. S., Idoyaga-Vargas, V., and Sellinger, O. Z., 1971, A comparison of the ATPase activity of the glial cell fraction and the neuronal perikaryal fraction isolated in bulk from rat cerebral cortex, *J. Neurochem.* **18**:1599–1603.

Meyer, I., and Meyer, P., 1964, Enzyme histochemistry of the growing and adult oligodendrocyte, *Acta Neurol. Scand.* **40**:89–90.

Mikoshiba, K., Aoki, E., and Tsukada, Y., 1980, 2′,3′-Cyclic nucleotide-3′-phosphohydrolase activity in the central nervous system of a myelin deficient mutant (shiverer), *Brain Res.* **192**:195–204.

Miyamoto, E., and Kakiuchi, S., 1974, *In vitro* and *in vivo* phosphorylation of myelin basic protein by exogenous and endogenous adenosine 3′:5′-mono-phosphate-dependent protein kinases in brain, *J. Biol. Chem.* **249**:2769–2777.

Mori, S., and LeBlond, C. P., 1970, Electron microscopic identification of three classes of oligodendrocytes and a preliminary study of their proliferative activity in the corpus callosum of young rats, *J. Comp. Neurol.* **139**:1–30.

Nagata, Y., Mikoshiba, K., and Tsukada, Y., 1974, Neuron cell body enriched and glial cell enriched fractions from young and adult rat brains: Preparation and morphological and biochemical properties, *J. Neurochem.* **22**:493–503.

Naidoo, D., 1962, The activity of 5′-nucleotidase determined histochemically in the developing rat brain, *J. Histochem. Cytochem.* **10**:421–434.

Naidoo, D., and Pratt, O. E., 1954, The development of adenosine 5′-phosphatase activity with the maturation of the rat cerebral cortex, *Enzymologia* **16**:298–304.

Nishizawa, Y., Kurihawa, T., and Takahashi, Y., 1981, Immunohistochemical localization of 2′,3′-cyclic nucleotide-3′-phosphodiesterase in the central nervous system, *Brain Res.* **212**:219–222.

Norton, W. T., 1980, Myelin enzymes: Indicators of non-insulating functions, in: *Search for the Cause of Multiple Sclerosis and Other Chronic Diseases of the CNS* (A. Boese, ed.), pp. 64–75, Verlag Chemie, Weinheim.

Norton, W. T., and Cammer, W., 1984, Isolation and characterization of myelin, in: *Myelin,* 2nd ed. (P. Morell, ed.), Plenum Press, New York (in press).

Olafson, R. W., Drummond, G. I., and Lee, J. F., 1969, Studies on 2′,3′-cyclic nucleotide 3′-phosphohydrolase from brain, *Can. J. Biochem.* **47**:961–966.

Ord, M. G., and Thompson, R. H. S., 1952, Pseudo-cholinesterase activity in the central nervous system, *Biochem. J.* **51**:245–251.

Parthe, V., 1981, Histochemical localization of carbonic anhydrase in vertebrate nervous tissue, *J. Neurosci. Res.* **6**:119–131.

Pevzner, L., 1979, *Functional Biochemistry of the Neuroglia,* Consultant Bureau, New York, 306 pp.

Pevzner, L., 1982, Oligodendrocytes, in: *Handbook of Neurochemistry,* Vol. 1, 2nd ed. (A. Lajtha, ed.), pp. 357–395, Plenum Press, New York.

Pleasure, D., Abramsky, O., Silberberg, D., Quinn, B., Parris, J., and Saida, T., 1977, Lipid synthesis by an oligodendroglial fraction in suspension culture, *Brain Res.* **134**:377–382.

Pleasure, D., Lichtman, C., Eastman, S., Lieb, M., Abramsky, O., and Silberberg, D., 1979, Acetoacetate and D-(−)-β-hydroxybutyrate as precursors for sterol synthesis by calf oligodendrocytes in suspension culture: Extramitochondrial pathway for acetoacetate metabolism, *J. Neurochem.* **32**:1447–1450.

Poduslo, S. E., 1975, The isolation and characterization of a plasma membrane and a myelin fraction derived from oligodendroglia of calf brain, *J. Neurochem.* **24**:647–654.

Poduslo, S. E., and Norton, W. T., 1972, Isolation and some chemical properties of oligodendroglia from calf brain, *J. Neurochem.* **19**:727–736.

Poduslo, S. E., Miller, K., and McKhann, G. M., 1978, Metabolic properties of maintained oligodendroglia purified from brain, *J. Biol. Chem.* **253**:1592–1597.

Pope, A., 1960, Quantitative histochemistry of the cerebral cortex, *J. Histochem. Cytochem.* **8**:425–430.

Potanos, J. N., Wolfe, A., and Cowen, D., 1959, Cytochemical localization of oxidative enzymes in human nerve cells and glia, *J. Neuropathol. Exp. Neurol.* **18**:627–635.

Radin, N. S., Brenkert, A., Arora, R. C., Sellinger, O. Z., and Flangas, A. L., 1972, Glial and neuronal localization of cerebroside-metabolizing enzymes, *Brain Res.* **39**:163–169.

Reddy, J. K., 1973, Possible properties of microbodies (peroxisomes): Microbody proliferation and hypolipidemic drugs, *J. Histochem. Cytochem.* **21**:967–971.

Reiss, D. S., Lees, M. B., and Sapirstein, V. S., 1981, Is Na + K ATPase a myelin-associated enzyme?, *J. Neurochem.* **36**:1418–1426.

Roessmann, V., and Friede, R. L., 1966, Changes in butyrylcholinesterase activity in reactive glia, *Neurology* **16**:123–129.

Romanul, F., and Cohen, R. B., 1960, A histochemical study of dehydrogenases in the central and peripheral nervous systems, *J. Neuropathol. Exp. Neurol.* **19**:135–136.

Roussel, G., Delaunoy, J.-P., Nussbaum, J.-L., and Mandel, P., 1979, Demonstration of a specific localization of carbonic anhydrase C in the glial cells of rat CNS by an immunohistochemical method, *Brain Res.* **160**:47–55.

Salganicoff, L., and Koeppe, R. E., 1968, Subcellular distribution of pyruvate carboxylase, diphosphopyridine nucleotide and triphosphopyridine nucleotide isocitrate dehydrogenases, and malate enzyme in rat brain, *J. Biol. Chem.* **243**:3416–3420.

Sapirstein, V. S., Lees, M. B., and Trachtenberg, M. C., 1978, Soluble and membrane bound carbonic anhydrases from rat CNS: Regional development, *J. Neurochem.* **31**:283–287.

Scarpelli, D. G., and Pearse, A. G. E., 1958, Physical and chemical protection of cell constituents and the precise localization of enzymes, *J. Histochem. Cytochem.* **6**:369–376.

Schubert, P., Reddington, M., and Kreutzberg, G. W., 1979, On the possible role of adenosine as a modulatory messenger in the hippocampus and other regions of the CNS, in: *Development and Chemical Specificity of Neurons* (M. Cuenod, G. W., Kreutzberg, and F. E. Bloom, eds.), pp. 149–165, Elsevier, New York.

Scott, T. G., 1965, The specificity of 5′-nucleotidase in the brain of the mouse, *J. Histochem. Cytochem.* **13**:657–667.

Seligman, A. M., and Rutenburg, A. M., 1951, The histocemical demonstration of succinic dehydrogenase, *Science* **113**:317–320.

Silver, A., 1974, *The Biology of Cholinesterases,* American Elsevier, New York, 595 pp.

Sinha, A. K., and Rose, S. P. R., 1971, Bulk separation of neurones and glia: A comparison of techniques, *Brain Res.* **33**:205–217.

Snyder, D. S., and Whitaker, J. N., 1983, Postnatal changes in cathepsin D in rat neural tissue, *J. Neurochem.* **40**:1161–1170.

Snyder, D. S., Raine, C. S., Farooq, M., and Norton, W. T., 1980, The bulk isolation of oligo-dendroglia from whole rat forebrain: A new procedure using physiologic media, *J. Neurochem.* **34:**1614–1621.

Snyder, D. S., Zimmerman, T. R., Jr., Farooq, M., Norton, W. T., and Cammer, W., 1983, Carbonic anhydrase, 5'-nucleotidase and 2',3'-cyclic nucleotide-3'-phosphodiesterase activities in oligodendrocytes, astrocytes and neurons isolated from the brains of developing rats, *J. Neurochem.* **40:**120–127.

Solyom, A., and Trams, E. G., 1972, Enzyme markers in characterization of isolated plasma membranes, *Enzyme* **13:**329–372.

Spicer, S. S., Stoward, P. J., and Tashian, R. E., 1979, The immunohistolocalization of carbonic anhydrase in rodent tissues, *J. Histochem. Cytochem.* **27:**820–831.

Sprinkle, T. J., and McDonald, T. F., 1982, Immunofluorescence in oligodendrocytes treated with anti-CNP antisera, *Trans. Am. Soc. Neurochem.* **13:**172.

Sprinkle, T. J., Baker, M. D., and McDonald, T. F., 1981, Immunocytochemical localization of CNP in adult bovine optic nerve, *Trans. Am. Soc. Neurochem.* **12:**209.

Stahl, W. L., and Broderson, S. H., 1976, Localization of Na,K-ATPase in brain, *Fed. Proc. Am. Soc. Exp. Biol.* **35:**1260–1265.

Stefanovic, V., Mandel, P., and Rosenberg, A., 1975, Concanavalin A inhibition of ecto-5'-nucleotidase of intact cultured C6 glioma cells, *J. Biol. Chem.* **250:**7081–7083.

Stekhoven, F. S., and Bonting, S. L., 1981, Transport adenosine triphosphatase: Properties and functions, *Physiol. Rev.* **61:**1–76.

Sternberger, N. H., Itoyama, Y., Kies, M. W., and Webster H. de F., 1978, Myelin basic protein demonstrated immunocytochemically in oligodendroglia prior to myelin sheath formation, *Proc. Natl. Acad. Sci. U.S.A.* **75:**2521–2524.

Sternberger, N. H., Quarles, R. H., Itoyama, T., and Webster, H. de F., 1979, Myelin-associated glycoprotein demonstrated immunocytochemically in myelin and myelin-forming cells of developing rat, *Proc. Natl. Acad. Sci. U.S.A.* **76:**1510–1514.

Stoffyn, A., Stoffyn, P., Farooq, M., Snyder, D. S., and Norton, W. T., 1981, Sialosyltransferase activity and specificity in the biosynthesis *in vitro* of sialosylgalactosylceramide (G_{M4}) and sialosyllactosylceramide (G_{M3}) by rat astrocytes, neuronal perikarya, and oligodendroglia, *Neurochem. Res.* **6:**1149–1157.

Szuchet, S., Stefansson, K., Wollmann, R. L., Dawson, G., and Arnason, B. G. W., 1980, Maintenance of isolated oligodendrocytes in long-term culture, *Brain Res.* **200:**151–164.

Tholey, G., Roth-Schechter, B. F., and Mandel, P., 1980, Development of glial cells in primary cultures: Energy metabolism and lactate dehydrogenase isozymes, *Neurochem. Res.* **5:**847–854.

Vercelli-Retta, J., Silveira, R., Dajas, F., and Rodriquez, D., 1976, Enzyme histochemistry of rat interfascicular oligodendroglia, with special reference to 5'-nucleotidase, *Acta Anat.* **96:**514–516.

Waehneldt, T. V., Matthieu, J.-M., and Neuhoff, V., 1977, Characterization of a myelin-related fraction (SN 4) isolated from rat forebrain at two developmental stages, *Brain Res.* **138:**29–43.

Waelsch, H., Berl, S., Rossi, C. A., Clarke, D. D., and Purpura, D. P., 1964, Quantitative aspects of CO_2 fixation in mammalian brain *in vivo*, *J. Neurochem.* **11:**717–728.

Wiggins, R. C., Miller, S. L., Benjamins, J. A., Krigman, M. R., and Morell, P., 1976, Myelin synthesis during postnatal nutritional deprivation and subsequent rehabilitation, *Brain Res.* **107:**257–273.

Winick, M., 197, Nutrition and cell growth, *Fed. Proc. Am. Soc. Exp. Biol.* **29:**1510–1515.

Wood, J. G., Jean, D. H., Whitaker, J. N., McLaughlin, B. S., and Albers, R. W., 1977, Immu-
  nocytochemical localization of the sodium, potassium activated ATPase in knifefish brain,
  J. Neurocytol. **6:**571–581.
Yandrasitz, J. R., Ernst, S. A., and Salganicoff, L., 1976, The subcellular distribution of carbonic
  anhydrase in homogenates of perfused rat brain, *J. Neurochem.* **27:**707–715.
Zimmerman, T. R., Jr., and Cammer, W., 1982, ATPase activities in myelin and oligodendro-
  cytes from the brains of developing rats and from bovine brain white matter, *J. Neurosci.*
  Res. **8:**73–81.

OLIGODENDROCYTE DEVELOPMENT IN CULTURE SYSTEMS

STEVEN E. PFEIFFER

1. INTRODUCTION

1.1. The Oligodendrocyte as a Model Cell Biological System

The oligodendrocyte has as its primary recognized function the task of producing a prodigious amount of membrane, possibly unequaled by any other cell

Abbreviations used in this chapter: (ARA-C) cytosine arabinoside; (BUdR) 5-bromo-2'-deoxyuridine; (CA) carbonic anhydrase; (CGalT) UDP-galactose:ceramide galactosyl transferase (cerebroside galactosyl transferase); (CNP) 2',3'-cyclic nucleotide 3'-phosphohydrolase; (CST) 3'-phosphoadenosine-5'-phosphosulfate cerebroside sulfate transferase (cerebroside sulfotransferase); (DIC) day(s) in culture; (EAE) experimental allergic encephalomyelitis; (EM) electron microscope, e.-microscopic, e. microscopy; (GalCer) galactosylceramide (galactocerebroside); (GalCer sulfate) galactosylceramide sulfate (sulfatide); (GFAP) glial fibrillary acidic protein; (GPDH) glycerol-3-phosphate dehydrogenase; (GS) glutamine synthetase; (HMG-CoA) β-hydroxy-β-methylglutaryl-coenzyme A; ([^{3}H]-TdR) tritiated thymidine; (IgG) immunoglobulin G; (LDH) lactate dehydrogenase; (LM) light microscope, l.-microscopic, l. microscopy; (MAG) myelin-associated glycoprotein; (MBP) myelin basic protein; (MS) multiple sclerosis; (PAGE) polyacrylamide gel electrophoresis, p. g. electrophoretic; (PLP) proteolipid protein; (RIA) radioimmunoassay; (sulfatide) GalCer sulfate; (W1, W1a, W1b, W3 proteins) Wolfgram proteins (see Section 2.3.2c).

STEVEN E. PFEIFFER ● Department of Microbiology, University of Connecticut Health Center, Farmington, Connecticut 06032 type, and maintaining it for a lifetime. Morell and Norton (1980) estimate that during development, these otherwise rather diminutive cells produce several times their mass in myelin membrane each day. Additional interest is occasioned by the manner in which oligodendrocytes send multiple copies of this specialized membrane a substantial distance from their cell bodies before amplifying it into vast sheets that become wrapped and compacted around qualified axons (Peters, 1964; M. B. Bunge *et al.,* 1962; Hirano, 1968; R. P. Bunge, 1968). Thus, oligodendrocytes engage in membrane biogenesis on a scale to intrigue the membrane biochemist.

In the process of effecting this feat, oligodendrocytes receive critical signals from other cells that stimulate and modulate the substantial degree of intrinsic information that oligodendrocytes seem to acquire at an early age (below). Both cellular and humoral factors appear to contribute to the stimulation and maintenance of oligodendrocyte differentiated function. Some of these factors have been identified as known hormones or nutrients, while others herald new communication signals the molecular natures and modes of action of which can be only guessed at present. These factors promise a fascinating field of study to the cell biologist interested in cellular sociology, while simultaneously calling on the skill of the biochemist and molecular biologist to expound mechanisms.

Finally, the completed product, myelin, is remarkable not only for its morphological symmetry, but also for the conservation of energy and space it provides in assisting neuronal conduction. Indeed, the failure to produce or maintain this critical product quickly leads to a seriously impaired level of physiological function. Here is an arena in which morphologists, physiologists–biophysicists, and physicians find an opportunity to mix their talents.

1.2.   Myelinogenesis in Culture

This chapter will analyze the impact (both established and projected) of *in vitro* culture systems on these various aspects of oligodendrocyte differentiation. Throughout, the term *myelinogenesis* will be used to denote the whole process of oligodendrocyte development and differentiation (Figure 1), with the recognition that this term is being used in a broader sense than is usual.

This process is visualized as a series of individual events that occur approximately sequentially (allowing for periods of possible simultaneous parallel expression) and that are postulated, until proved otherwise, to be independently regulated by a plethora of factors. In this view, these regulatory phenomena are derived from signals originating both intrinsically and extrinsically to the oligodendrocytes. A stem or precursor cell first becomes committed to its future at a genetic level. These precursors are then recruited in a stepwise manner along the path to myelin formation during a period of proliferation

Commitment of myelinogenic precursor cells		
Recruitment to become functional "oligodendroglia"		Induction
Oligodendroglial proliferation and maturation		
Synthesis and intracellular transport of myelin membrane components		Assembly
Assembly of components into a membrane		
Formation of oligodendroglial processes		
Process–axon interaction		
Wrapping of axon by oligodendrocyte membrane		Morphogenesis
Myelination Formation of a multilamellar membrane around axon		
Compaction of the myelin membranes		
Myelin maintenance		Maintenance and repair
Remyelination		

FIGURE 1. A conceptual scheme for the sequence of events in myelinogenesis.

and maturation that is expressed phenotypically by the appearance and accumulation of a number of myelin-specific (or at least enriched) "markers." This period of commitment and initiation of specific myelinogenic gene expression can conveniently be brought under the heading of myelinogenic *induction.*

The synthesis and intracellular transport of these components allow their *assembly* into an immature myelin membrane, of which oligodendrocyte-process formation may be an early example.

The interaction of the processes with axons, the initial wrapping of the axons, and finally the formation of a multilamellar membrane and its subsequent compaction can be combined under the heading of *myelin morphogenesis.* The latter aspects of this period constitute "myelination" *per se.*

Finally, mechanisms must exist to maintain the integrity of the myelin sheath, for biochemical turnover of myelin is a certainty, and along with such renewal, the possibility of remyelinogenesis and ultimately remyelination must be considered.

1.3. Experimentally Critical Aspect of Cell-Specific Markers

Certain identification of neuroglial cells as either astrocytes or oligodendroglia is at least as difficult in tissue culture as it is in fixed and stained material when viewed through the light or electron microscope
WINDLE (1958)

The difficulty is not with cells which are morphologically similar to those described in classical anatomy, but, rather, with the many intermediate forms present
BORNSTEIN AND MURRAY (1958)

It would be difficult to overestimate the value of specific markers for
identifying and quantitating the different cell types present in
heterogeneous cultures and for studying the properties of individual
cells
RAFF *et al.* (1979*b*)

Three main criteria for oligodendrocyte identification and function have been used in studies of their development in culture. First, light-microscopic (LM) and ultrastructural characterizations have utilized the descriptions from analyses of oligodendrocytes *in vivo* (e.g., Privat, 1975; Skoff *et al.*, 1976*a, b*) [for *in vitro* examples, see also Berg and Schachner (1981), Sarlieve *et al.* (1981), and other papers discussed in Section 2]. While these criteria have been applied with some success, particularly at the ultrastructural level, such identification is often fraught with uncertainty. This is particularly true in dissociated cultures of mixed cell type in which normal histiotypic relationships have been purposely disrupted; at the LM level, small, round cells with processes may just as easily prove to be neurons as oligodendrocytes. Add an additional confounding agent such as an antiserum, toxin, or genetic mutation, and further uncertainty can intrude.

Second, immunocytochemical identification has become increasingly useful over the past half dozen years or so (Table 1) (also see Chapter 4). Thus, it is becoming increasingly unnecessary or even unacceptable to depend *solely* on morphology for the identification of oligodendrocytes. This situation results from recognition of biochemical markers specific for, or at least highly enriched in, different cell types. These markers and their recognition by serological tech-

TABLE 1.   Some Cell Markers in Current Use in Studies of Myelinogenesis in
Central Nervous System Culture Systems

Oligodendrocytes
    Galactosylceramide (GalCer)
    Sulfatide (GalCer sulfate)
    2′,3′-Cyclic nucleotide 3′-phosphohydrolase (CNP), Wolfgram proteins W1a and W1b
    Carbonic anhydrase (CA)
    Myelin basic protein (MBP)
    Proteolipid protein (PLP)
    Myelin-associated glycoprotein (MAG)
    Lactate dehydrogenase (LDH)
Neurons
    Tetanus toxin (specificity now doubtful)
    Neuron-specific enolase
    Thy-1
    A2B5 (specificity now doubtful)
Astrocytes
    Glial fibrillary acidic protein (GFAP)
    Glutamine synthetase (GS)

---

niques have made possible the routine identification and quantification of mye-linogenic processes in a mixed cell population, allowing one to express the data on a "per-specific-cell-type" basis. Insofar as a case can be made for the cell being closer to a true "biological unit" than is a milligram of cellular protein, such an analysis becomes of more than passing interest.

Third, immunological reagents used in a quantitative subcellular fashion [e.g., radioimmunoassay (RIA)], biochemical analyses, and enzymatic assays for cell-type-specific markers constitute another level of quantification.

A combination of serological cell identification and biochemical analysis allows one to distinguish between population and individual cell phenomena in development (e.g., Barbarese and Pfeiffer, 1981). That is, an increase in the specific activity of a myelinogenic marker may be due either to an increase in the number of cells expressing that marker or to an increase in the level of activity per cell, or both.

With no attempt to do justice to the cunning that has led to the delineation of these molecules as cell-type-specific markers, a brief note on the origins of these conclusions may be in order. To some extent, the assignment of a bio-chemical entity (e.g., an enzymatic activity, structural protein, or surface anti-gen) to a given cell type has depended on a correspondence between, for exam-ple, the immunofluorescence staining and the morphological peculiarities of that cell type. This is, however, only a part of the process of making an assign-ment, and the process, where possible, profits markedly from the demonstration of serological–structural relationships in normal tissue sections.

At least as valuable in the process is the use of previously determined biochemical and physiological data, particularly in the case of most of the markers for oligodendrocytes. The presence of myelin basic proteins (MBPs), for example, does not identify oligodendrocytes because antisera against MBPs stain cells previously suspected, on morphological grounds, to be oligodendro-cytes. Rather, the connection can be made fairly because MBPs have been shown to be specific components of myelin, and myelin is made by cells defined as oligodendrocytes.

Taken together, these reagents and methodologies allow a wide latitude in the study of oligodendrocytes in culture. In particular, using immunological tools: (1) not only can general cell types be recognized by analysis of "differ-entiation antigens" (Boyse and Old, 1969), but also further refinement of anti-sera specificity can lead to the identification of subclasses of cells; (2) specific cell types can be isolated from single-cell suspensions (e.g., Campbell *et al.,* 1977), or cells can be selectively eliminated by antibody-mediated cytotoxicity (Brockes *et al.,* 1979); (3) the subcellular distribution of antigens can be mapped (e.g., Sternberger *et al.,* 1978*a, b*); (4) specific molecules can be iso-lated by immunoaffinity chromatography and analyzed (e.g., Drummond and Dean, 1980); and (5) cellular functional properties can be modified (e.g., Diaz *et al.,* 1978). The relationship of the development of this area to a similar one for the immune system should be noted (Cantor and Boyse, 1977; Parkhouse and Cooper, 1977).

Several markers are in current use for studies of oligodendrocytes in culture (Table 1) (see Chapters 4 and 6 for additional references). Galactosylceramide [galactosylcerebroside (GalCer)] is one of the first of the identified oligodendrocyte markers to appear on the cell surface. Its sulfated analogue, GalCer sulfate (sulfatide), also appears early in oligodendrocyte development. The recognition of several enzyme activities associated with myelin and oligodendrocytes has led to additional serological markers. These include glycerol-3-phosphate dehydrogenase (GPDH), carbonic anhydrase (CA), lactate dehydrogenase (LDH), and 2',3'-cyclic nucleotide-3'-phosphohydrolase (CNP). Finally, the major proteins of myelin, myelin basic protein (MBP), proteolipid protein (PLP), and the Wolfgram proteins, are also useful markers for oligodendrocytes. A relatively minor constituent, myelin-associated glycoprotein (MAG), also shows promise as a marker.

Several markers for nonoligodendrocytes have also proved particularly useful in studies of oligodendrocytes in culture, especially when examined by double-label techniques in conjunction with an oligodendrocyte marker. *Neuron-specific enolase* (14-3-2) (Cicero *et al.,* 1970; Schmechel *et al.,* 1978) and *Thy-1 antigen* (Mirsky and Thompson, 1975; Morris, 1982) have utility as neuronal markers. *Tetanus toxin,* which recognizes gangliosides GD_{1b} and GT_1 (van Heyningen, 1963), binds to the surfaces of neurons in cultures of both PNS and CNS tissue (Dimpfel *et al.,* 1975, 1977; Mirsky *et al.,* 1978; Fields *et al.,* 1978). Monoclonal antibody A2B5, which reacts with one of the GQ gangliosides, and possibly with others, identifies chick neurons (Eisenbarth *et al.,* 1979). The identification of populations of certain glial cells and their progenitors that are also recognized by these "neuronal" markers is described in Section 3.3.

Astrocytes are frequently identified immunocytochemically by staining with *glial fibrillary acidic protein* (GFAP) antisera (Eng *et al.,* 1971; Raff *et al.,* 1979*a,b*). *Glutamine synthetase* (GS) has also shown substantial promise as an astrocytic marker (Norenberg and Martinez-Herandez, 1979; Schousboe, 1982).

With the advent of monoclonal antibodies (Kohler and Milstein, 1976), additional cell-specific markers with increased specificity will be available (e.g., Sommer and Schachner, 1981; Ranscht *et al.,* 1982). Thus, this approach will continue to be a cornerstone for studies of the type outlined below, not only for oligodendrocytes, but also for an increasing number of other classes and subclasses of the nervous system.

1.4. Schwann Cells vs. Oligodendrocytes: Differences in the Extent of Intrinsically Derived Regulation of Myelinogenic Function

Given the structural and functional similarities of myelin from the PNS and CNS [although critical differences are well recognized (R. P. Bunge, 1968; Webster, 1975)], one might suspect that Schwann cells and oligodendrocytes are close developmental cousins and that it would be appropriate to discuss their differentiation in culture together in this chapter. This view would seem to be strengthened by the substantial degree of interchangeability of Schwann cells and oligodendrocytes seen in studies of experimental myelination. For example, CNS oligodendrocytes can myelinate PNS axons (Aguayo *et al.,* 1978; Weinberg and Spencer, 1979; Wood *et al.,* 1980; Bray *et al.,* 1981); conversely, PNS Schwann cells can myelinate CNS axons (Blakemore, 1977; B. M. Harrison, 1980). Even species differences do not necessarily constitute a barrier, for human Schwann cells will myelinate mouse axons (Aguayo *et al.,* 1977). However, a closer look discloses that these two cells are very different, operating under very different regulatory requirements. Cell-culture techniques have in recent years contributed substantially to establishing these differences.

Developmental studies suggest that oligodendrocytes are derived from neural epithelium (Schaper, 1897) and Schwann cells from neural crest (R. G. Harrison, 1924; Detweiler and Kehoe, 1939; Weston, 1963). Whereas an oligodentrocyte can produce many segments of myelin on more than one axon at a time, and as a result often remain at some distance from the myelinated segments (Maturana, 1960; Peters, 1960; R. P. Bunge *et al.,* 1965; Peters *et al.,* 1976; Sternberger *et al.,* 1978*a*), a Schwann cell has a one-to-one correspondence with a myelinated segment and is intimately associated physically with that segment (Geren, 1954) [see figures on pages 92 and 99 in Morell and Norton (1980)]. While there are some notable shared biochemical markers between CNS and PNS myelin, and thus between oligodendrocytes and Schwann cells (e.g., MBPs, GalCer and sulfatide, and CNP), important differences exist as well [e.g., PLP in oligodendrocyte myelin, P_0 glycoprotein in Schwann-cell myelin (e.g., Everly *et al.,* 1974), RAN-1 Schwann-cell surface antigen (Fields *et al.,* 1975, 1978; Brockes *et al.,* 1977)].

The extent of the intrinsic informational content and the extrinsic regulatory requirements of oligodendrocytes and Schwann cells also differ markedly (Gould *et al.,* 1982; Varon and Manthorpe, 1982). It has been demonstrated by several laboratories in a variety of ways that neurons are mitogenic for Schwann cells. One very graphic example of this is found in the studies of Wood and Bunge (Wood and Bunge, 1975; Wood, 1976) [see also R. P. Bunge and M. B. Bunge (1981) and Chapter 1]. In their system, essentially pure populations of sensory ganglionic neurons or Schwann cells are developed. Using tritiated thymidine ($[^3H]$-TdR) uptake into DNA and autoradiography to assay for cell cycling and mitotic activity, they found that Schwann cells placed in close association with neurons were dividing, whereas Schwann cells in a region devoid of neurons were not. Subsequent work by Salzer and colleagues (Salzer and Bunge, 1980; Salzer *et al.* (1980*a,b*) has provided evidence that the mitogenic factor may be a neurite surface protein (see also DeVries *et al.,* 1982; Manthorpe *et al.,* 1980). This is an example of an extrinsic regulatory factor for Schwann cells. From experiments such as these, it appears that Schwann cells have a strong requirement for *continued* interactions, quite possibly direct contact, with neurons for mitotic activity. There are also humoral mitogens for Schwann cells, such as those found in pituitary extracts (Raff *et al.,* 1978*a,b;* Brockes *et al.,* 1980*a*).

Neurons also send clear signals to Schwann cells for myelination. One of the most graphic experimental approaches that shows this involves nerve grafting (Aguayo *et al.,* 1976*a,b;* Weinberg and Spencer, 1975, 1976). Briefly, peripheral nerves can be cut and reconnected with other nerves or introduced as a grafted segment into another nerve. The axons regrow and invade the distal stump, in which the cut axons have become degraded, but in which the Schwann cells have been retained and have in fact proliferated. The invading, regenerating axons are eventually remyelinated. The importance of axonal signals in this remyelination process is demonstrated by the following cross-anastomosis experiment. Some nerves, such as the cervical sympathetic trunk, are normally not myelinated. However, if a cervical sympathetic nerve segment is grafted into a phrenic nerve, which normally is myelinated, the regenerating phrenic nerves that invade the graft are remyelinated. The conclusion is made, after consideration of a variety of appropriate control studies, that Schwann cells of the cervical sympathetic trunk are competent to myelinate, but do not receive the correct signal from their axons. That signal is provided by phrenic axons.

Actual myelination is, of course, a very stringent and complex process of differentiation. Are neuronal signals also required for Schwann cells to start myelinogenesis, for example, by synthesizing myelin-specific lipids and proteins? The requirement for continued neuronal stimulation appears to extend to early Schwann-cell expression of myelin-related differentiated function as well. *In vivo,* Schwann cells accumulate MBPs and P_0 glycoprotein only after they have received the signal to myelinate. This phenomenon is paralleled in culture. When rat sciatic-nerve Schwann cells from 5-day-old rat pups are grown in culture, they *initially* express several myelin-related properties. However, within days, this expression is largely lost (Figure 2) (see also Brockes *et al.,* 1979; Raff *et al.,* 1978*c,* 1979*b;* Kennedy *et al.,* 1980; Ranscht *et al.,* 1982). Thus, the expression of surface GalCer and sulfatide (as assessed by immu-

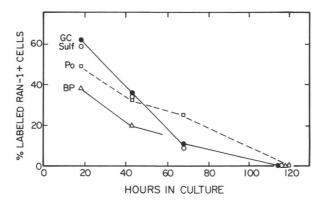

FIGURE 2. Rat sciatic-nerve Schwann cells in culture. The curves show the percentages of Schwann cells [identified by immunofluorescent staining with anti-RAN-1 surface antigen (Fields, 1979)] that also stained positively with anti-GalCer (GC), -sulfatide (Sulf), -P_0 protein (P_0), or -MBP (BP). Adapted from Mirsky et al. (1980) and Brockes et al. (1980b).

nofluorescence) and MBP and P_0 protein [as measured by polyacrylamide gel electrophoresis (PAGE)] drops to undetectable levels over a period of a few days. In addition, M. B. Bunge et al. (1980) have also presented evidence that neuronal stimulation is needed for Schwann-cell basal-lamina formation. While it seems clear that a major proportion of myelinogenic function is lost, it may not be absolute. For example, Fryell (1980) found continued Schwann-cell synthesis of sulfatide when the sensitive $^{35}SO_4$ incorporation assay was used. Whether this "contradiction" is due to relative assay sensitivities, or whether the sulfatide is not transported to the cell surface [as appears to be the case with the oligodendroglioma cell lines G26-20 and -24 (Pfeiffer et al., 1981a; Steck and Perruisseau, 1980)], is not clear. On the other hand, Brockes et al. (personal communication, 1982) have used a sensitive RIA to confirm the dramatic reduction of P_0 protein. Nevertheless, the Schwann cells are still highly differentiated, for they continue to express the RAN-1 surface antigen (Mirsky et al., 1980) and S100 protein (Moore, 1965), both of which are apparently intrinsic Schwann-cell properties. Therefore, the neuronal stimulation required for myelin-specific properties is not only profound, but also rather specific.

We find quite a different story when oligodendrocytes are grown in culture (see below). Even in the absence of any substantial neuronal population (as judged by the absence of tetanus-toxin-binding cells), they continue to express myelinogenic function for months, even after passage (Mirsky et al., 1980; Berg and Schachner, 1981). An interesting control experiment demonstrates this difference between oligodendrocytes and Schwann cells even in mixed cultures of the two (Kennedy et al., 1980; Mirsky et al., 1980).

2. CULTURE SYSTEMS

Oligodendrocytes have been studied in a variety of culture systems that are organized and presented here on the basis of increasing cellular disaggregation or, conversely, decreasing normal histiotypic relationships among cells.

In analyzing the contributions made by the various culture approaches, emphasis will be given to the data with regard to four main periods of oligodendrocyte differentiation (Figure 3). Point A represents the time at which an oligodendrocyte marker first becomes detectable in the population of maturing oligodendrocytes. The determination of this time point is a function not only of the biologically interesting issues of gene regulation and product stability, but also of the sensitivity of the assays. B, represented in Figure 3 as a slope and a duration, measures the product of B_1, the number of cells recruited from the immediately preceding precursor pool to express the marker in question, and B_2, the average level of the marker per recruited cell. C recognizes the optimal level of B attained, i.e., the product of C_1, the ultimate number of cells recruited, and C_2, the maximal steady-state level achieved per cell. D is the time at which down-regulation occurs, the reverse of the processes that contribute to B and C, and E assesses the time–course and extent of this down-regulation. Figure 3 provides a framework within which early oligodendrocyte differentiation in culture can be considered and compared to patterns observed *in vivo*. A comparison of these parameters among markers may lead to some insights regarding the extent to which the various steps are obligatorily sequential or, in contrast, the extent to which they are under parallel regulation and thus susceptible to parallel shifting by experimental (or pathological) intervention.

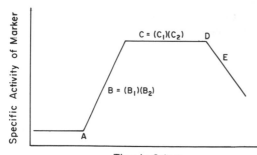

FIGURE 3. Critical experimental points in the analysis of oligodendrocyte development in culture. (A) Time of first appearance of a marker activity; (B) development of expression of the marker activity; [(B_1)] cellular recruitment or proliferation of recruited cells (or both), i.e., number of active cells; [(B_2)] cellular expression, i.e., level of marker activity per recruited cell; (C) maximal level of marker specific activity achieved; [(C_1)] number of active cells; [(C_2)] average activity per active cell; (D) temporal extent of maintenance of maximal levels; (E) down-regulation, rate and extent.

2.1. Explant Cultures

It seems, therefore, justifiable to hope that with practice and with some technical improvements, as for instance in respect of nutrient media, it may be possible to provide an easily made and easily handled experimental system upon which biochemical studies . . . can be made directly.
LUMSDEN AND POMERAT (1951)

The original technique for introducing brain tissue into culture for the study of myelination, a technique that continues to enjoy wide usage, involves the maintenance of small pieces of tissue, generally about 0.5–1 mm^2 in a rich medium. The fragment size is chosen to be small enough to allow adequate exchanges with the environment, yet large enough to maintain some element of histiotypic organization, at least initially. Substantial cellular reorganization and outward migration occur in culture, but these rearrangements are largely accomplished in the tissue's own way and time [contrast with dissociated cultures (Sections 2.2 and 2.3)]. Of particular experimental interest is that despite the isolation of the tissue from systemic influences present in the animal, oligodendrocyte maturation and substantial myelination occur. In addition, since there appear to be few if any barriers to the entry of radioactive precursors, drugs, sera, and other substances into the CNS explants, and since the chemical environment is under direct experimental control, a variety of experimental inquiries into the mechanism of myelin synthesis and maintenance have been possible. A review of some of the milestones in the development of the myelinating explants follows, and additional specific examples of their contributions to the field are discussed later.

Peterson (1950) and Peterson and Murray (1955a,b) developed methods for maintaining chick dorsal-root ganglia in Maximow chambers and first described the formation of myelin sheaths in culture. They demonstrated thereby that one of the more complex intercellular relationships of the nervous system, the interaction of Schwann cells and axons, was able to develop, apparently normally, in an isolated culture environment.

At about the same time, Pomerat and co-workers (Pomerat *et al.,* 1950; Pomerat, 1951; Lumsden and Pomerat, 1951; Pomerat and Costero, 1956) were pursuing studies of growth patterns of kitten cerebellum cultured on coverslips in roller tubes. They noted the survival of a variety of cell types, including "pulsating" oligodendrocytes. Hogue (1953), meanwhile, had demonstrated success in maintaining fragments of human brain obtained from fetal or postnatal autopsy material (up to 33 years of age) in hanging drops and roller-tube cultures. Again, oligodendrocytes were identified by LM. Wolfgram and Rose (1957) also observed oligodendrocytes in kitten corpus callosum explants.

Hild (1957, 1963*a,b*) extended the description of myelin formation to explants of mammaliam CNS grown on coverslips in roller tubes ("flying coverslips"). He noted that the original histiotypic organization of an explant is not maintained intact in culture, as might have been predicted *a priori,* but rather that "the architectural plan of the tissue . . . becomes progressively rearranged as a result of readjustments essential to the *in vitro* experience."

Bornstein (1958) and Bornstein and Murray (1958) pursued the culture of newborn rat and kitten cerebellum using the Maximow-chamber technique. This allowed serial observations of the same culture over a long-term. They demonstrated that newborn-rat cerebellar explants maintained on a glucose-rich medium underwent a 2-week period of cellular outgrowth and (re)organization that led to myelination during the 3rd week (Bornstein and Murray, 1958; Murray, 1959, 1964, 1965).

These observations were extended by Ross and Bornstein (1962) using the electron microscope (EM) and helped to establish the notion that myelinogenesis in cultured mammalian CNS involved "the participation of a neuroglial cell contributing its external membrane to the formation of the multilamellated myelin sheath."

These results and conclusions have subsequently been amply verified and extended for cerebellum of chick, rodent, cat, and guinea pig (Perier, 1959; Hild and Tasaki, 1962; Piper, 1962; Geiger, 1963; Bornstein, 1964; Wolf, 1964; Field and Hughes, 1965, 1969; Field *et al.,* 1968; Allerand and Murray, 1968; Storts and Koestner, 1969; Crain and Bornstein, 1972; Bornstein, 1973; Kim and Tunicliff, 1974; Hauw *et al.,* 1974; Raine and Bornstein, 1974; Silberberg, 1975; Aparicio *et al.,* 1976; Seil, 1979), spinal cord of chick, rodent, and human (Peterson *et al.,* 1965; R. P. Bunge *et al.,* 1965; Boyde *et al.,* 1968; Kim *et al.,* 1972; R. P. Bunge and Wood, 1973), brainstem and cerebral cortex (Hild, 1966), and hippocampus (Beach *et al.,* 1982). In addition, there have been occasional reports of myelinated neuronal *soma* in cultures of rodent brain (Hild, 1963*a;* Field *et al.,* 1968; Kim, 1970; Kim and Tanaka, 1971).

These early studies appropriately concentrated on morphological examinations of the cultured explants to ascertain the extent to which maturation *in vitro* resembled or faithfully reproduced the course of normal cellular differentiation, tissue organization, and myelination (Murray, 1965, 1971; Lumsden, 1965; Varon, 1970). Nevertheless, the power of these culture models was at the same time being emphasized through the elucidation of certain nutritional requirements for myelination (e.g., Peterson and Murray, 1960) (also see Section 3.1).

Starting in the late 1960s, myelinating rodent spinal cord and brain explants have been analyzed for an increasing variety of biochemical parameters, often those that characterize the myelin sheath, with a view toward developing a quantitative assay for the extent of myelin formation. These studies have complemented the morphological findings in supporting the notion that maturation in culture is similar to that seen in the animal (Lehrer and Bornstein, 1968; Seil and Herndon, 1970; Wolf, 1970; Lehrer *et al.*, 1970*a,b;* Silberberg *et al.*, 1972; Lehrer, 1973), a point we will return to in Section 4.1. For example, Lehrer *et al.* (1970*a,b*) examined the development of the activities of several enzymes of glucose metabolism. The greatest rates of change were between 8 and 15 days in culture (DIC), the time when other studies indicated that myelination began.

Histochemical methods were also used to study enzymatic activities related to carbohydrate metabolism in newborn-rat cerebellar explants (Yonezawa *et al.*, 1962*a,b*). These workers found important changes in enzymatic activity and subcellular distribution in oligodendrocytes (and other cell types). Succinate dehydrogenase and NAD and NADP dehydrogenases diaphorases were especially active in supporting cells during myelin formation (Yonezawa *et al.*, 1962*b*) and declined again once the myelin sheath reached completion.

Sulfatide synthesis was measured in cultures of 13- to 14-day fetal mouse spinal cord (Fry *et al.*, 1972, 1973). The rate of incorporation of ^{35}S-labeled sulfate increased markedly between 8 and 12 DIC and more slowly thereafter. This synthetic activity was correlated temporally with the appearance of myelin. In similar measurements with newborn-rat cerebellar cultures, some of the labeled sulfatide was recovered in a sucrose-gradient fraction with the density properties of myelin (Silberberg *et al.*, 1972). Latovitzki and Silberberg (1973, 1975, 1977) studied galactolipid levels and galactosyltransferase activity, as well as the activity of 2′,3′-cyclic nucleotide-3′-phosphohydrolase (CNP) in newborn rat cerebellar cultures. Galactolipid levels began to rise after 10 DIC, later than *in vivo,* but at about the time when myelin could first be detected by LM. Variability among cultures of the same age could be correlated to the extent of myelin production determined morphologically. Galactosyl- and glucosyltransferase activities were studied in control cultures and in cultures undergoing antiserum-induced demyelination. Galactosyltransferase activity increased with age in culture over the 16 DIC of the experiment; at 16 DIC, the activity was 22% of whole rat brain of similar age. CNP activity followed a nearly identical time course, increasing from 2 DIC onward to a value at 16 DIC of 0.8 μmole/min per mg protein. When these experiments were repeated under conditions of antiserum-induced demyelination, galactosyltransferase and CNP activities were also reduced, suggesting that these activities may be specific characteristics of oligodendrocytes.

Sterol synthesis and CNP activity were studied in cultures of newborn-mouse spinal cord (Pleasure and Kim, 1976*a,b;* Kim and Pleasure, 1978). The specific activity of CNP rose rapidly until 15 DIC, then rose more slowly to 1.3 μmoles/min per mg protein (Pleasure and Kim, 1976*a*) or continuously to 30 DIC to 2.5 μmoles/min per mg protein (Pleasure and Kim, 1976*b*), paralleling the time of onset *in vivo* quite closely. Hydroxymethylglutaryl-CoA reductase activity rose sharply between 5 and 11–15 DIC, a pattern delayed by about 10 days compared to that *in vivo*. Similarly, the rate of incorporation of labeled acetate into sterol was greatest at 12 DIC.

Myelin basic protein accumulation in fetal-mouse spinal-cord ex-plants began at 8 DIC and increased throughout the experiment (20 DIC) to a low level of 9 pmoles/mg protein (recalculated) (Sheffield and Kim, 1977). CNP activity began to rise slightly ahead of MBP accumulation, though both approximately paralleled the appearance of visible myelin formation.

Membrane fractions prepared by centrifugation from newborn-rat cere-bellar cultures and noncultured littermate cerebella have been compared by Bradbury (1977, 1978) and Bradbury and Lumsden (1979). The myelinlike material from culture, despite a normal myelin ultrastructural appearance in the explants, was deficient in galactolipids at early times compared to *in vivo*. CNP activity was also somewhat reduced, though to a lesser degree. The pro-portion of galactolipids did slowly increase in the myelin fractions from these cultures between 21 and 60 DIC.

The composition of myelin isolated from cultures initiated from 14- to 16-day fetal-rat spinal cord was studied by Fagg *et al.* (1979). PAGE analysis of the myelin proteins isolated from these cultures suggested that the myelin from explants closely resembled that isolated from rat spinal cord, although there appeared to be less basic protein and more Wolfgram protein. Further, the developmental patterns for the proteolipid protein (PLP), Wolfgram proteins, and DM-20 protein were somewhat different than *in vivo,* although the final amounts accumulated were not too different.

Returning to a study of myelin production as determined by morphology, Seil, Blank, and co-workers (Seil *et al.,* 1979, 1980*b;* Blank *et al.,* 1980; Seil and Blank, 1981) used cytosine arabinoside (ARA-C) to eliminate oligoden-drocytes, or kainic acid to eliminate neurons capable of being myelinated, from mouse cerebellar explants. In neither type of treated explant could any sub-stantial myelin formation be observed. Nevertheless, when the two types of deficient explants were cocultured in apposition, myelin was formed in the ARA-C-treated (neuron-retaining) explant. Presumably, oligodendrocytes from kainic-acid-treated explants migrated into the other explant and associ-ated with the neurons.

At this point, a brief summary of the state of the explant culture model is in order, leaving for later the description of additional experiments using explants to elucidate aspects of myelinogenic growth factors (Section 3.1), mechanisms of demyelination (Section 3.2), and mutations that affect myeli-nation (Section 3.4).

Explant cultures of chick and rodent brain are generally maintained in Maximow chambers or on coverslips in roller tubes. Cerebellum and spinal cord have been the favored materials, though cortex and brainstem can also be cultured. Certainly, by morphological standards, interesting amounts of myelin are made in these cultures over a reasonably short period of time (e.g., 2–3 weeks in culture for rodent cerebellum). The existing data suggest that with some exceptions, biochemical development occurs in an amount and a time–course quite similar to those observed *in vivo*. Some of these measurements have been attempts to quantify the amount of morphologically identifiable myelin by correlating it with the level of accumulation of a biochemical activity. Although generally this correlation has appeared to be good, these biochemical parameters also develop in dissociated cultures in which little or no actual myelin is formed (see below), so the significance of this correspondence may be somewhat illusory.

2.2. Dissociated–Reaggregated Cell Cultures

Turning to dissociated–reaggregated cell cultures, we find the investigator in a slightly perverse position; having wreaked histiotypic havoc on the tissue, the investigator then asks the cells to put themselves back together again. Nevertheless, this technique has the potential for being a powerful tool for the study of cellular interactions important in development, including the analysis of genetic and biochemical phenomena that underlie morphogenesis. There is a substantial body of experimental work on the reaggregation of a variety of embryonic tissues (Moscona, 1965a,b; Steinberg, 1963). The embryonic tissue is first dissociated to a single-cell suspension by either enzymatic or mechanical means. The cells are then placed in a small flask that is rotated continuously so as to form a gentle vortex, encouraging cellular interactions and aggregation. Typically, after a period of reaggregation and recovery, the cells sort themselves out according to type in reproducible, orderly ways (Steinberg, 1963). Cells from embryonic organs can form complex histiotypic patterns in aggregates (Moscona, 1965a,b; Garber, 1967; Orr, 1968), the outcome being dependent on the extent of embryonic development of the organ at the time of dissociation (Moscona, 1965a,b; Garber, 1967). The mechanisms that mediate the sorting out of cells and formation of a characteristic histiotypic organization have spawned considerable interest and controversy (Moscona, 1968; Steinberg, 1963). Specific aggregation-enhancement factors have been sought and in some cases found (Moscona, 1968; Lilien, 1968).

DeLong (1970) and Sidman (1970) extended this background to the developing mouse CNS, in particular hippocampus and isocortex. Again, a remarkable degree of histiotypic organization was obtained in the aggregates over a period of days to weeks. As with other tissues, the potential for morphogenetic reorganization was critically dependent on the developmental age of the dissociated tissue [see also Stefannelli *et al.* (1977) concerning studies of chick-retina reaggregation].

The reaggregating-culture model received additional credibility with the studies of Seeds (1971, 1973, 1975) (see also Seeds and Gilman, 1971; Seeds and Hafke, 1978). They showed that reaggregating cultures of 16- to 18-day fetal-mouse brain, dissociated by a combination of enzymatic and mechanical treatments, underwent a biochemical (i.e., neurotransmitter-related enzymatic activity) differentiation pattern similar to that in the developing mouse brain. EM was used in characterizing the development of morphologically mature synapses and myelinated axons in these cultures (Seeds and Vatter, 1971; Seeds, 1973). Cell aggregation was largely completed in 24 hr, resulting in apparently random collections of loosely packed cells. A "sorting-out" phase then occurred over the next 1–7 DIC, after which morphological and biochemical differentiation ensued (DeLong, 1970; Seeds, 1971, 1975; Honegger and Richelson, 1976).

The development of myelinogenic activity in reaggregation cultures initiated from 7-day embryonic chick brain was examined by Schmidt (1975). CNP activity increased between 6 and 16 DIC and reached a second peak at 28 DIC in the experiment presented and then declined. The peak CNP activity was about 5% of that *in vivo*. The rate of sulfatide synthesis increased between 0 and 16 DIC and then also declined. After 35–40 DIC, both activities were minimal.

Honegger and Richelson (1976) eschewed the enzymatic treatment during dissociation in favor of mechanical sieving of the brain. Their initial studies concentrated on the expression of a number of enzymatic activities of neurotransmitter metabolism. Tissue less than 2 days of age after birth was required for aggregate formation, and the pattern of enzyme-activity development varied with the age of the starting tissue. The highest levels of specific activity for the neuron-specific enzymes were found after 3–4 weeks in culture when fetal brain was used.

The culture system of Honegger and Richelson (1976) has been used for a number of investigations of myelinogenesis. In reaggregating cultures from 17-day fetal rats and mice, Sheppard *et al.* (1978) found that CNP activity began at 15–20 DIC and reached substantial levels of 6–7 μmoles/min per mg protein at 35 DIC. 3'-Phosphoadenosine-5'-phosphosulfate cerebroside sulfate transferase [cerebroside sulfotransferase (CST)] activity began at 16–20 DIC and attained a peak at 24 DIC. Matthieu *et al.* (1978, 1979, 1980), Matthieu and Honegger (1979), Bourre *et al.* (1979), and Trapp *et al.* (1979) studied cultures initiated from 15- to 16-day-old fetal-rat brains. Myelin, which was not found by EM analysis at 19 DIC, was present at 26 DIC. However, the amount of myelin found in the aggregates was much lower than that observed at the corresponding age *in vivo* (Trapp *et al.,* 1979). In addition, myelin compaction was sometimes abnormal, with the "axons only loosely wrapped with poorly compacted myelin lamellae . . . in the vicinity of normally myelinated axons." This coexistence of normal and abnormal would seem to suggest a cell-by-cell variability in the cultures, rather than a general ("systemic") defect of the medium. Glycolipid accumulation in these cultures was rather low, comparable to those of a 12- to 13-day-old rat (Bourre *et al.,* 1979). Nevertheless, the increase that did occur corresponded to the somewhat delayed appearance of myelin. Sulfatide synthesis (as measued by $^{35}SO_4$ incorporation) began *after* (the exact point being indeterminate from the data) 18 DIC (Matthieu *et al.,* 1978; Matthieu and Honegger, 1979), from 20 to 40 DIC (Bourre *et al.,* 1979). MBP accumulation began after (see Section 2.1) 20 DIC and rose to a very low value of 7–15 pmoles/mg protein (recalculated) at 40 DIC. UDP-galactose:ceramide galactosyl transferase [cerebroside galactosyl transferase (CGalT)], CST, and CNP activities all began to rise rather early after 6–8 DIC, equivalent to postnatal day 1, and attained maximal levels by 20–30 DIC (CGalT), 30 DIC (CST), or 40–50 DIC [CNP (0.5–3 μmoles/min per mg protein)]. By 40 DIC, severe degradation was evident in the aggregates (including a substantial increase in cholesterol esters) and myelinated axons were no longer found. Possibly the degenerative phase can be reduced through the modification of media components (Trapp *et al.,* 1978).

Membrane fractions were isolated from similar 33- and 50-day-old cultures (Matthieu *et al.,* 1979, 1980). CNP activity was about 3 μmoles/min per mg protein in 33 DIC homogenates and about 2 μmoles/min per mg protein in 50 DIC material. In an isolated membrane, however, the CNP activity reached levels of 20 μmoles/min per mg protein, comparable to that of myelin. PAGE analyses of the myelin fraction from these cultures revealed all the major myelin proteins. When the amount of protein was approximated by Fast Green dye binding (spectrophotometric gel scanning), the ratio of the relative amounts of MBP to PLP was similar to that in myelin from young animals. This result, coupled with data on the yield of myelinlike membrane, the increased levels of high-molecular-weight proteins, the very low levels of cerebroside (Bourre *et al.,* 1979), and the persistence of the apparent higher-molecular-weight form of the major fucose-labeled glycoprotein, led the authors to conclude that the membrane fraction was similar to immature myelin characteristic of 15-day-old rat brain. The conclusion of retarded myelin maturation in culture elicits memories of similar "slow myelin maturation" discussed by Bradbury (1977) and Fagg *et al.* (1979) in explant cultures. Nevertheless, the ratio of the amount of small and large MBPs, another indicator of myelin maturation, was similar in the cultures to that *in vivo* [as also found more recently by Barbarese and Pfeiffer (1981) for dissociated–attached cultures].

Fetal-rat-brain aggregates have been cultivated in a chemically defined medium consisting of Dulbecco's Modified Eagle's Medium supplemented with insulin, triiodothyronine, hydrocortisone, transferrin, and trace elements (Honegger *et al.,* 1979; Honegger and Matthieu, 1980). There was some retardation in cellular growth and differentiation in the defined medium compared to that supplemented with 15% fetal calf serum. Nevertheless, aggregation did occur in defined medium, and myelinated axons were sent by 30 DIC, although myelin-sheath compaction was often incomplete. CST activity began to increase at 6 DIC, peaked at 11 DIC, and then declined. CNP activity increased between 6 and 16 DIC, lagging slightly compared to CST, and then remained at about 2.2 μmoles/min per mg protein.

The development of glycerol-3-phosphate dehydrogenase (GPDH) activity was studied in reaggregating cell cultures of various brain areas from mice ranging in age from 12 gestational days to 6 days postnatal (Kozak *et al.,* 1977; Kozak, 1977). For example, GPDH activity in cerebellar aggregates initiated from 4-day-old mice began to increase on the *in vivo* schedule at about 5 DIC, reaching a plateau of activity by 30 DIC. The increase was due to the development of the adult isozyme activity.

In summary, reaggregating dissociated cell cultures of fetal and newborn mouse and rat brain have been characterized ultrastructurally and biochemically. Cellular reorganization is followed by the differentiation of neurons and glia. Some myelinlike membrane is formed, generally beginning after about 3 weeks in culture. Biochemical analyses have confirmed that a substantial degree of cellular differentiation, both neuronal and glial, takes place, including myelinogenic activity. Membrane fractions isolated from cultures with morphologically identifiable myelin reveal biochemical characteristics confirming a myelinlike identity, though it appears to be a relatively immature form. Depending on the marker studied and the exact technique used, marker expression is either on time relative to that *in vivo* or only moderately delayed. Generally, these time–courses are correlated with the appearance of myelin, although as also suggested for explant cultures (Section 2.1), this coincidence may be somewhat illusory, since dissociated–attached cultures (Section 2.3) also express myelinogenic marker development in the absence of compact myelin formation. After 40 DIC or so, reaggregated cultures begin to undergo degradative changes, including the loss of myelin.

The main advantage of reaggregated cultures would seem to be in the analysis of the mechanisms of cell interaction and reorganization and the determination of the importance of these mechanisms in the development of myelinogenic potential over relatively short periods of time (less than 30 DIC). What cell types are critical? What aspects of cell-surface integrity are important? Are there cell-type number ratio requirements?

2.3. Dissociated–Attached Cell Cultures

Dissociated–attached cell cultures will be defined to include those culture systems in which the tissue has been dissociated by mechanical or enzymatic means or both into single-cell suspensions or at least very small clumps of cells and grown as populations of mixed cell type attached to a solid substrate in at least a quasi two-dimensional state (see Figure 6A). Therefore, this designation rules out dissociated–reaggregated cell cultures, which allow a fair degree of opportunity for cells to reestablish normal histiotypic relationships (e.g., Garber, 1967) while being maintained in suspension as three-dimensional clumps. It also arbitrarily eliminates cultures of purified cell types, which are given separate consideration in Section 2.4. However, it does acknowledge and allow for the reaggregation of dissociated cells that routinely occurs to varying extents during the period between plating the cell suspension and attachment (e.g., Varon and Raiborn, 1969). The extent to which such aggregates are formed can be controlled somewhat by culture techniques that affect the rate of attachment of cells to the substrate. For example, coating the dishes with poly-L-lysine (Yavin and Yavin, 1974) enhances attachment and reduces the time available for preliminary reaggregation. The aforestated definition for dissociated–attached cell cultures also allows for postattachment cell-sorting and stratification that routinely occurs in cultures of this type, leading to multilayers consisting of a basal layer of astrocytes, fibroblasts, and occasional patches of ciliated ependymal cells, on top of which grow neurons and oligodendrocytes (Wiesmann *et al.,* 1975; McCarthy and de Vellis, 1980). Thus, the term "monolayer culture" occasionally applied to these cultures is more often than not a clear misnomer; clumps, aggregates, and layers represent elements of the norm.

2.3.1. Early Studies

The use of dissociated–attached cell cultures for studies of oligodendrocyte differentiation derived impetus from the early work of Sensenbrenner *et al.* (1971) and Werner *et al.* (1971) with chick embryo brain and from their work immediately following with chick, rat, mouse, and human embryonic material (Sensenbrenner *et al.,* 1972; Booher and Sensenbrenner, 1972; see also Bornstein and Model, 1972). These authors maintained dissociated (0.25% trypsin, or sieving) 8-day-old embryonic-chick brain or 9-day-old embryonic-rat brain in culture and noted over a period of a few weeks the survival and development of cells judged to be neurons and oligodendrocytes as well as other cells. The putative oligodendrocytes grew on top of a cellular matrix of polygonal cells and were often clustered around neurons and their processes. Brain extract added to the culture medium enhanced the number of oligodendrocytes (see Section 3.1). Occasional examples of myelin formation, as judged by phase-contrast microscopy, were also reported. If older embryos were used, neuronal development was restricted, but oligodendrocytes and astrocytes survived. These cellular identifications, although necessarily carried out by morphological criteria, have been amply confirmed more recently with the advent of cell-specific serological techniques (see Section 1.3). The authors correctly predicted that these cultures would be useful "in biochemical studies which involved hormones" (e.g., N. R. Bhat *et al.*, 1979), "proteins" (e.g., Barbarese and Pfeiffer, 1981), or "drugs" (e.g., Siegrist *et al.*, 1980) "which affect the central nervous system" and noted that "factors involved in promoting neuronal and glial differentiation can be applied and their action analyzed during the reorganization and evolution of the cultures" (Booher and Sensenbrenner, 1972).

Numerous studies with dissociated–attached brain-cell cultures have noted, on morphological and intuitive grounds, the presence of "oligodendrocytes" (Varon and Raiborn, 1969; Grosse and Lindner, 1970, 1972; Sensenbrenner *et al.*, 1971; Booher and Sensenbrenner, 1972; Bornstein and Model, 1972; Yavin and Menkes, 1973; Yavin and Yavin, 1974, 1977; Korinkova and Lodin, 1977; Noël-Courtney and Heinen, 1977; Sensenbrenner, 1977; Fedoroff, 1977, 1978; McCarthy and de Vellis, 1978, 1980; Haugen and Laerum, 1978; Rioux *et al.*, 1980; Lodin *et al.*, 1978a,b; Hansson *et al.*, 1980). Varon and Raiborn noted as recently as 1969 that "the culture of dissociated cells from neural tissue has hardly been explored" and set out on a logical controlled course of studies of dissociated chick brain to remedy the situation.

2.3.2. Biochemical and Serological Studies

Subsequent studies have increasingly stressed biochemical and serological analyses of specific myelin products produced by dissociated cultures as a function of time in culture ("in development"). In the majority of cases, the experiments have been designed to provide information on either (1) biochemical parameters such as enzyme activities per culture or per mg protein or (2) the number of cells expressing a biochemical marker by serological analysis. Only rarely have these two pieces of data been gathered for the same cultures and the biochemical data expressed per cell.

2.3.2a. Sulfatide Synthesis. Historically, sulfatide and other lipids have been the earliest to be examined in detail (see also Chapter 5). Wiesmann *et al.* (1975) carefully examined net sulfatide synthesis via $^{35}SO_4$ incorporation into trypsin-dissociated cultures of newborn mouse brain. Synthesis began at 6–8 DIC and rose to a peak at 17 DIC. More recent reports from this laboratory, using mechanically dissociated newborn mouse brain, found an earlier period of sulfate incorporation (initiation at 3 DIC, peak at 11 DIC) in addition to the later pattern (Siegrist *et al.*, 1981). These investigators also reported corresponding patterns of development for several related enzymatic activities. Amonn *et al.* (1978) found that high concentrations of certain antibiotics depressed the rate of sulfatide synthesis (as measured by $^{35}SO_4$ incorporation).

Sulfatide synthesis and related enzymatic activities have also been nicely studied in newborn and fetal mouse brain in culture by Sarlieve *et al.* (1980*a*) and N. R. Bhat *et al.* (1979, 1981). Although the cultures initiated from 15-day embryos developed the activities under consideration more slowly than did cultures started from one-day-postnatal brain, the former developed much higher specific activities. Sulfatide synthesis began at 24 DIC, rapidly reached a maximum at 32 DIC, and then decreased. Later studies by this laboratory using apparently similar cultures showed more rapid developmental kinetics (N. R. Bhat *et al.*, 1981). Sulfatide synthesis began at 5–10 DIC, but did not peak until 40 DIC. Further characterization of these cultures, including analyses of morphological changes and neuronal content, have also appeared (Sarlieve *et al.*, 1980*b*, 1981).

Pfeiffer *et al.* (1981*b*) examined the onset and maintenance of sulfatide synthesis (again using $^{35}SO_4$ incorporation) into cultures started from 19- to 21-day fetal rat brain. Synthesis began at around 8 DIC and peaked at 20 DIC, that is, on essentially the same schedule as occurs *in vivo* (Davison and Gregson, 1962; McKhann and Ho, 1967). These results have recently been confirmed by analyses of sulfatide accumulation, using high-performance liquid chromatography (Singh and Pfeiffer, 1983).

All these studies indicate a proclivity by dissociated rodent cultures for the initiation and rapid development of sulfatide synthesis.

2.3.2b. Galactosylceramide Synthesis. The synthesis of galactosylceramide (GalCer), the immediate biochemical precursor of sulfatide, has not been studied extensively by biochemical techniques in dissociated cultures. However, the identification of oligodendrocytes by anti-GalCer immunocytochemistry (Figure 4) has gained wide use, so much so that a GalCer$^+$ cell has to some extent become a definition for an oligodendrocyte in culture (Raff *et al.*, 1978*c*).

Raff *et al.* (1979*b*) found that about 5% of the cells in optic-nerve or corpus-callosum cultures of rat pups became GalCer$^+$, a percentage somewhat greater than that found in cultures of cerebellum and cerebral cortex. Large membranous expansions were made visible by the immunofluorescent staining. Small GalCer$^+$ cells were found in newborn-rat optic-nerve cultures as early as 1 DIC (Mirsky *et al.*, 1980).

Cultures initiated from adult-rat optic nerve dissociated enzymatically also contained GalCer$^+$ cells, although only 0.1% of the total cells were so labeled (Kennedy and Lisak, 1980). The authors asked an interesting question: What is the relationship of the surviving cultured GalCer$^+$ cells to those oli-

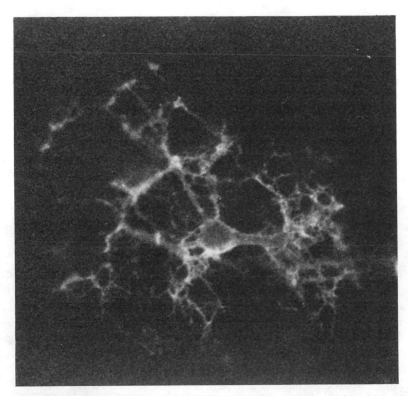

FIGURE 4. Oligodendrocyte in a culture of dissociated 19- to 21-day fetal-rat brain after 22 DIC stained by immunofluorescence with anti-GalCer. ×526.

godendrocytes involved in myelination *in vivo* at the time of isolation? They also demonstrated that human oligodendrocytes can be stained with GalCer antisera (Kennedy *et al.,* 1980).

The number of GalCer$^+$ cells increased during 7–14 DIC before attaining a steady state in cultures of unspecified, but presumably newborn (Sandru *et al.,* 1980), mouse brain (Bologa-Sandru *et al.,* 1981*a*).

Abney *et al.* (1981) used cultures initiated from either 10- or 13-day embryonic-rat brain; GalCer$^+$ cells first appeared at 13–14 DIC or 10–11 DIC, respectively. Therefore, they concluded that glial cells develop (with regard to GalCer expression) on schedule in culture, retaining cognizance of their embryonic history prior to dissociation.

Ranscht *et al.* (1982) studied 15-day fetal-, or newborn-, rat-brain cultures with a monoclonal antibody to GalCer and a rabbit antibody to sulfatide. GalCer$^+$ cells appeared prior to sulfatide-positive cells. At 6 DIC (fetal) or 1 DIC (newborn), few GalCer$^+$ cells were noted, and less than 30% of them were weakly sulfatide-positive. At 5 DIC later, "more" GalCer$^+$ cells were seen, 60–80% of which were sulfatide-positive. After a further 9 DIC, 95% of an unspecified number of GalCer$^+$ cells were also sulfatide-positive. These data confirm the culture's knowledge of its embryonic history (Abney *et al.,* 1981) and suggest that GalCer is expressed prior to sulfatide on the surface of developing oligodendrocytes (as might be predicted on biochemical-pathway grounds). Antibody sensitivity must of course be considered before a definitive conclusion can be made in this case.

These studies all seem to agree that oligodendrocytes in dissociated–attached cell cultures synthesize and accumulate GalCer readily on their surfaces with a time–course very similar to that occurring in normal *in vivo* development.

2.3.2c. Wolfgram Proteins and 2′,3′-Cyclic Nucleotide 3′-Phosphohydrolase Activity. The class of relatively high-molecular-weight proteins (43,000–60,000 daltons) described by Wolfgram (1966) can be resolved into multiple bands by PAGE, the two most predominant bands of which were designated W2 and W3 by Wiggins *et al.* (1974), but W1 and W2 by Nussbaum *et al.* (1977) (Figure 5). Subsequently, Waehneldt and Malotka (1980) labeled a closely spaced doublet W1 and W2. Although these authors were apparently attempting to follow the earlier terminology of Nussbaum *et al.* (1977), it appears that in fact their W1 and W2 are a resolved doublet of the Nussbaum *et al.* (1977) W1, while a higher-molecular-weight band tentatively identified as tubulin ("TUB") corresponds to W2 of Nussbaum *et al.* (1977). Shortly thereafter, Sprinkle *et al.* (1980) and Drummond and Dean (1980) defined the relationship of Wolfgram proteins and CNP. Sprinkle *et al.* (1980) used the Waehneldt and Malotka terminology, calling the resolved doublet W1 and W2, and related these bands to CNP species called, correspondingly, CNP1 and CNP2. Drummond and Dean (1980) also resolved the W1 of Nussbaum *et al.* (1977) into a doublet, termed the bands W1a and W1b, and related them to two components with the same electrophoretic mobility previously identified as CNP and labeled CNa and CNb. The terminology of Nussbaum *et al.* (1977) and Drummond and Dean (1980) seems to have predominated, and one can refer to the doublet bands in question as W1a and W1b, and to the corresponding CNP species as CNPa and CNPb (lower- and higher-molecular-weight species, respectively). At present, published studies of Wolfgram protein and CNP in dissociated cultures have not evaluated the development of the subspecies by electrophoretic methods.

Labourdette *et al.* (1979) introduced trypsin-dissociated (newborn?)-rat cerebral hemispheres into culture and maintained them up to 5 months. Using antiserum prepared against Wolfgram protein (W1), they noted small W1$^+$ cells that were not labeled with anti-glial fibrillary acidic protein (GFAP) sera. They reported that when calf serum was used as a supplement, in contrast to

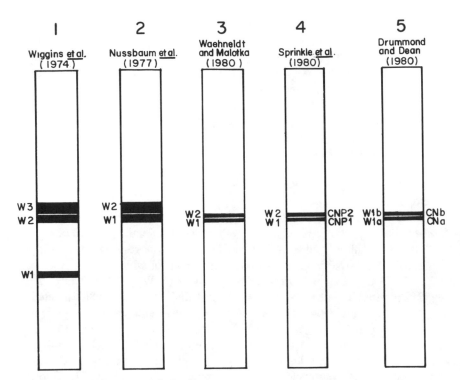

FIGURE 5. Comparison of some of the variations used to denote the Wolfgram–CNP doublet. Slightly modified from a drawing contributed by Dr. T. Sprinkle, Atlanta.

fetal calf serum, up to 46% of the cells were "small cells," judged to be oligo-dendrocytes on the basis of their labeling with anti-W1 serum (unfortunately, the *percentage* of these small cells positive for W1 is not given). It is curious that cultures thought to be so rich in "oligodendrocytes" proved to be so poor in CNP activity (0.8 μmole/min per mg protein after 45 DIC). Subsequent experiments (Labourdette *et al.*, 1980) emphasized the importance of high plating densities, thereby eliminating the calf serum–fetal calf serum differences (were the same lots of fetal calf serum used?). In these latter experiments, "some" W1$^+$ small cells were seen at 10 DIC, and "most but not all" small cells were W1$^+$ at 20 DIC. Unfortunately, in these experiments, the fraction of the total cell number that was small cells was not stated. When cells were plated at high density, a peak of CNP activity was observed at 20 DIC (1.3 μmoles/min per mg protein), a much more rapid development than seen in their earlier work. A further paper by this group (Roussel *et al.*, 1981) reporting studies on a similar culture system found no W1$^+$ cells at 6 DIC, "some" at 8 DIC, about "50 percent of small cells" $W1^+$ at 16 DIC, and "most small cells" $W1^+$ at 28 DIC.

A protein band comigrating with Wolfgram protein (PAGE) and low levels of CNP activity were observed in extracts of cultures of 16-day embryonic rat cerebral hemispheres (Richter-Landsberg and Yavin, 1979).

CNP activity was also examined in dissociated cultures of 15-day embryonic mouse (Sarlieve *et al.*, 1980*a*). Specific activities began to increase from the start and were still rising at 40 DIC (1 μmole/min per mg protein).

In 19- to 21-day fetal-rat-brain cultures, the initial appearance and increase in CNP activity were nearly identical to those for sulfatide synthesis; i.e., the increase started at 8–10 DIC and rapidly reached a maximum (6–7 μmoles/min per mg protein) at 21 DIC, a level maintained thereafter throughout the experiment (to 60 DIC) (Pfeiffer *et al.*, 1981*b*) (Figure 6).

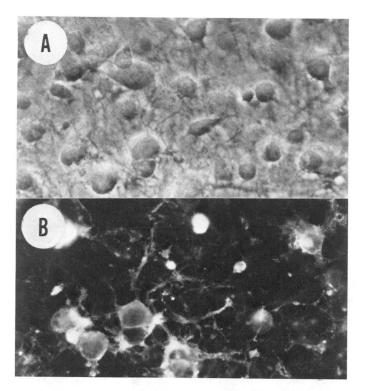

FIGURE 6. Dissociated 19- to 21-day fetal-rat-brain culture after 21 DIC. (A) Phase-contrast. (B) Oligodendrocytes stained by immunofluorescence with rabbit anti-bovine CNP. ×526.

Although CNP activity can appear early in cultures of rodent brain, there appears to be more variability among the results from various laboratories than for sulfatide synthesis. This suggests that the regulation of CNP may be more sensitive to environmental modifications introduced through brain dissociation and culture.

2.3.2d. Myelin Basic Protein. Several laboratories have used antisera raised against MBP to identify oligodendrocytes in cultures and assess their myelinogenic development. Labourdette et al. (1979) and Roussel et al. (1981) followed the appearance of MBP$^+$ cells in conjunction with their studies of Wolfgram protein (see Section 2.3.2c) in dissociated newborn mouse brain. The general appearance of the two markers was similar.

MBP$^+$ cells in cultures of newborn-rat optic nerve were found after 5 DIC, later than the first appearance of GalCer$^+$ cells at 1 DIC (see Section 2.3.2b) (Mirsky et al., 1980).

In adult-rat optic-nerve cultures, Kennedy and Lisak (1980) found that all GalCer$^+$ cells were also MBP$^+$ and vice versa. In cultures of 20-week fetal-human spinal cord, 50% of the GalCer$^+$ cells were also MBP$^+$; in contrast, none of the GalCer$^+$ cells in human optic-nerve cultures were MBP$^+$ (Kennedy et al., 1980).

Bologa-Sandru et al. (1981a) studied MBP in dissociated mouse brain in their experiments in conjunction with GalCer. MBP$^+$ cells appeared only after 14 DIC [in contrast to GalCer$^+$ cells, which appeared at 7 DIC (see Section 2.3.2b)] and slowly increased. At 28 DIC, only about 3% of the GalCer$^+$ cells were also MBP$^+$; on the other hand, all MBP$^+$ cells were GalCer$^+$. It would be interesting to learn what happens to the MBP$^+$/GalCer$^+$ ratio at times greater than 28 DIC.

Barbarese and Pfeiffer (1981) combined immunofluorescent identification of MBP$^+$ cells with RIA of MBP in developing cultures initiated from 19- to 21-day rat embryos. MBP accumulation began after 20 DIC and reached a peak (300 pmoles/mg protein) at 34 DIC before declining. The number of MBP$^+$ cells increased 20-fold during this period. Combining these data, they determined that MBP accumulated at the rate of 0.2 fmole/oligodendrocyte per day, with each oligodendrocyte having on the average 1 fmole/cell at all times examined. Thus, the accumulation of MBP in the cultures between 20 and 35 days was due primarily to an increase in the number of oligodendrocytes that contained MBP, rather than to continued increases in the amount of MBP per cell. These rates of accumulation per cell are comparable to those calculated to occur in vivo. Subsequent to the peak activity, the amount of MBP declined over the next 30 DIC to a new level (100 pmoles/mg protein) that was stable until the end of the experiment at 120 DIC. In immunofluorescent studies (Figure 7), it was also noted that although morphologically identifiable myelin was not produced, the oligodendrocytes elaborated a com-

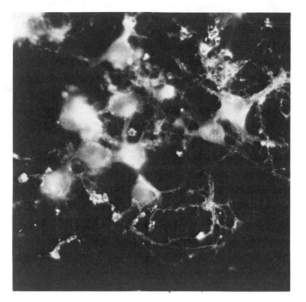

FIGURE 7. Oligodendrocytes in a dissociated 19- to 21-day fetal-rat-brain culture after 21 DIC. Stained by immunofluorescence with anti-MBP (rhodamine-labeled second antibody). ×526.

plex network of MBP$^+$ processes and sheets similar to those seen with anti-GalCer immunofluorescence (e.g., Mirsky *et al.,* 1980). Unlike the situation *in vivo,* in which MBP is present in oligodendrocyte cell bodies only during the early period of myelination and subsequently becomes restricted to the myelin sheath (Sternberger *et al.,* 1978a,b; Hartman *et al.,* 1979), in culture, MBP remained distributed in the perikarya, processes, and membranous sheets throughout the period of culture. Finally, the development of the four molecular forms of MBP (Barbarese *et al.,* 1978) was examined by the immunoblot technique of Towbin *et al.* (1979). Although the normal ratios of the four forms were eventually achieved, the ratios among them were modulated somewhat differently during development in culture. From these studies, the authors concluded that the accumulation, modulation of the molecular forms, and insertion of MBP into the membrane can occur in the absence of myelin formation, but that continued metabolic stability, subcellular sequestration, and fine control of the relative proportions of the different forms of MBP may be dependent on myelin morphogenesis. In subsequent work from this laboratory (Pfeiffer *et al.,* 1981b), the onset of MBP accumulation was compared with that of sulfatide synthesis and CNP activity. Unlike the latter markers, which followed the *in vivo* schedule, MBP was substantially delayed in its expression. It is noteworthy that once started, however, the rate of development is comparable to that seen *in vivo* (and parallels that for the other two markers). That is, the delay is specifically in the time of *initiation* of MBP accumulation in the cultures. Since this accumulation is determined largely by the number of cells that have become MBP$^+$, the delay can be said to be attributable to delay in recruitment of cells for this phase of myelinogenesis.

These studies allow the conclusion that oligodendrocytes in culture readily synthesize and maintain high levels of MBP, but that its regulation is more affected by the rigors of dissociated culture than are sulfatide synthesis and CNP activity.

2.3.2e. Proteolipid Protein.   The accumulation of PLP has been studied in dissociated cultures of 19- to 21-day-old fetal brain (Macklin and Pfeiffer, 1983). PLP was detected by both electroblotting and immunofluorescence as early as 10 DIC. The number of PLP-containing cells assayed by immunofluorescence reached 5×10^4 cm^2 by 30 DIC. The time–course of accumulation of PLP$^+$ cells preceded by 7–10 days that for the accumulation of MBP. Thus, the accumulations of PLP and MBP in these cultures appear to be under separate temporal regulation.

2.3.2f. Cholesterol Ester Hydrolase.   The expression of this enzyme activity (Eto and Suzuki, 1973) in cultures of 19- to 21-day fetal rat brain was low until 21 DIC before rising to a peak at 31 DIC (S. Bhat and Pfeiffer, 1981). Thus, it follows the delayed pattern of expression seen for MBP.

2.3.2g. Carbonic Anhydrase.   Carbonic anhydrase (CA) II was used as a biochemical and immunochemical marker to study the influence of adult-brain extract on oligodendrocytes (see Section 3.1.4) in cultures of newborn-rat cerebral hemispheres (Sensenbrenner *et al.*, 1980*b*, 1982; Pettman *et al.*, 1980; Delaunoy *et al.*, 1980). The most active period of CA II activity was between 13 and 23 DIC.

CA II was also examined in cultures of 14- to 15-day embryonic-mouse brain (Sarlieve *et al.*, 1981). An increase in the specific activity of CA II was seen after 4–8 DIC, and a steady-state level was attained by at least 20 DIC.

2.3.2h. Summary of Dissociated–Attached Cell Cultures.   Study of dissociated cultures of rodent brain, optic nerve, and spinal cord has been actively pursued in recent years. Although these cultures generally do not produce actual compact myelin (exceptions are noted in Section 3.5), they do produce substantial membrane elaborations that can be visualized to best advantage via immunofluorescent staining. Nevertheless, the cultures do become highly differentiated with regard to myelinogenic function (e.g., GalCer, sulfatide, CNP–W1, and MBP) and can remain so for months. In fact, the absence of myelin formation *per se* has proved to have some interesting experimental advantages for biochemical analyses, one of which is that the accumulation of a large, increasing background pool of myelin-associated products is avoided, which thereby allows one to look more easily at what the oligodendrocyte cell bodies are doing.

Several general conclusions can be drawn: First, the expression of at least several myelinogenic markers can occur in dissociated–attached cell cultures in the absence of compact myelin formation, perhaps in excess of what might have been presupposed on the basis of histiotypic organization and morphological grounds. Second, the environmental signals that regulate the onset of the gene expression relevant to GalCer, sulfatide, CNP–W1, and probably PLP are different from those for MBP and cholesterol ester hydrolase. Thus, the *approximately* coordinate regulation of these myelin markers that occurs *in vivo* has been further dissociated *in vitro*. In other words, myelinogenesis appears to involve multiple parallel, but distinct, biochemical regulatory pathways. Of these, those related to MBP accumulation and cholesterol ester hydrolase activity must be more stringently dependent on the normal *in vivo* environment. However, asynchrony in the appearance of the various parameters has been noted even *in vivo* (Detering and Wells, 1976).

Dissociated–attached cell cultures appear frequently in later sections of this review, further emphasizing their substantial utility in the analysis of oligodendrocyte development and maintenance of function.

2.4. Isolated Oligodendrocytes

> *... viable oligodendrocytes are relatively easy to obtain from brain in high yield and purity, ...*
> NORTON (1983)

All the systems described to this point consist of a mixture of cells, the types and proportions of which depend on a number of experimental parameters. However, to assess definitively the extent of developmental information truly intrinsic to oligodendrocytes, it will be necessary to isolate and grow them in pure culture. Similarly, to ascertain the cellular source of many extrinsically derived factors that impinge on oligodendrocytes, it will be necessary to develop methods for the isolation and growth of various types of neurons, astrocytes, and other cells. Thus, it is no surprise that substantial effort has gone into developing methods of cellular isolation (e.g., Varon and Raiborn, 1969). The list of papers studying various parameters of isolated oligodendrocytes has grown long. Most of these studies have analyzed the cells immediately on isolation, some have studied biological processes over a period of hours to a few days, and relatively few have more recently examined oligodendrocyte development in long-term cultures. At this point, it is fair to say that enrichment of oligodendrocytes has been achieved, often dramatically so, but that absolute purity is still a goal, especially in long-term culture situations, in which overgrowth by a more vigorously proliferating population can readily occur.

Furthermore, it must be kept in mind that any cell-isolation method has the potential for yielding only a subpopulation of cells on the one hand, or mixing disparate populations on the other (e.g., as a function of brain region) (similar problems exist, of course, for dissociated mixed cell cultures). Nevertheless, Norton (1983) has provided rough estimates that current methods can yield a large enough fraction of the total oligodendrocytes to presume representative populations.

The isolation procedures fall into three main categories: (1) so-called "bulk" isolation directly from brain or white matter, (2) serologically assisted isolation from brain or culture, and (3) isolation by differential-shaking release from cultures (partial enrichments in cultures based on various nutritional or other culture techniques are discussed in Sections 2.1–3 and 3.1).

Bulk isolation has followed a basic pattern of dissociation by either mechanical or enzymatic means or both followed by a centrifugation step in a gradient (either step or continuous, generally in sucrose, Ficoll, or Percoll). The background, technical concepts, and modifications of this area have recently been thoroughly reviewed by Norton (1983) (see also Henn, 1980; Nagata and Tsukada, 1978). In light of the orientation of this chapter toward the extended culture of oligodendrocytes [and the view that even short-term studies profit from (require?) such long-term maintenance to avoid very real concerns about cell viability and thus metabolic stability], only those studies that demonstrate relatively long-term culture will be discussed in further detail.

Szuchet and co-workers have isolated oligodendrocytes from 3- to 6-month-old lamb brain and maintained them in culture for long periods (Szuchet et al., 1980; Szuchet and Stefansson, 1980; Mack and Szuchet, 1981; Mack et al., 1981; Wollman et al., 1981). The level of CNP activity at isolation was 1.9–2.0 μmoles/min per mg protein. The cells stained with anti-GalCer (75% GalCer$^+$ at 11–15 DIC) and anti-MBP (>90% MBP$^+$ at 21 DIC). After an initial inferred "dedifferentiation" characterized both by a loss of certain morphological characteristics and reduced levels of myelinogenic biochemical activities, the cultured oligodendrocytes synthesized GalCer (maximum level attained at about 20 DIC and maintained until 45 DIC), sulfatide (peak at 20 DIC, reduced synthetic rates thereafter), and gangliosides. Process and membrane formation were noted throughout the culture period. Recently, it has been reported that oligodendrocytes isolated by this method can myelinate fetal rat dorsal-root-ganglion neurons in culture (Wood et al., 1983).

Gebicke-Harter et al. (1981) used an enzymatic perfusion-Percoll centrifugation procedure to isolate oligodendrocytes from 8- to 12-week cat-brain white matter. They reported, on the basis of ultrastructural analysis and staining with anti-GalCer, that 95% of the isolated cells were oligodendrocytes and that this value remained approximately constant for 2–10 weeks of culture.

Oligodendrocytes isolated by a trypsin–Percoll gradient centrifugation method have also been cultured for a period of weeks (Lisak *et al.,* 1981). The population was 95% GalCer$^+$ at 1 DIC and 30–40% at 21 DIC. Anti-MBP stained 50–60% of the cells at 1 DIC and also 30–40% at 21 DIC (a result consistent with a delayed accumulation of MBP as discussed in Section 2.3). Astrocytes (immunofluorescence with anti-GFAP) constituted the main contaminant cell type.

Oligodendrocytes were also isolated from adult-bovine white matter using a trypsinization–buffer incubation–sucrose gradient approach (Farooq *et al.,* 1981; Norton, 1983). The population was considered by morphological and immunochemical criteria to be 95% oligodendrocytes at the time of isolation. The cells could be maintained in culture for over a month; in time, the oligodendrocytes tended to grow on top of a rapidly proliferating layer of fibroblasts.

McCarthy and de Vellis (1980) have reported a method for isolating oligodendrocytes from primary cultures of newborn-rat brain that makes use of (1) the stratification that occurs in such cultures whereby oligodendrocytes (and neurons) grow on top of other cell types, especially astrocytes, and (2) the differential adhesion among cell types in these cultures. Thus, vigorous shaking at 10 DIC released the oligodendrocytes, which could then be replaced and maintained for long periods. Oligodendrocytes prepared in this way had characteristic morphologies, CNP activities of about 0.6 μmole/min per mg protein at isolation [i.e., at 10 DIC, near the beginning of CNP activity development (see Section 2.3)], and GPDH activities of around 40 nmoles/min per mg protein.

The McCarthy and de Vellis (1980) procedure was adapted to enrich for oligodendrocytes from dissociated cultures of 19- to 21-day fetal-rat brain, adding the buffer lysis step of Snyder *et al.* (1980) to limit contamination by neurons (and astrocytes), which are substantially more plentiful in cultures derived from fetal brain (for a discussion, see McCarthy and de Vellis, 1980) (S. Bhat *et al.,* 1981). The cells could be cultured for at least 60 days, and when assayed after 29 DIC had high levels of CNP (7.1 μmoles/min per mg protein), sulfatide synthesis (nominally about 170 pmoles/hr), and MBP (about 1000 pmoles/mg protein). More recent experiments have demonstrated that a contaminating population of Thy-1-negative but tetanus-toxin-receptor-positive cells is present in these preparations, presumably similar to the tetanus-toxin-receptor-bearing cells described by Raff *et al.* (1983) as oligodendrocyte–astrocyte progenitor cells (see Section 3.3).

The culture systems described above can be expected to continue to improve and will allow additional types of investigations of both humoral and cellular regulation of oligodendrocyte function.

2.5. Clonal Lines

The development of clonal lines of biochemically differentiated cells growing in culture offers the possibility of providing permanently established, functionally and genetically homogeneous, viable populations of normal specified cell types that can be produced in quantities sufficient for biochemical studies.

PFEIFFER *et al.* (1981*a*)

The goals and experimental advantages expressed in the statement above are sufficiently seductive to have led many laboratories to try to produce clonal lines of the cell type of particular interest to their area of investigation. While the clonal-line approach has enjoyed success in some areas, this seems not to have been the case to date for oligodendrocytes. Since many aspects of clonal glial lines have been reviewed fairly recently (e.g., Pfeiffer *et al.*, 1977, 1981*a*; Benda, 1978), only a few additional comments will be made here.

Several lines of cells have in fact been developed that express some myelinogenic characteristics, in particular CNP activity or sulfatide synthesis or both [e.g., C_6 (Benda *et al.*, 1968); G26-20,-24 (Sundarraj *et al.*, 1975)]. However, MBP accumulation beyond minimal levels has not been demonstrated in clonal lines (McDermott and Smith, 1978; Pfeiffer *et al.*, 1981*a*, Table II). While disappointing, this negative result is perhaps instructive, for it is consistent with the concept discussed earlier (Section 2.3.2d) that MBP synthesis is under more stringent control than, for example, that of CNP. This situation also offers the experimenter the possibility of discovering the key missing element needed to activate MBP accumulation.

In a recent approach, McMorris *et al.* (1981) have combined the bulk-isolated oligodendrocyte and the clonal-line approaches by producing cell hybrids of isolated bovine oligodendrocytes and the C_6 glioma line (Benda *et al.*, 1968). One of the hybrid lines in particular (CO-13-7) expressed CNP activity (1.4–4.1 μmoles/min per mg protein) and GPDH activity (330 nmoles/min per mg protein, inducible by hydrocortisone), activities that were also present in the C_6 parent, as well as GalCer and sulfatide, and MBP. Again, however, MBP levels were very low (5–6 pmoles/mg protein). Still, the results are encouraging insofar as the latter three markers have not been detected in C_6 cells. This work is continuing with *rat* oligodendrocyte–rat clonal-line hybrids to minimize possible cross-species regulation problems (McMorris, personal communication).

For the present, to paraphrase Pfeiffer *et al.* (1977), the most useful type of inquiry that can be carried out using clonal lines to study oligodendrocytes may be the elucidation of specific biochemical events already known to occur during myelinogenesis *in vivo* in an environment free of normal interactions among different cell types and organismic regulation, and optimally open to experimental control of the external environment. Excellent examples of this use of clonal lines can be found in Chapter 8 and in the studies of CNP-activity regulation of McMorris (1977), to cite just two sources. Nevertheless, in all such investigations, there will be present the spectre of possible malignant transformation-induced changes in the regulatory mechanisms.

Whether clonal lines will realize their theoretical potential for studies of oligodendrocyte development, and in particular myelination, is yet to be seen. In view of the expansion of techniques for primary culture and isolated oligo-dendrocytes, the urgency for developing additional clonal lines is perhaps waning a bit. Nevertheless, the potential benefits will continue to beckon, and attempts to isolate a more generally useful myelinogenic line will continue.

3. SOME SPECIFIC AREAS OF INVESTIGATION

The culture systems described in Section 2, although in some respects still not completely characterized, have been used as one approach in the study of several areas of myelinogenesis. In this section, the approach and contribution of the various culture systems to some specific questions are considered.

3.1. Nutrition and Growth Factors

Speaking specifically about established clonal lines, it was observed in a previous review article (Pfeiffer *et al.*, 1981*a*) that a principal thread that "runs throughout cell culture history has been the gradual accumulation of knowledge regarding the specific nutritional requirements of cells. As these requirements have been better elucidated, cell cultures have become increasingly useful as experimental tools." Some applications of brain-cell cultures to studies of nutritional requirements for myelinogenesis are considered next.

3.1.1. Glucose

High glucose consumption is a characteristic feature of nervous tissue, and in particular, it increases considerably during the period of myelinogenesis (Murray, 1965). Thus, it is no surprise that glucose is an essential nutritional factor in cultures of nervous tissue, especially for myelinogenesis (Bornstein and Murray, 1958; Hild, 1957) and myelin maintenance (Bornstein and Appel, 1961). One of the earliest contributions of explant cultures (Murray *et al.*, 1962; Murray, 1965) was to confirm and define this requirement more carefully. For example, optimal myelin formation occurred in explant cultures of newborn-rat cerebellum maintained in the presence of 11–33 mM glucose (2–6 g/liter). Nearly all studies of myelinogenesis have used media with the glucose concentration in this range, generally between 25 and 33 mM (4.5–6 g/liter) (see also Lodin et al., 1978a,b). Higher glucose concentrations can be toxic.

3.1.2. Serum

All culture systems to date have required a serum supplement (generally fetal calf, calf, or horse serum) to support normal compact-myelin formation, although this may be about to change [for example, Honegger et al. (1979) obtained somewhat abnormal myelin formation in reaggregates maintained in a defined medium (see below)]. Murray et al. (1962) and Murray (1965) compared the effectiveness of serum supplements ranging from 10 to 50% of the medium. Using newborn cerebellar explants in Eagle's basal medium, they found that with 10% serum, glial outgrowth occurred but neuronal development was absent. Increasing the serum concentration to 25% (or using 30% chick embryo extract) allowed a minimal amount of neuronal maturation and myelination. Only with the use of 50% serum, or a very complex medium consisting of serum as well as whole-egg ultrafiltrate, did they obtain approximately normal neuronal differentiation and myelination. Bornstein (1973a) and Kim (1975, 1976) found that serum, but not chick embryo extract, was necessary for myelination.

When cultures of newborn-mouse cerebellar explants were fed with 7.5% serum in the medium, only 50% of the cultures showed morphological evidence of myelin at 10 days in culture (DIC) and 75% at 20 DIC and the activites of $2',3'$-cyclic nucleotide $3'$-phosphohydrolase (CNP) and β-hydroxy-β-methyl-glutaryl (HMG)-CoA reductase were reduced (Kim and Pleasure, 1978). In contrast, when a 15 or 30% serum concentration was used, the majority of the cultures were already heavily myelinated at 12–14 DIC.

A question of obvious interest is what the critical components present in serum are. We (Pfeiffer et al., 1981a) have previously commented that "whereas the growth requirements for amino acids, salts, vitamins, etc. have been at least approximately known since the 1950s, the components of the blood sera traditionally used to supplement these basal media are for the most part only now being identified." We noted further that it has been suggested by Sato (1975) "that the role of sera in cell culture is to provide panels of hormones which, if identified, could be used in place of complex and undefined serum components." This hypothesis has received increasing support as a variety of nutritive requirements have been identified, many clearly components of normal sera, that, when appropriately combined into hormonally defined, serum-free media, support proliferation or the expression of differentiated function or both (e.g., Bottenstein et al., 1979; Barnes and Sato, 1980; Gospodarowicz and Moran, 1976).

The idea of chemically defined media has found expression in studies of myelinogenesis through the work of Honegger *et al.* (1979) and Honegger and Matthieu (1980). They cultured 15- to 16-day fetal-rat brain in a medium consisting of Dulbecco's Modified Eagle's Medium, insulin, hydrocortisone, triiodothyronine, transferrin, and trace elements. Although there was some retardation in cellular growth and the development of biochemical differentiation, suggesting that additional necessary factors are still missing, the aggregates underwent substantial myelinogenic development to myelin sheaths at 30 DIC (although with some abnormalities present).

Some of the key components are therefore known factors (see Section 3.1.3), while others [e.g., those derived from brain extracts (see Section 3.1.4)] await identification.

3.1.3. Hormones

Several well-known hormones have proved to have particular interest for myelinogenesis (see Chapter 8). Cell culture has helped to elucidate some aspects of their effects.

For example, Barnett (1948) noted that myelination in the CNS was severely inhibited in hypothyroid animals, and subsequent work in several laboratories confirmed an important role for thyroid hormones in a number of aspects of nerve-cell development. Hamburgh and Bunge (Hamburgh and Bunge, 1964; Hamburgh, 1966) found that rat cerebellar explant cultures supplemented with thyroxine (1.5 μg/ml) underwent more rapid myelin formation {from 8 to 9 DIC, compared to 12–14 DIC in controls [Figure 3 of Hamburgh and Bunge (1964) and Figure 4 of Hamburgh (1966)]} even though the cultures were grown in a very rich, serum-containing medium (balanced salt solution, beef serum ultrafiltrate, placental serum, and chick embryo extract) that might have been expected to provide saturating amounts of the hormone [see N. R. Bhat *et al.* (1979) (discussed below)].

The influence of thyroid hormones on some aspects of myelinogenesis in cultures derived from 15-day-old mouse embryos was studied by N. R. Bhat *et al.* (1979, 1981) and by Pieringer *et al.* (1980). They showed that triiodothyronine and thyroxine stimulated the synthesis of galactosylceramide (GalCer), GalCer sulfate (sulfatide), and monogalactosyldiacylglycerol sulfate (the latter two through the stimulation of the appropriate sulfotransferase activity; sulfated mucopolysaccharide synthesis was not affected). CNP activity was also stimulated by these hormones. These hormone effects occurred in serum-free medium as well.

Breen and de Vellis (1975) (see also Chapter 8) used explant cultures of 20- to 21-day fetal-rat-brain areas to demonstrate that hydrocortisone induced the activity of cytoplasmic glycerol-3-phosphate dehydrogenase.

3.1.4. Growth Factors

It has become clear, often through experiments utilizing cell culture, that there is a complex mixture of growth and differentiation factors that are required for the normal development of the nervous system (e.g., Varon and Bunge, 1978). Some of these are humoral factors found outside the nervous system, such as nerve growth factor present in submaxillary gland (Levi-Montalcini, 1966), while others have their origins within the nervous system (e.g., Lim *et al.*, 1977; Barde *et al.*, 1978; see also Pfeiffer *et al.*, 1981*a*), in which case both humoral and cellular activities can be expected (for additional references, see Schachner and Willinger, 1979).

Sensenbrenner and co-workers have studied the effects of brain extracts on brain-cell development in culture. Dissociated newborn-rat cerebral hemispheres were seeded at a high cell density favoring oligodendrocyte survival (Labourdette *et al.*, 1979, 1980). They found that extracts of adult-rat brains (and chick brains) stimulated the proliferation of the presumptive oligodendrocytes and approximately doubled the specific activity (per milligram protein) of CA II in mixed cultures (Sensenbrenner *et al.*, 1972, 1980*b*, 1982; Pettman *et al.*, 1980; Delaunoy *et al.*, 1980). A good correlation between the number of oligodendrocytes in the cultures and the level of CA II was reported. Extracts from older animals had stronger effects. However, even in the presence of the brain extracts, the CA II activity was low compared to that observed *in vivo*. While the contribution of various cell types is not known at present, the probability of neuronal involvement seems high (e.g., Hanson *et al.*, 1982*a,b*).

This is still a fledgling field within the area of nervous-system differentiation, and of myelinogenesis in particular. The identification, isolation, and characterization of a plethora of factors can be expected in the years ahead. Throughout this endeavor, cell-culture systems will undoubtedly play prominent roles as both sources of and targets for such factors.

3.2. Experimental Myelinogenic Pathology

3.2.1. Serum Factors

One of the most vigorously pursued uses of cultures in studies of myelinogenesis is that of serum-induced demyelination (for a review, see Seil, 1982). Serum from patients with multiple sclerosis (MS), serum (or sensitized lymph-node cells) from animals immunized with whole CNS tissue, white matter, or purified myelin [experimental allergic encephalomyelitis (EAE) sera], and anti-GalCer have all been shown to demyelinate mature CNS explant cultures in the presence of complement. Newborn-rat cerebellar cultures demyelinated with EAE serum had only 28% of the cerebroside galactosyl transferase (CGalT) activity found in control cultures (Latovitzki and Silberberg, 1975). Whereas demyelination by EAE sera is thought to be antibody-related, most of the demyelinating activity of MS sera may be caused by nonimmunoglobulin factors (Lebar *et al.,* 1976; Grundke-Iqbal *et al.,* 1981); this activity has been found at significant levels in control human sera as well (see Bornstein and Hummelgard, 1976; Traugott *et al.,* 1979; Booe *et al.,* 1980).

In the absence of complement, white-matter-induced EAE sera and anti-GalCer sera did not cause demyelination in culture, but produced a swelling of myelin lamellae with a doubling of the intraperiod line to 22 nm and the formation of a four-leaflet structure (Bornstein and Raine, 1976; Grundke-Iqbal and Bornstein, 1979). Administration of these sera without complement resulted in an exaggerated production of oligodendrocyte processes and abnormal myelin formation (Raine *et al.,* 1978). Complement-inactivated EAE serum components (white-matter-induced) bound to oligodendrocytes and to the intraperiod line of the swollen myelin (Johnson *et al.,* 1979). Whereas both immunoglobulin G (IgG) and non-IgG immunoglobulins were found to mediate complement-dependent demyelination (Grundke-Iqbal *et al.,* 1981), it appeared that only the IgG immunoglobulins were involved in the myelin swelling and oligodendrocyte-process exaggeration in the absence of complement. The process is reversible, for the removal of the EAE serum results in a return to a normal myelin configuration. In both the induction of the abnormality and the recovery, the morphological changes appeared to proceed from external to internal lamellae.

When EAE or anticerebroside sera with or without complement activity were added to CNS explant cultures (generally fetal-mouse spinal cord or rodent cerebellum) *prior to* myelin formation, normal myelin formation was inhibited (Bornstein and Raine, 1970, 1980; Fry *et al.,* 1972, 1973, 1974; Latovitzki and Silberberg, 1975; Dorfman *et al.,* 1976, 1978, 1979; Hruby *et al.,* 1977; Raine *et al.,* 1978; Diaz *et al.,* 1978). Concentrations of antiserum too low to demyelinate (when complement was included) could still inhibit myelin formation. Nevertheless, many oligodendrocytes differentiated, but formed numerous cell processes and exaggerated amounts of morphologically abnormal myelin that was only rarely associated with axons. These results have led to the suggestion that the antisera block an axonal–oligodendrocyte signal (Bornstein and Raine, 1980). In contrast, neurons, astrocytes, and other cell types seemed to have developed normally. The phenomenon was again reversible, even after long-term inhibition, with the removal of the serum leading to fairly prompt, although reduced, myelination (Bornstein and Raine, 1970; Dorfman *et al.,* 1976).

These studies have been substantiated by the addition of biochemical data. For example, Fry *et al.* (1972, 1973, 1974) noted that the incorporation of

$^{35}SO_4$ into sulfatide and the development of CNP activity in explant cultures were markedly depressed when EAE serum or anti-GalCer serum was present. Again, the removal of the EAE serum resulted in a resumption of the development of these myelinogenic properties. In contrast, no such effects of EAE serum were observed on the activities of glucose-6-phosphate dehydrogenase, NADP-isocitrate dehydrogenase, or three lysosomal enzymes, and arylsulfatase A activity was only slightly reduced. Latovitzki and Silberberg (1975) inhibited myelinogenesis of newborn-rat cerebellar cultures with 2% EAE serum (with complement) and found a concurrent 10-fold reduction in CGalT activity.

Since anti-GalCer is a component of EAE serum, and since its removal by absorption prevents the inhibition of myelinogenesis in culture (Fry et al., 1974), it is reasonable to conclude that either GalCer or some other galactose-containing surface molecule may be the active target of the EAE serum component. However, the possible effects of antisera on other *surface* antigens have apparently not been tested. It has been demonstrated, however, that antibodies to MBP, proteolipid protein, and myelin-associated glycoprotein generally have no antimyelin activity in explant cultures (Kies et al., 1973; Lebar et al., 1976; Yonezawa et al., 1976; Johnson and Bornstein, 1978; Seil and Agrawal, 1980; Seil et al., 1968, 1973, 1975a,b, 1980a, 1981; Raine et al., 1981). In contrast, demyelination in fetal rat brain reaggregates exposed to anti-MBP was reported by Matthieu et al. (1980).

The absence of a requirement for complement activity in association with the serum-induced inhibition of oligodendrocyte differentiation suggests that a more specific interference with differentiation is occurring, rather than simply cell killing. The cells undergoing myelinogenesis on removal of the inhibitory sera are thought to preexist at the time of inhibitory release (Dorfman et al., 1976, 1978).

3.2.2. Drugs

The effects of several drugs on myelinogenesis and demyelination have also been assessed in culture systems. Demyelination in cultures has been effected with thiamine antimetabolites (Yonezawa and Iwanami, 1966) and methyl mercuric acetate (Kim, 1971). Hexachlorophene inhibited sulfatide synthesis in cerebellar explants, apparently due to a reduction in the level of phosphoadenosine phosphosulfate (Pleasure et al., 1974), although Matthieu et al. (1980) found that cerebroside sulfotransferase (CST) activity itself was inhibited in fetal-rat-brain reaggregated cultures exposed to hexachlorophene. Other drug effects that have been studied in explants include the degeneration of myelinated axons induced by the nonmetabolizable amino acid, 1-amino-cyclopentane-1-carboxylic acid (Nixon et al., 1976) and retarded myelin formation following inhibition of cholesterol biosynthesis by AY9944 [*trans*-1,4-*bis*(2-chlorobenzylaminomethyl)cyclohexane] (Kim, 1975). In dissociated cultures, the addition of theophylline resulted in reduced levels of HMG-CoA reductase and of CST (Siegrist *et al.,* 1980).

3.3. Oligodendrocyte Proliferation and Early Development

Many of the culture systems and experiments described in the preceding sections have dealt either explicitly or indirectly with the developmental biology of oligodendrocytes. In this section, a number of additional papers are considered that are concerned with the proliferation and concomitant differentiation of oligodendrocyte precursor cells and immature oligodendrocytes.

As discussed in Section 1.4 and in Chapter 1, oligodendrocytes are thought to arise from neuroectoderm, specifically from cells of the subependymal layer. Subventricular cells develop into immature glial-cell precursors that migrate, proliferate, and eventually differentiate into mature oligodendrocytes (e.g., Altman, 1969; Privat and Leblond, 1972; Privat, 1975). Oligodendrocytes have been catalogued into three main morphological subtypes based on the density of cytoplasmic staining in transmission EM. The light, medium, and dark oligodendrocytes appear in that order during development (Mori and Leblond, 1970; Paterson *et al.,* 1973; Imamoto *et al.,* 1978; Nadler, 1978). Examples of these types have been inferred in cell cultures as well by some of the authors discussed in Section 2.

The interplay between cell cycling (cell division) and differentiation has been a recurrent point of interest in developmental biology. In the nervous system, experiments utilizing autoradiographic "birthdating" and morphological examinations have indicated multiple periods of cellular proliferation and complex developmental family trees (see Jacobson, 1978; Sturrock, 1982; also see Chapter 1). Of particular interest to our present purposes are the numerous studies showing that oligodendrocytes proliferate prior to the onset of myelin formation (e.g., Skoff *et al.,* 1976*a,b*; Vaughn, 1969; Imamoto *et al.,* 1978; Mitrova, 1967), with the earliest-maturing oligodendrocytes becoming postmitotic in the rat at around 5 postnatal days and the majority completing their proliferative phases between 7 and 17 postnatal days. For optic nerve, at least, it appears that substantial oligodendrocyte proliferation and development continue after the onset of myelin formation (Vaughn, 1969; Hirose and Bass, 1973; Skoff *et al.,* 1976*a,b*) [also see further references and discussion in Norton (1983) and in Chapter 1], and Sturrock and McRae (Sturrock and McRae, 1980; Sturrock, 1981, 1982) found dark-staining oligodendrocytes (characterized by EM) connected to myelin sheaths in various phases of mitosis. The question of the extent and timing of oligodendrocyte proliferation has been pursued in cell cultures as well (see Fedoroff, 1977, 1978).

Both astrocytic and oligodendrocytic proliferation have been reported in cultures derived from embryonic chick and mammalian (including adult) brain (Sensenbrenner *et al.,* 1980*a*; Hugosson *et al.,* 1968; Choi and Lapham, 1974; Courtney and Bassleer, 1967; Hansson and Sourander, 1964; Lumsden and Pomerat, 1951; Pomerat, 1958; Wolfgram and Rose, 1957). Manuelidis and Manuelidis (1971) studied [^{3}H]-TdR incorporation into cultures derived from 15-day fetal-mouse or -rat spinal cord. They found a peak in proliferative activity between 7 and 12 DIC, prior to myelination. Ultrastructural analyses led them to conclude that "young" oligodendrocytes, but not those closely associated with myelin sheaths, proliferated.

Experiments designed to determine critical periods of oligodendroglial proliferation during their development *in vitro* have been carried out (Silberberg *et al.,* 1972, 1980; Younkin and Silberberg, 1973, 1976; Latovitzki and Silberberg, 1975, 1977; Dorfman *et al.,* 1976; Dorfman, 1977). The authors used a combination of autoradiography, morphological identification of oligodendrocytes and myelin, biochemical assays for myelinogenic markers, and drugs to study these phenomena in explants of newborn-rat cerebellum and spinal cord. There was one peak of proliferation in cerebellar cultures at 5–6 DIC and a second at 9–10 DIC, both prior to myelination, which began (LM identification) after 13 DIC. Exposing cultures between 2 and 12 DIC to [^{3}H]-TdR led in all cases to labeled oligodendrocytes associated with myelinated axons by 15 DIC.

Holtzer and co-workers (Holtzer, 1970) have developed the idea of a "quantal cell cycle," conceived theoretically as one in which the daughter cells have genetic options different from those of the mother cell. Experimentally, such a developmentally critical cell division has been identified by the sensitivity of such cells to the incorporation of 5-bromo-2′-deoxyuridine (BUdR) into their DNA (Abbott *et al.,* 1972; Holtzer *et al.,* 1972). In contrast, a developmentally inconsequential "proliferative cell cycle" would be insensitive to BUdR incorporation, but still sensitive to inhibitors of DNA synthesis such as cytosine arabinoside (ARA-C) (Graham and Whitmore, 1970).

In the experiments cited above, Silberberg and colleagues inhibited cell proliferation (via inhibition of DNA synthesis and thus cell cycling) with ARA-C and observed an asynchronously dividing population of precursor cells with a peak again at 5 DIC. Overall, the period from 1 to 15 DIC was particularly sensitive to the effects of the drug, with the most sensitive period occurring from 5 to 7 DIC.

Similar experiments using BUdR produced consistent results. Again, a sensitive period at 5–7 DIC (2–4 DIC for spinal cord) was found and interpreted as representing a cell division critical to oligodendrocyte development. They found that activities of both CNP and CGalT, but not of UDP-glucose:ceramide glycosyl transferase, were reduced by BUdR treatment during this critical period. The BUdR inhibition was reversible by a mechanism apparently requiring DNA synthesis.

Taken together, these experiments suggest that oligodendrocytes divide after birth but prior to producing myelin, probably at least several times, and that one of these divisions is critical for development of myelinogenic-specific functions, but not for general survival functions.

Finally, using BUdR incorporation and ARA-C inhibition of DNA synthesis to assess oligodendrocyte proliferation, this group concluded that the inhibition of myelinogenesis by EAE serum or anti-GalCer serum (see Section 3.1.2) did not occur via a block to the critical premyelination cell proliferation, which apparently proceeded unimpeded (of course, if the BUdR-sensitive cell cycle occurred before the cells became GalCer$^+$, the lack of interference by anti-GalCer is only to be expected). Nor was proliferation required on removal of the blocking antiserum for (delayed) myelination to proceed. Thus, these workers suggest that this delayed myelination was the product of a pool of "covertly differentiated" oligodendrocytes that were already postmitotic, but that were not yet expressing detectable levels of myelinogenic end products.

The appearance of oligodendrocytes identified by LM and scanning and transmission EM in cultures started from mechanically dissociated 14-day fetal-mouse tel- and diencephalon was studied by Rioux et al. (1980). They reported that the density of the "oligodendrocytelike" cells increased especially between 9 and 16 DIC, comparable to 3–10 days postnatal. These data were reinforced by [^{3}H]-TdR incorporation studies. Therefore, within the confines of morphological identification of oligodendrocytes, these data also suggest that mouse oligodendrocytes in culture proliferate postnatally and prior to myelination.

Wiesmann et al. (1980) have stated that "putative oligodendrocytes" (identified morphologically) in cultures initiated from dissociated newborn mouse brain divide between 8 and 12 DIC, forming "microclones."

Abney et al. (1981) cultured 10-day fetal rat brain and reported that after 14–15 DIC (2–3 days postnatal), less than 5% of the GalCer$^+$ cells were labeled in a 24-hr exposure to [^{3}H]-TdR. It is not clear whether or not this represents a contradiction to other data cited above, for (1) only those cells that had become GalCer$^+$ at 14–15 DIC were being considered and (2) the autoradiographs were exposed for only 2 days. Taken at face value, these data would suggest that GalCer$^+$ cells are postmitotic cells arising from previously proliferated GalCer$^-$ precursors. Pruss et al. (1982) used similar methods to study oligodendrocytes in cultures of dissociated neonatal rat CNS and came to the same conclusion; i.e., GalCer$^+$ cells were "rarely if ever seen to incorporate" [^{3}H]-TdR. GalCer$^+$ cells plated on irradiated 3T3 monolayers did divide, however.

A limiting dilution analysis was used to estimate the presence and number of oligodendrocyte precursor cells prior to the time they express currently known oligodendrocyte markers (Barbarese *et al.,* 1983). This analysis suggested that there are at least 300–500 surviving oligodendrocyte progenitor cells per 19- to 21-day fetal-rat brain introduced into culture. Comparisons of this number with estimates of the number of oligodendrocytes in "mature" cultures at 38 DIC of adult-rat brain suggested further that this stem-cell population must undergo approximately 10 divisions to generate the population of oligodendrocytes.

An example of another approach to identifying oligodendrocytes (or their precursors) at a stage prior to the time at which they express a known myelinogenic marker is seen in the work of Schachner and co-workers (Sommer and Schachner, 1981; Schachner *et al.,* 1981). They have developed monoclonal antibodies to oligodendrocytes, some of which recognize only $GalCer^+$ cells (anti-O1, O2), others of which recognize not only $GalCer^+$ cells but also a class of $GalCer^-$ cells (anti-O3, O4). One enticing conclusion is that the anti-O3$^+$ or -O4$^+$/anti-GalCer$^-$ cells are immediate precursors to the $GalCer^+$ cells. If one could identify an antibody that stains, for example, O_3^+ cells *and in addition* a population of O_3^- cells, one could, in principle, detect increasingly early stages of oligodendrocyte development. Monoclonal antibody A2B5 identifies chick neurons (Eisenbarth *et al.,* 1979) and a small population of astrocytes and oligodendrocytes (Schnitzer and Schachner, 1982). Recently, cells thought to be progenitors of oligodendrocytes (and a type of astrocyte) have been shown to also bind both tetanus toxin and A2B5, as well as antiserum O4 (Raff *et al.,* 1983). Thus, the possibility of studying earlier stages in oligodendrocyte development (pre-GalCer-positive cells) has arisen.

In summary, while relatively little has been done at this time using cell cultures to understand the very early events of oligodendrocyte development, the tools would appear to be in place. Substantial contributions to this area can be expected in the near future.

3.4. Genetic Mutants of Myelinogenesis

> *Thus, study of these mutations will provide the means to compile a catalogue, so to speak, of the genetic instructions for making and maintaining the CNS myelin sheath.*
> BILLINGS-GAGLIARDI AND WOLF (1982)

Numerous mutations that affect neurological structure and function are known in mice, including several that lead to defective myelin formation (Sidman *et al.,* 1965; Billings-Gagliardi and Wolf, 1982). Culture systems offer an especially useful approach for the study of these hypomyelination mutants. Introducing mutant brain into culture isolates the tissue from systemic influences and thereby allows one to distinguish between intrinsic and extrinsic tissue factors that influence the development of the phenotypic defect. By mixing mutant and normal tissue, the relative influence of cell-localized vs. diffusible trophic or toxic factors can be assessed, and the specific cell type at risk can be determined (see reviews by Billings-Gagliardi and Wolf, 1982; Wolf and Billings-Gagliardi, 1983).

Studies of hypomyelination mutants have to date concentrated on the "jimpy," an X-linked recessive [jp (Phillips, 1954; Sidman *et al.,* 1964, 1965)] and its allele "jimpy-msd" [jp^{msd} (Meier and MacPike, 1970)]; "quaking," an autosomal recessive [qk (Sidman *et al.,* 1964, 1965)]; and "shiverer," also an autosomal recessive [shi (Biddle *et al.,* 1973; Chernoff *et al.,* 1974)]. The characteristics of these and other myelination mutants are discussed in the reviews cited above. Briefly, all result in animals that are severely deficient in CNS myelin formation and that have concomitant neurological distresses such as tremors, jimps, quakes, shivers, and perhaps convulsions.

In a series of experiments dating back to 1969, Wolf, Billings-Gagliardi, and co-workers have carefully studied mouse mutants in culture (Wolf and Holden, 1969; Wolf, 1974, 1977; Billings-Gagliardi *et al.,* 1976, 1980; Wolf *et al.,* 1981; Billings-Gagliardi and Wolf, 1982; Wolf and Billings-Gagliardi, 1983). Using explants of the newborn cerebellum (Section 2.1), they found that jimpy, jimpy-msd, and quaking were all deficient in myelin in culture just as they are *in situ*. Of the three, quaking made the most myelin (although it was not visible at the LM level, possibly because of an abnormal lipid composition), jimpy-msd was intermediate, and jimpy had the least. Their morphological analyses suggested that jp and jp^{msd} myelin, although of course very limited in quantity, was normal. In contrast, qk appeared to make larger quantities of abnormal myelin. Throughout these studies, the authors stressed and demonstrated the importance of (1) having closely linked marker genes to allow identification of mutant animals at a preclinical stage and (2) the potential influence of the animal's genetic background on the expression of the mutation. Overall, they found that the *in situ* hypomyelinating defect was reproduced in culture, thus suggesting a defect intrinsic to nervous tissue. Since coculturing mutant and control explants in close proximity did not alter the outcome, they concluded that cell-bound factors rather than diffusible agents were most likely involved. Finally, careful coculture of mutant-cerebellum with normal optic-nerve explants resulted in increased myelin formation in the case of both jp^{msd} and qk cerebellum. Therefore, axons in mutant explants are apparently myelination-competent, and the primary defect is most likely localized in the oligodendrocytes.

Compared to normal controls, jimpy explants grown under high oxygen tension incorporated $^{35}SO_4$ into sulfatide at a lower rate, had decreased levels of CST, higher rates of sulfatide degradation, and correspondingly lower levels of total sulfatide (Wiesmann *et al.*, 1979, 1980). Coculturing of normal and jimpy brain explants had no corrective effect on the deficient sulfatide metabolism.

Sandru and colleagues (Sandru *et al.*, 1980; Bologa-Sandru *et al.*, 1981*b*) have carried out a series of experiments on cultures of newborn dissociated jimpy mouse brain. Jimpy cultures developed GalCer$^+$ cells at around 7 DIC, similar to control cultures, but developed only 5% as many MBP$^+$ cells by 18 DIC. It is not clear from this experiment whether the extent or time–course of the appearance of MBP$^+$ cells is delayed. They suggest that the jimpy mutation affects a second phase of myelinogenesis that includes MBP expression and myelin formation.

Little or no myelin was formed in either jimpy or quaking explants in roller-tube cultures. CNP rose to only 0.3 μmole/min per mg protein at 14 DIC (compared to 1.4–1.7 in normal controls), and MBP was not detectable (Kim and Pleasure, 1980). HMG-CoA reductase was moderately depressed at 14 DIC.

In cerebellar explant cultures of quaking mice, myelin formation was very poor, while Purkinje cell development, for example, appeared normal (Mikoshiba *et al.*, 1979). Conditioned medium from quaking-mouse cultures had no effect on control cultures. The investigators suspected that the quaking defect was intrinsic to the oligodendrocytes, as opposed, for example, to an astrocytic hypertrophy. Subsequently, they used similar methods to study shiverer mice (Mikoshiba *et al.*, 1980). No myelin was found, but CNP activity did develop to a level of 1.3 μmoles/min per mg protein at 20 DIC.

In cerebellar explants of shiverer mice, only small amounts of poorly compacted myelin were synthesized (Hauw *et al.*, 1980). No obvious abnormalities in the oligodendrocytes were found by EM examination.

Clearly, the tip of the iceberg of this particularly critical area of research has appeared.

3.5. Myelin-Membrane Synthesis

The formation of myelin compacted around axons has been rather routinely observed in expertly manipulated explant cultures (e.g., Hild, 1957; Bornstein and Murray, 1958) (see Sections 2.1 and 3.1–4). Similarly, when brain cells first dissociated by mechanical or enzymatic means or both have been encouraged to reaggregate in suspension prior to their further development as "neoexplants," some myelin has also been observed after 4 weeks or more (e.g., Seeds and Vatter, 1971) (see Section 2.2). Nevertheless, for both explants and reaggregates, evidence has appeared that suggests that myelin matures more slowly *in vitro* than *in vivo* (e.g., Bradbury, 1977; Bradbury and Lumsden, 1979; Fagg *et al.*, 1979; Matthieu *et al.*, 1979), and normal-appearing myelin may be side-by-side with various abnormalities (e.g., Matthieu *et al.,* 1980).

In contrast to explants and reaggregates, myelin formation has generally been absent in dissociated–attached cell cultures in which reaggregation phenomena are minimized (Section 2.3), although a variety of myelinogenic biochemical activities do develop. Nevertheless, membrane elaborations are commonly in evidence (e.g., Sarlieve *et al.,* 1980*a*; Szuchet and Stefansson, 1980; Barbarese and Pfeiffer, 1981; Berg and Schachner, 1981; Sommer and Schachner, 1981; Macklin and Pfeiffer, 1983), and exceptions have been reported.

For example, Kim (1972) reported that myelination, observed by LM, was seen after 24 DIC in dissociated cultures of 11-day chick embryo spinal cord, i.e., delayed relative to the time–course in comparable explants. They suggested that the extra time required reflected the need for cells to reestablish appropriate histiotypic relationships (Seeds and Vatter, 1971). Bornstein and Model (1972) found myelination in some of the larger aggregates of cultures initiated from 13- to 14-day fetal-mouse CNS after 3 weeks of culture. Booher and Sensenbrenner (1972) and Sensenbrenner *et al.* (1972) also found occasional examples of myelin formation (phase-contrast microscopy) in cultures of dissociated embryonic chick or rat brain. Bird and James (1975) reported the formation of some myelin after 21 DIC in dissociated 18- to 19-day fetal mouse spinal cord studied by LM and EM. Yavin and Yavin (1977) dissociated 16-day fetal rat cerebral hemispheres and cultured them in polylysine-coated dishes. They reported EM evidence for myelin formation as early as 8 DIC. Often, the myelin was formed around a bundle of fibers.

Of course, the search is on for the necessary conditions under which dissociated cultures could routinely be encouraged to produce copious amounts of real myelin. This may be as "simple" as supplementing the culture with the right neurons, as in the work of Wood *et al.* (1980), who observed the formation of CNS myelin by 2 weeks in culture when optic-nerve explants were cocultured with Schwann-cell-depleted dorsal-root-ganglion neurons. On the other hand, the possible importance of the histiotypic integrity present in explants, which is at least partially reestablished in dissociated–reaggregated cell cultures and possibly in dissociated–attached cell cultures as well, is of interest with respect not only to signals mediated by direct cell contact but also to microenvironmental modification through secreted factors.

4. SOME CONCLUSIONS

4.1. Comparison of Myelinogenesis in Culture Systems and *in Vivo*

Questions are often raised regarding the extent to which cultured cells are "normal." The optimist asks how many normal activities can be carried out by cells in culture. Margaret Murray (1977), an apparent optimist, has suggested that "anything a cell does in culture must be included among its possibilities." The pessimist, on the other hand, asks how artifactual culture systems are. While the two questions are opposite sides of the same coin, the perspective from which the questions are asked can determine one's subsequent experimental course.

To phrase the problem a bit differently, one can: (1) compare the course and extent of development in a culture system to that observed *in vivo* and then modify the culture system as required to get it as close to the *in vivo* pattern as possible—this approach seems possible with explants of cerebellum and spinal cord; or (2) note, and even encourage, differences between *in vitro* and *in vivo* growth and development and attempt to interpret the differences in some useful way—this approach is being used especially with dissociated cultures.

The latter approach in effect emphasizes that cells from the CNS growing in culture are *not* normal and that we can profit from the abnormalities. The differences present in a culture system can be considered in terms of induced "mutations" of tissue phenotype. Consider the example of dissociated embryonic CNS cell cultures, specifically with regard to oligodendrocyte development; similar analyses could be made with variations for other culture systems as well. The act of dissociation creates a "mutation" of histiotypic organization. A three-dimensional structure is reduced to a semi-two-dimensional array of cells. Cell contacts and interactions are at least temporarily disrupted. This fortuitous situation thus allows one to assess the importance of these physical parameters in oligodendrocyte development. Existing studies suggest that the onset of synthesis of galactosylceramide, sulfatide, proteolipid protein, and 2′, 3′-cyclic nucleotide 3′-phosphohydrolase is largely impervious to these insults. In contrast, the appearance of MBP-positive cells and the increase of cholesterol ester hydrolase activity are delayed by these culture-induced "mutations." On the other hand, once the process of MBP$^+$ cell recruitment is initiated, the rate of recruitment and the level of MBP attained per cell are apparently normal.

Finally, we can ask whether any of the culture systems allow, in whole or in part, truly normal myelinogenic development. The best candidate here would seem to be organotypic, or explant, cultures of cerebellum or spinal cord. As reviewed in Section 2.1, myelinated axons develop in such cultures at approximately the same time as they would *in vivo* [Murray (1965) and many others since]. Still, there are somewhat conflicting conclusions in the literature that are based, not so much on conflicting data, but rather on the type of data considered and on points of view. For example, Billings-Gagliardi and Wolf (1982) comment on the different perspectives of the experimental morphologist and biochemist with regard to myelin formation and how this affects their relative conclusions. Thus, a perusal of Section 2 reveals that several laboratories have noted that myelin-membrane formation in explants "faithfully reproduces the events as they were known to occur *in vivo*" (e.g., Raine and Bornstein, 1979), and Silberberg *et al.* (1980) commented that "all the evidence to date suggests that biochemical events which characterize myelin *in vivo* occur as well in the myelinating organotropic culture system." Nevertheless, Latovitzki and Silberberg (1973) noted that galactolipid content *in vivo* "rose earlier and more rapidly than *in vitro*," and Bradbury and Lumsden (1979) commented on the "slow myelin maturation" *in vitro*. Similarly, Fagg *et al.* (1979) and Barbarese and Pfeiffer (1981) found that while myelin protein composition was in the end quite similar, there may be different patterns at earlier times.

In conclusion, normality *in vitro* is a bit capricious and must be judged relative not only to a platonic form of the normal (more mundanely, to *in vivo* realities), but also to one's perspective and the goals of the experiment.

4.2. Prospectus

The reader most likely has already inferred, the author discovered the hard way, and the editor undoubtedly noted with some concern that a review of myelinogenesis in culture systems spans very nearly the entire field. While this has undoubtedly caused some problems for the aforenamed triumvirate, it bodes well for the utility of cultures in this area of research. The various culture systems have been rigorously challenged by basic morphological and biochemical characterization and experimental modification and have shown substantial promise.

ACKNOWLEDGMENTS

It is a pleasure to acknowledge helpful suggestions made in regard to content and style by my colleagues R. Bansal, E. Barbarese, S. Bhat, J. Carson, A. Edgar, W. Macklin, H. Singh, and F. Woodiel. Special thanks are due to Ms. Janice Seagren for manuscript preparation. This effort was supported by Grants NS 10861 from the National Institutes of Health and RG 1213 from the National Multiple Sclerosis Society.

5. REFERENCES

Abney, E. R., Bartlett, P. P., and Raff, M. C., 1981, Astrocytes, ependymal cells, and oligodendrocytes develop on schedule in dissociated cell cultures of embryonic rat brain, *Dev. Biol.* **83:**301–310.

Abbott, J., Mayne, R., and Holtzer, H., 1972, Inhibition of cartilage development in organ cultures by the thymidine analogue 5-bromo-2-deoxyuridine, *Dev. Biol.* **28:**430–442.

Aguayo, A. J., Charron, L., and Bray, G. M., 1976*a*, Potential of Schwann cells from unmyelinated nerves to produce myelin: A quantitative ultrastructural and radiographic study, *J. Neurocytol.* **5:**565–573.

Aguayo, A. J., Epps, J., Charron, L., and Bray, G. M., 1976*b*, Multipotentiality of Schwann cells in cross-anastomosed and grafted myelinated and unmyelinated nerves: Quantitative microscopy and radioautography, *Brain Res.* **104:**1–20.

Aguayo, A. J., Kasarjian, J., Skamene, E., Konghavn, P., and Bray, G. M., 1977, Myelination of mouse axons by Schwann cells transplanted from normal and abnormal human nerves, *Nature (London)* **268:**753–755.

Aguayo, A. J., Dickson, R., Trecarten, J., Attiwell, M., Bray, G. M., and Richardson, P. R., 1978, Ensheathment and myelination of regenerating PNS fibers by transplanted nerve glia, *Neurosci. Lett.* **9:**97–104.

Allerand, C. D., and Murray, M. R., 1968, Myelin formation *in vitro:* Endogenous influences on cultures of newborn mouse cerebellum, *Arch. Neurol.* **19:**292–301.

Altman, J., 1969, DNA metabolism and cell proliferation, in: *Handbook of Neurochemistry,* Vol. 2 (A. Lajtha, A., ed.), pp. 137–182, Plenum Press, New York.

Amonn, F., Baumann, U., Wiesmann, U. N., Hofmann, K., and Herschkowitz, N., 1978, Effects of antibiotics on the growth and differentiation in dissociated brain cell cultures, *Neuroscience* **3:**465–468.

Aparicio, S. R., Bradbury, K., Bradbury, M., and Howard, L., 1976, Organ cultures of nervous tissues, in: *Organ Culture in Biomedical Research,* British Society of Cell Biology Symposium I (M. Balls and M. Monnickendam, eds.), pp. 309–354, Cambridge University Press, Cambridge.

Barbarese, E., and Pfeiffer, S. E., 1981, Developmental regulation of myelin basic protein in dispersed cultures, *Proc. Natl. Acad. Sci. U.S.A.* **78:**1953–1957.

Barbarese, E., Carson, J. H., and Braun, P. E., 1978, Accumulation of the four basic proteins in mouse brain during development, *J. Neurochem.* **31:**779–782.

Barbarese, E., Pfeiffer, S. E., and Carson, J. H., 1983, Progenitors of oligodendrocytes: Limiting dilution analysis in fetal rat brain culture, *Dev. Biol.* **96:**84–88.

Barde, Y. A., Lindsay, R. M., Monard, D., and Thoenen, H., 1978, New factor released by cultured glioma cells supporting survival and growth of sensory neurones, *Nature (London)* **274:**818.

Barnes, D., and Sato, G. G., 1980, Methods for growth of cultured cells in serum-free media, *Anal. Biochem.* **102:**255–270.

Barnett, R. J., 1948, Some aspects of the experimental cretin-like animal, Thesis, Yale University School of Medicine, New Haven, Connecticut.

Beach, R. L., Bathgate, S. L., and Cotman, C. W., 1982, Identification of cell types in rat hippocampal slices maintained in organotypic cultures, *Dev. Brain Res.* **3:**3–20.

Benda, P., 1978, Rodent glial lines, in: *Dynamic Properties of Glia Cells* (E. Schoffeniels, G. Franck, L. Hertz, and D. B. Tower, eds.), pp. 67–81, Pergamon Press, Oxford.

Benda, P., Lightbody, J., Sato, G. H., Levine, L., and Sweet, H., 1968, Differentiated rat glial cell strain in tissue culture, *Science* **161:**370–371.

Berg, G., and Schachner, M., 1981, Immunoelectron microscopic identification of O-antigen-bearing oligodendroglial cells *in vitro, Cell Tissue Res.* **219:**313–325.

Bhat, N. R., Sarlieve, L. L., Subba Rao, G., and Pieringer, R. A., 1979, Investigations on myelination *in vitro, J. Biol. Chem.* **254:**9342–9344.

Bhat, N. R., Subba Rao, G. S., and Pieringer, R. A., 1981, Investigations on myelination *in vitro:* Regulation of sulfolipid synthesis by thyroid hormone in cultures of dissociated brain cells from embryonic mice, *J. Biol. Chem.* **256:**1167–1171.

Bhat, S., and Pfeiffer, S. E., 1981, Cholesterol ester hydrolases in primary cultures of fetal rat brain, *Trans. Am. Soc. Neurochem.* **12:**252.

Bhat, S., Barbarese, E., and Pfeiffer, S. E., 1981, Requirement for nonoligodendrocyte cell signals for enhanced myelinogenic gene expression in long-term cultures of purified rat oligodendrocytes, *Proc. Natl. Acad. Sci. U.S.A.* **78:**1283–1287.

Biddle, R., March, E., and Miller, J. R., 1973, *Mouse News Lett.* **48:**24.

Billings-Gagliardi, S., and Wolf, M. K., 1982, CNS hypomyelinated mice: Morphological and tissue culture studies, *Adv. Cell. Neurobiol.* **3:**275–307.

Billings-Gagliardi, S., Suva, M., and Wolf, M. K., 1976, Organotypic culture studies of myelin-deficient quaking mutant mice: A progress report, *In Vitro* **12:**321–322.

Billings-Gagliardi, S., Adcock, L. H., Schwing, G. B., and Wolf, M. K., 1980, Hypomyelinated mutant mice. II. Myelination *in vitro, Brain Res.* **200:**135–150.

Bird, M., and James, D. W., 1975, Myelin formation in cultures of previously dissociated mouse spinal cord, *Cell Tissue Res.* **162:**93–105.

Blakemore, W. F., 1977, Remyelination of CNS axons by Schwann cells transplanted from the sciatic nerve, *Nature (London)* **266:**68–69.

Blank, N. K., Seil, F. J., and Herndon, R. M., 1980, Cytosine arabinoside induced ultrastructural alterations in developing cerebellum in tissue culture, *J. Neuropathol. Exp. Neurol.* **39:**341.

Bologa-Sandru, L., Siegrist, H. P., Z'Graggen, A., Hofmann, K., Weissman, U., Dahl, D., and Herschkowitz, J., 1981*a,* Expression of antigenic markers during the development of oligodendrocytes in mouse brain cell cultures, *Brain Res.* **210:**217–229.

Bologa-Sandru, L., Zalc, B., Herschkowitz, N., and Baumann, N., 1981*b,* Oligodendrocytes of Jimpy mice express galactosylceramide: An immunofluorescence study on brain sections and dissociated brain cell cultures, *Brain Res.* **225:**425–430.

Booe, I. M., Joseph, B. S., Walsh, M. J., Potvin, A. R., and Tourtellotte, W. W., 1980, Multiple sclerosis serum and cerebrospinal fluid immunoglobulin binding to Fc receptors of oligodendrocytes, *Ann. Neurol.* **9:**371–377.

Booher, J., and Sensenbrenner, M., 1972, Growth and cultivation of dissociated neurons and glial cells from embryonic chick, rat, and human brain in flask cultures, *Neurobiology* **2:**97–105.

Bornstein, M. B., 1958, Serial observations of growth patterns, myelin formation, maintenance and degeneration in cultures of newborn rat and kitten cerebellum, *Anat. Rec.* **130:**275.

Bornstein, M. B., 1964, Morphological development of neonatal mouse cerebral cortex in tissue culture, in: *Neurological and Electroencephalographic Correlative Studies in Infancy* (P. Kellaway and I. Peterson, eds.), pp. 1–10, Grune and Stratton, New York.

Bornstein, M. B., 1973, Organotypic mammalian central and peripheral nervous tissue, in: *Tissue Culture Methods and Applications* (P. F. Kruse, Jr., and M. K. Patterson, Jr., eds), pp. 86–92, Academic Press, New York,

Bornstein, M. B., and Appel, S. H., 1961, The application of tissue culture to the study of experimental "allergic" encephalomyelitis. I. Patterns of demyelination, *J. Neuropathol. Exp. Neurol.* **20:**141–157.

Bornstein, M. B., and Hummelgard, 1976, Multiple sclerosis: Serum induced demyelination in tissue culture, in: *Etiology and Pathogenesis of the Demyelinating Diseases* (H. Shiraki, T. Yonezawa, and Y. Kuroiwa, eds.), pp. 341–350, Japan Science Press, Tokyo.

Bornstein, M. B., and Model, P. G., 1972, Development of synapses and myelin in cultures of dissociated embryonic mouse spinal cord, medulla, and cerebrum, *Brain Res.* **37:**287–293.

Bornstein, M. B., and Murray, M. R., 1958, Serial observations on patterns of growth, myelin formation, maintenance and degeneration in cultures of newborn rat and kitten cerebellum, *J. Biophys. Biochem. Cytol.* **4**:499–505.

Bornstein, M. B., and Raine, C. S., 1970, Experimental allergic encephalomyelitis antiserum inhibition of myelination *in vitro, Lab. Invest.* **23**:536–542.

Bornstein, M. B., and Raine, C. S., 1976, The initial structural lesion in serum-induced demyelination *in vitro, Lab. Invest.* **35**:391–401.

Bornstein, M. B., and Raine, C. S., 1980, Antiserum-induced alterations of myelinogenesis in cultured CNS and PNS tissues, in: *Tissue Culture in Neurobiology* (E. Giacobinni, A. Vernadakis, and A. Shahar, eds.), pp. 427–440, Raven Press, New York.

Bottenstein, J., Hayashi, I., Hutchings, S., Masui, H., Mather, J., McClure, D. B., Ohasa, S., Rizzino, A., Sato, G., Serrero, G., Wolfe, R., and Wu, R., 1979, The growth of cells in serum-free hormone-supplemented media, in: *Methods in Enzymology 58* (W. B. Jakoby and I. H. Pastan, eds.), pp. 94–110, Academic Press, New York.

Bourre, J.-M., Honegger, P., Daudu, O., and Matthieu, J.-M., 1979, The lipid composition of rat brain aggregating cell cultures during development, *Neurosci. Lett.* **11**:275–278.

Boyde, A., James, D. W., Tresman, R. L., and Willis, R. A., 1968, Outgrowth from chick embryo spinal cord *in vitro* studied with the scanning electron microscope, *Z. Zellforsch.* **90**:1–18.

Boyse, E. A., and Old, L. D., 1969, Some aspects of normal and abnormal cell surface genetics, *Ann. Rev. Genetics* **3**:269–290.

Bradbury, K., 1977, Myelin maturation: Evidence from organ cultures of cerebellum, *Biochem. Soc. Trans.* **5**:1775–1777.

Bradbury, K., 1978, Abnormal myelin maturation *in vitro:* The role of cerebrosides, *Adv. Exp. Med. Biol.* **100**:171–178.

Bradbury, K., and Lumsden, C. E., 1979, The chemical composition of myelin in organ cultures of rat cerebellum, *J. Neurochem.* **32**:145–154.

Bray, G. M., Rasminsky, M., and Aguayo, A. J., 1981, Interactions between axons and their sheath cells, *Annu. Rev. Neurosci.* **4**:127–162.

Breen, G. A. M., and de Vellis, J., 1975, Regulation of glycerol phosphate dehydrogenase by hydrocortisone in rat brain explants, *Exp. Cell Res.* **91**:159–169.

Brockes, J. P., Fields, K. L., and Raff, M. C., 1977, A surface antigenic marker for rat Schwann cells, *Nature (London)* **266**:364–366.

Brockes, J. P., Fields, K. L., and Raff, M. C., 1979, Studies on cultured rat Schwann cells. I. Establishment of peripheral nerve, *Brain Res.* **165**:105–118.

Brockes, J. P., Lemke, G. E., and Balzer, D. R., Jr., 1980*a*, Purification and preliminary characterization of a glial growth factor from the bovine pituitary, *J. Biol. Chem.* **255**:8374–8377.

Brockes, J. P., Raff, M. C., Nishiguchi, D. J., and Winter, J., 1980*b*, Studies on cultured rat Schwann cells. III. Assays for peripheral myelin proteins, *J. Neurocytol.* **9**:67–77.

Bunge, M. B., Bunge, R. P., and Pappas, G. D., 1962, Electron microscopic demonstrations of connection between glial and myelin sheath in the developing mammalian nervous system, *J. Cell Biol.* **12**:448–453.

Bunge, M. B., Williams, A. K., Wood, P. M., Uitto, J., and Jeffrey, J. J., 1980, Comparison of nerve cell and nerve cell plus Schwann cell cultures, with particular emphasis on basal lamina and collagen formation, *J. Cell Biol.* **84**:184–202.

Bunge, R. P., 1968, Glial cells and the central myelin sheath, *Physiol. Rev.* **48**:197–251.

Bunge, R. P., and Bunge, M. B., 1981, Cues and constraints in Schwann cell development, in: *Studies in Developmental Neurobiology* (W. M. Cowan, ed.), pp. 322–353, Oxford University Press, Oxford.

Bunge, R. P., and Wood, P., 1973, Studies of the transplantation of spinal cord tissue in the rat. I. The development of a culture system for hemisections of embryonic spinal cord, *Brain Res.* **57:**261–276.

Bunge, R. P., Bunge, M. B., and Peterson, E. R., 1965, An electron microscope study of cultured rat spinal cord, *J. Cell Biol.* **24:**163–191.

Campbell, G. Le M., Schachner, M., and Sharrow, S. O., 1977, Isolation of glial cell-enriched and -depleted populations from mouse cerebellum by density gradient centrifugation and electronic cell sorting, *Brain Res.* **127:**69–86.

Cantor, H., and Boyse, E. A., 1977, Regulation of the immune response by T cell sub-classes, *Contemp. Top. Immunobiol.* **7:**47–67.

Chernoff, G., March, E., and Miller, J. R.,1974, *Mouse News Lett.* **48:**24.

Choi, B. H., and Lapham, B. W., 1974, Autoradiographic studies of migrating neurons and astrocytes of human fetal cerebral cortex *in vitro, Exp. Mol. Pathol.* **21:**204–217.

Cicero, T. J., Cowan, W. M., Moore, B. W., and Suntzeff, V., 1970, The cellular localization of the two brain specific proteins S-100 and 14-3-2, *Brain Res.* **18:**25–34.

Courtney, B., and Bassleer, R., 1967, Etude histoautoradiographique de l'incorporation de thymidine, d'uridine, et de leucine tritiées dans des cellules nerveuses d'embryon de poulet isolées et cultivées *in vitro, C. R. Acad. Sci. Paris* **264:**497–499.

Crain, S. M., and Bornstein, M. B., 1972, Organotypic bioelectric activity in cultured reaggregates of dissociated rodent brain cells, *Science* **176:**182–184.

Davison, A. N., and Gregson, N. A., 1962, The physiological role of cerebron sulphuric acid (sulphatide) in the brain, *Biochem. J.* **85:**558–568.

Delaunoy, J. P., Hog, F., Devilliers, G., Bansart, M., Mandel, P., and Sensenbrenner, M., 1980, Developmental changes and localization of carbonic anhydrase in cerebral hemispheres of the rat and in rat glial cell cultures, *Cell. Mol. Biol.* **26:**235–240.

DeLong, G. R., 1970, Histogenesis of fetal mouse isocortex and hippocampus in reaggregating cell cultures, *Dev. Biol.* **22:**563–583.

Detering, N. K., and Wells, M. A., 1976, The non-synchronous synthesis of myelin components during early stages of myelination in the rat optic nerve, *J. Neurochem.* **26:**253–257.

Detweiler, S. R., and Kehoe, K., 1939, Further observations on the origin of the sheath cells of Schwann, *J. Exp. Zool.* **81:**415–435.

DeVries, G., Salzer, J. L., and Bunge, R. P., 1982, Axolemma-enriched fractions isolated from PNS and CNS are mitogenic for cultured Schwann cells, *Dev. Brain Res.* **3:**295–299.

Diaz, M., Bornstein, M. B., and Raine, C. S., 1978, Disorganization of myelinogenesis in tissue culture by anti-CNS antiserum, *Brain Res.* **154:**231–239.

Dimpfel, W., Neale, J. H., and Haberman, E., 1975, ^{125}I-labelled tetanus toxin as a neuronal marker in tissue cultures derived from embryonic CNS, *Naunyn-Schmiedeberg's Arch. Exp. Pathol. Pharmakol.* **290:**329–333.

Dimpfel, W., Huang, R. T. C., and Haberman, E., 1977, Gangliosides in nervous tissue cultures and binding of ^{125}I-labelled tetanus toxin—a neuronal marker, *J. Neurochem.* **29:**329–334.

Dorfman, S., 1977, Perturbation of oligodendroglial function and myelination *in vitro* by myelination inhibition antisera, *Diss. Abstr. Int.* **38:**03-B (Order no. AAD77-19842).

Dorfman, S. H., Holtzer, H., and Silberberg, D. H., 1976, Effect of 5-bromo-2'-deoxyuridine or cytosine-β-D-arabinofuranoside hydrochloride on myelination in newborn rat cerebellum cultures following removal of myelination inhibiting antiserum to whole cord or cerebroside, *Brain Res.* **104:**283–294.

Dorfman, S. H., Fry, J. M., Silberberg, D. H., Grose, C., and Manning, M. C., 1978, Cerebroside antibody titers in antiserums capable of myelination inhibition and demyelination, *Brain Res.* **147:**410–415.

Dorfman, S. H., Fry, J. M., and Silberberg, D. H., 1979, Antiserum induced myelination inhibition *in vitro* without complement, *Brain Res.* **177**:105–114.

Drummond, R. J., and Dean, G., 1980, Comparison of 2′,3′-cyclic nucleotide 3′-phosphodiesterase and the major component of Wolfgram protein W1, *J. Neurochem.* **35**:1155–1165.

Eisenbarth, G. S., Walsh, F. S., and Nirenberg, M., 1979, Monoclonal antibody to a plasma membrane antigen of neurons, *Proc. Natl. Acad. Sci. U.S.A.* **76**:4913–4917.

Eng, L. F., Vanderhaeghen, J. J., Bignami, A., and Gerstl, B., 1971, An acidic protein isolated from fibrous astrocytes, *Brain Res.* **28**:351–354.

Eto, Y., and Suzuki, K., 1973, Cholesterol ester metabolism in rat brain, *J. Biol. Chem.* **268**:1986–1991.

Everly, J. L., Brady, R. O., and Quarles, R. H., 1974, Evidence that the major protein in rat sciatic nerve myelin is a glycoprotein, *J. Neurochem.* **21**:329–334.

Fagg, G. E., Schipper, H. I., and Neuhoff, V., 1979, Myelin protein composition in the rat spinal cord in culture and *in vivo:* A developmental comparison, *Brain Res.* **167**:251–258.

Farooq, M., Cammer, W., Synder, D. S., Raine, C. S., and Norton, W. T., 1981, Properties of bovine oligodendroglia isolated by a new procedure using physiologic conditions, *J. Neurochem.* **36**:431–440.

Fedoroff, S., 1977, Tracing glial cell lineages by colony formation in primary cultures, in: *Cell, Tissue, and Organ Cultures in Neurobiology* (S. Fedoroff and L. Hertz, eds.), pp. 215–221, Academic Press, New York.

Fedoroff, S., 1978, The development of glial cells in primary cultures, in: *Dynamic Properties of Glial Cells* (E. Schoffeniels, G. Franck, D. B. Tower, and L. Hertz, eds.), pp. 83–92, Pergamon Press, New York.

Field, E. J., and Hughes, D., 1965, Toxicity of motor neuron disease serum for myelin in tissue culture, *Br. Med. J.* **2**:1399–1401.

Field, E. J., and Hughes, D., 1969, A comparison of toxicity of serum from multiple sclerosis and motor neurone disease on myelin *in vitro, Int. Arch. Allergy Appl. Immunol.* **36** (Suppl.):563–567.

Field, E. J., Hughes, D., and Raine, C. S., 1968, Electron microscopic observations on the development of myelin in cultures of neonatal rat cerebellum, *J. Neurol. Sci.* **8**:49–60.

Fields, K. L., 1979, Cell-type specific antigens of cells of the central nervous system and peripheral nervous system, *Curr. Topics Dev. Biol.* **13**(Pt. 1):237–257.

Fields, K. L., Gosling, C., Megson, M., and Stern, P. L., 1975, New cell surface antigens in rat defined by tumors of the nervous system, *Proc. Natl. Acad. Sci. U.S.A.* **72**:1286–1300.

Fields, K. L., Brockes, J. P., Mirsky, R., and Wendon, L. M. B., 1978, Cell surface markers for distinguishing different types of rat dorsal root ganglion cells in culture, *Cell* **14**:43–51.

Fry, J. M., Lehrer, G. M., and Bornstein, M. R., 1972, Sulfatide synthesis: Inhibition by experimental allergic encephalomyelitis serum, *Science* **175**:192–194.

Fry, J. M., Lehrer, G. M., and Bornstein, M. B., 1973, Experimental inhibition of myelination in spinal cord cultures: Enzyme assays, *J. Neurobiol.* **4**:453–459.

Fry, J. M., Weissbarth, S., Lehrer, G. M., and Bornstein, M. B., 1974, Cerebroside antibody inhibits sulfatide synthesis and myelination and demyelinates in cord tissue cultures, *Science* **183**:540–542.

Fryell, K. J., 1980, Synthesis of sulfatide by cultured rat Schwann cells, *J. Neurochem.* **35**:1461–1464.

Garber, B., 1967, Aggregation *in vivo* of dissociated cells. I. Role of developmental age in tissue reconstruction, *J. Exp. Zool.* **164**:339–350.

Gebicke-Harter, P. J., Althaus, H.-H., Schwartz, P., and Neuhoff, V., 1981, Oligodendrocytes from postnatal cat brain in cell culture. I. Regeneration and maintenance, *Dev. Brain Res.* **1**:497–518.

Geiger, R. S., 1963, The behavior of adult mammalian brain cells in culture, *Int. Rev. Neurobiol.* **5**:1–52.

Geren, B. B., 1954, The formation of myelin from the Schwann cell surface of myelin in the peripheral nerves of chick embryos, *Exp. Cell Res.* **7**:558–562.

Gospodarowicz, D., and Moran, J. S., 1976, Growth factors in mammalian cell culture, *Annu. Rev. Biochem.* **45**:531–558.

Gould, R. M., Matsumoto, D., and Mattingly, G., 1982, The Schwann cell, in: *Handbook of Neurochemistry,* Vol. 1, 2nd ed. (A. Lajtha, ed.), pp. 397–414, Plenum Press, New York.

Graham, F. L., and Whitmore, G. F., 1970, The effect of 1-β-D-arabinofuranosylcytosine on growth, viability, and DNA synthesis of mouse L-cells, *Cancer Res.* **30**:2627–2635.

Grosse, G., and Lindner, G., 1970, Untersuchungen zur Differenzierung isolierter Nerven und Gliazellen des zentralnervösen Gewebes von Hühnerembryonen in der Zellkultur, *J. Hirnforsch.* **12**:207–215.

Grosse, G., and Lindner, G., 1972, Untersuchungen zur Differenzierung disaggregierter Zellen des Telencephalon von Hühnerembryo in Langzeit Zellkulturen, *Z. Mikrosk. Anat. Forsch. Leipzig* **85**:438–448.

Grundke-Iqbal, I., and Bornstein, M. B., 1979, Multiple sclerosis: Immunochemical studies on the demyelinating serum factor, *Brain Res.* **160**:489–503.

Grundke-Iqbal, I., Raine, C. S., Johnson, A. B., Brosnan, C. F., and Bornstein, M. B., 1981, Experimental allergic encephalomyelitis—characterization of serum factors causing demyelination and swelling of myelin, *J. Neurol. Sci.* **50**:63–79.

Hamburgh, M., 1966, Evidence for a direct effect of temperature and thyroid hormone on myelinogenesis *in vitro, Dev. Biol.* **13**:15–30.

Hamburgh, M., and Bunge, R. P., 1964, Evidence for a direct effect of thyroid hormone on maturation of nervous tissue grown *in vitro, Life Sci.* **3**:1423–1430.

Hanson, G. R., Iverson, P. L., and Partlow, L. M., 1982*a*, Preparation and partial characterization of highly purified primary cultures of neurons and non-neuronal (glial) cells from embryonic chick cerebral hemispheres and several other regions of the nervous system, *Dev. Brain Res.* **3**:529–545.

Hanson, G. R., Partlow, L. M., and Iverson, P. L., 1982*b*, Neuronal stimulation of non-neuronal (glial) cell proliferation: Lack of specificity between different regions of the nervous system, *Dev. Brain Res.* **3**:547–555.

Hansson, II. A., and Sourander, P., 1964, Studies on cultures of mammalian retina, *Z. Zellforsch.* **62**:26–47.

Hansson, E., Sellstrom, A., Persson, L. I., and Ronnback, L., 1980, Brain primary culture—a characterization, *Brain Res.* **188**:233–246.

Harrison, B. M., 1980, Remyelination by cells introduced into a stable demyelinating lesion in the central nervous system, *J. Neurol. Sci.* **46**:63–81.

Harrison, R. G., 1924, Neuroblast versus sheath cell in the development of peripheral nerves, *J. Comp. Neurol.* **37**:123–205.

Hartman, B. K., Agrawal, H. C., Kalmbach, S., and Shearer, W. T., 1979, A comparative study of the immunocytochemical localization of basic protein to myelin and oligodendrocytes in rat and chicken brain, *J. Comp. Neurol.* **188**:273–290.

Haugen, A., and Laerum, O. D., 1978, Induced glial differentiation of fetal rat brain cells in culture: An ultrastructural study, *Brain Res.* **150**:225–238.

Hauw, J.-J., Boutry, J.-M., Crosnier-Smith, N., and Robineau, R., 1974, Morphology of cultured guinea pig cerebellum, *Cell Tissue Res.* **152**:141–164.

Hauw, J.-J., Boutry, J.-M., and Jacque, C., 1980, Tissue culture study of the shiverer mutant mouse: Preliminary results, in: *Neurological Mutations Affecting Myelination* (N. Baumann, ed.), INSERM Symposium No. 14, pp. 475–480, Elsevier/North-Holland, Amsterdam.

Henn, F. A., 1980, Separation of neuronal and glial cells and subcellular constituents, in: *Advances in Cellular Neurobiology* (S. Federoff and L. Hertz, eds.), pp. 373–403, Academic Press, New York.

Hild, W., 1957, Myelinogenesis in cultures of mammalian central nervous tissue, *Z. Zellforsch.* **46:**71–95.

Hild, W., 1963*a*, Myelin formation around central neurons *in vitro, Tex. Rep. Biol. Med.* **21:**207–213.

Hild, W., 1963*b*, Myelinogenesis in cultures of mammalian central nervous tissue, *Z. Zellforsch.* **46:**71–85.

Hild, W., 1966, Cell types and neuronal connections in cultures of mammalian central nervous tissue, *Z. Zellforsch.* **69:**155–188.

Hild, W., and Tasaki, I., 1962, Morphological and physiological properties of neurons and glial cells in tissue culture, *J. Neurophysiol.* **25:**277–304.

Hirano, A., 1968, A confirmation of the oligodendroglial origin of myelin in the adult rat, *J. Cell Biol.* **38:**637–640.

Hirose, G., and Bass, N. H., 1973, Maturation of oligodendroglia and myelinogenesis in rat optic nerve: A quantitative histochemical study, *J. Comp. Neurol.* **152:**201–210.

Hogue, M. J., 1953, A study of adult human brain cells grown in tissue culture, *Am. J. Anat.* **93:**397–427.

Holtzer, H., 1970, Myogenesis, in: *Cell Differentiation* (O. Schjeide and J. de Vellis, eds.), pp. 476–503, Van Nostrand-Reinhold, Princeton, New Jersey.

Holtzer, H., Weintraub, H., Mayne, R., and Mochan, B., 1972, The cell cycle, cell lineages, and cell differentiation, *Curr. Top. Dev. Biol.* **7:**229–256.

Honegger, P., and Matthieu, J.-M., 1980, Myelination of aggregating fetal rat brain cell cultures grown in a chemically defined medium, in: *Neurological Mutations Affecting Myelination* (N. Baumann, ed.), INSERM Symposium No. 14, pp. 481–488, Elsevier/North-Holland, Amsterdam.

Honegger, P., and Richelson, E., 1976, Biochemical differentiation of mechanically dissociated mammalian brain in aggregating cell culture, *Brain Res.* **109:**335–354.

Honegger, P., Lenoir, D., and Favrod, P., 1979, Growth and differentiation of aggregating fetal brain cells in a serum-free defined medium, *Nature (London)* **282:**305–308.

Hruby, S., Alvord, E. C., Jr., and Seil, F. J., 1977, Synthetic galactocerebrosides evoke myelination-inhibiting antibodies, *Science* **195:**173–175.

Hugosson, R., Kallen, B., and Nilsson, O., 1968, Neuroglia proliferation studied in tissue culture, *Acta Neuropathol.* **11:**210–220.

Imamoto, K., Paterson, J. A., and Leblond, C. P., 1978, Radioautographic investigation of gliogenesis in the corpus callosum of young rats, I. Sequential changes in oligodendrocytes, *J. Comp. Neurol.* **180:**115–138.

Jacobson, M., 1978, *Developmental Neurobiology,* pp. 166–180, Plenum Press, New York.

Johnson, A. B., and Bornstein, M. B., 1978, Myelin-binding antibodies *in vitro*—Immunoperoxidase studies with experimental allergic encephalomyelitis, anti-galactosylcerebroside and multiple sclerosis sera, *Brain Res.* **159:**173–182.

Johnson, A. B., Raine, C. S., and Bornstein, M. B., 1979, Experimental allergic encephalomyelitis: Serum immunoglobulin binds to myelin and oligodendrocytes in cultured tissue—ultrastructural immunoperoxidase observations, *Lab. Invest.* **40:**568–575.

Kennedy, P. G. E., and Lisak, R. P., 1980, Astrocytes and oligodendrocytes in dissociated cell culture of adult rat optic nerve, *Neurosci. Lett.* **16:**229–233.

Kennedy, P. G. E., Lisak, R. P., and Raff, M. C., 1980, Cell type-specific markers for human glial and neuronal cells in culture, *Lab. Invest.* **43**:342–351.

Kies, M. W., Driscoll, B. F., Seil, F. J., and Alvord, E. C., Jr., 1973, Myelination inhibition factor: Dissociation from induction of experimental allergic encephalomyelitis, *Science* **179**:689–690.

Kim, S. U., 1970, Observations on cerebellar granule cells in tissue culture: A silver and electron microscopic study, *Z. Zellforsch.* **107**:454–465.

Kim, S. U., 1971, Electron microscopic study of mouse cerebellum in tissue culture, *Exp. Neurol.* **33**:237–246.

Kim, S. U., 1972, Formation of synapses and myelin sheaths in cultures of dissociated chick spinal cord, *Exp. Cell Res.* **73**:528–530.

Kim, S. U., 1975, Effects of cholesterol biosynthesis inhibitor AY9944 on organotypic cultures of mouse spinal cord: Retarded myelinogenesis and induction of cytoplasmic inclusions, *Lab. Invest.* **32**:720–728.

Kim, S. U., 1976, Effect of serum deprivation on myelinating mouse cerebellum cultures, *J. Neurosci. Res.* **2**:309–316.

Kim, S. U., and Pleasure, D. E., 1978, Tissue culture analysis of neurogenesis: Myelination and synapse formation are retarded by serum deprivation, *Brain Res.* **145**:15–25.

Kim, S. U., and Pleasure, D. E., 1980, Tissue culture of Jimpy and Quaking mouse mutants, in: *Neurological Mutations Affecting Myelination* (N. Baumann, ed.), INSERM Symposium No. 14, pp. 453–459, Elsevier/North-Holland, Amsterdam.

Kim, S. U., and Tanaka, Y., 1971, Myelinated neuronal soma in organized tissue culture of mouse central nervous tissue, *Exp. Neurol.* **30**:190–193.

Kim, S., and Tunnicliff, G., 1974, Morphological and biochemical development of chick cerebrum cultured *in vitro, Exp. Neurol.* **43**:515–526.

Kim, S. U., Oh, T. H., and Johnson, D. D., 1972, Developmental changes of acetylcholinesterase and pseudocholinesterase in organotypic cultures of spinal cord, *Exp. Neurol.* **35**:274–281.

Kohler, G., and Milstein, C., 1976, Derivation of specific antibody-producing tissue culture and tumour lines by cell fusion, *Eur. J. Immunol.* **6**:511–519.

Korinkova, P., and Lodin, Z., 1977, A transitional differentiation of glial cells of cultured corpus callosum caused by dibutyryl cyclic adenosine monophosphate, *Neuroscience* **2**:1113–1114.

Kozak, L. P., 1977, The transition from embryonic to adult isozyme expression in reaggregating cell cultures of mouse brain, *Dev. Biol.* **55**:160–169.

Kozak, L. P., Eppig, J. J., Dahl, D., and Bignami, A., 1977, Ultrastructural and immunohistological characterization of a cell culture model for the study of neuronal–glial interactions, *Dev. Biol.* **59**:206–227.

Labourdette, G., Roussel, G., Ghandour, M. S., and Nussbaum, J. L., 1979, Cultures from rat brain hemispheres enriched in oligodendrocyte-like cells, *Brain Res.* **179**:199–203.

Labourdette, G., Roussel, G., and Nussbaum, J. L., 1980, Oligodendroglia content of glial cell primary cultures, from newborn rat brain hemispheres, depends on the initial plating density, *Neurosci. Lett.* **18**:203–209.

Latovitzki, N., and Silberberg, D. H., 1973, Quantification of galactolipids in myelinating cultures of rat cerebellum, *J. Neurochem.* **20**:1771–1776.

Latovitzki, N., and Silberberg, D. H., 1975, Ceramide glycosyltransferase in cultured rat cerebellum: Changes with age, with demyelination, and with inhibition of myelination by 5-bromo-2'-deoxyuridine or experimental allergic encephalomyelitis serum, *J. Neurochem.* **24**:1017–1021.

Latovitzki, N., and Silberberg, N., 1977, UDP-galactose:ceramide galactosyltransferase and 2',3'-cyclic nucleotide 3'-phosphohydrolase activities in cultured newborn cerebellum: Association with myelination and concurrent susceptibility to 5-bromodeoxy-uridine, *J. Neurochem.* **29:**611–614.

Lebar, R., Boutry, J. M., Vincent, C. H., Robineaux, R., and Voisin, G. A., 1976, Studies on autoimmune encephalomyelitis in the guinea pig. II. An *in vitro* investigation of the nature, properties and specificity of the serum demyelinating factor, *J. Immunol.* **116:**1439–1446.

Lehrer, G. M., 1973, The tissue culture as a model for the biochemistry of brain development, in: *Progress in Brain Research,* Vol. 40, *Neurological Aspects of Maturating and Aging* (D. H. Ford, ed.), pp. 219–230, Elsevier, Amsterdam.

Lehrer, G. M., and Bornstein, M. R., 1968, Glucose metabolism in rat cerebellum tissue cultures as a function of age, *Trans. Am. Neurol. Assoc.* **93:**174–176.

Lehrer, G. M., Bornstein, M. B., Weiss, C., and Silides, D. J., 1970*a*, Enzymatic maturation of mouse cerebral neocortex *in vitro* and *in situ, Exp. Neurol.* **26:**595–606.

Lehrer, G. M., Bornstein, M. B., Weiss, C., Furnam, M., and Lichtman, C., 1970*b*, Enzymes of carbohydrate metabolism in the rat cerebellum developing *in situ* and *in vivo, Exp. Neurol.* **27:**410–425.

Levi-Montalcini, R., 1966, The nerve growth factor: Its mode of action on sensory and sympathetic nerve cells, *Harvey Lect.* **60:**217–259.

Lilien, J. E., 1968, Specific enhancement of cell aggregation *in vitro, Dev. Biol.* **17:**657–678.

Lim, R., Turriff, D. E., Troy, S. S., and Kato, T., 1977, Differentiation of glioblasts under the influence of glia maturation factor, in: *Cell, Tissue, and Organ Cultures in Neurobiology* (S. Fedoroff and L. Hertz, eds.), pp. 223–235, Academic Press, New York.

Lisak, R. P., Pleasure, D. E., Silberberg, D. H., Manning, M. C., and Saida, T., 1981, Long-term culture of bovine oligodendroglia isolated with a Percoll gradient, *Brain Res.* **223:**107–122.

Lodin, Z., Korinkova, P., Falton, J., and Fleischmannova, V., 1978*a*, Structure and ultrastructure of cultured glial cells from corpus callosum, *Acta Histochem.* **61:**165–183.

Lodin, Z., Korinkova, P., Falton, J., and Fleischmannova, V., 1978*b*, Differentiation of corpus callosum glial cells and factors influencing their maturation *in vitro, Acta Histochem.* **61:**184–191.

Lumsden, C. E., 1965, The clinical pathology of multiple sclerosis, in: *Multiple Sclerosis, A Reappraisal* (D. McAlpine, C. E. Lumsden, and E. D. Acheson, eds.), pp. 243–263, Livingstone, Edinburgh.

Lumsden, C., and Pomerat, C., 19651, Normal oligodendrocytes in tissue culture: A preliminary report on the pulsatile glial cells in tissue culture from the corpus callosum of the normal adult rat brain, *Exp. Cell Res.* **2:**103–114.

Mack, S. R., and Szuchet, S., 1981, Synthesis of myelin glycosphingolipids by isolated oligodendrocytes in tissue culture, *Brain Res.* **214:**180–185.

Mack, S. R., Szuchet, S., and Dawson, G., 1981, Synthesis of gangliosides by cultured oligodendrocytes, *J. Neurosci. Res.* **6:**361–368.

Macklin, W. B., and Pfeiffer, S. E., 1983, Myelin proteolipid protein time course in rat primary cultures of fetal rat brain, *Trans. Am. Soc. Neurochem.* **14:**212.

Manthorpe, M., Skaper, S., and Varon, S., 1980, Purification of mouse Schwann cells using neurite-induced proliferation in serum-free monolayer culture, *Brain Res.* **196:**467–482.

Manuelidis, L., and Manuelidis, E. E., 1971, An autoradiographic study of the proliferation and differentiation of glial cells *in vitro, Acta Neuropathol.* **18:**193–213.

Matthieu, J.-M., and Honegger, P., 1979, An *in vitro* model to study brain development: Brain aggregating cell cultures, in: *Models for the Study of Inborn Errors of Metabolism* (F. A. Hommes, ed.), pp. 259–277, Elsevier/North-Holland, Amsterdam.

Matthieu, J.-M., Honegger, P., Trapp, B. D., Cohen, S. R., and Webster, H. de F., 1978, Myelination in rat brain aggregating cell cultures, *Neuroscience* **3:**565–572.

Matthieu, J. M., Honeggar, P., Favrod, P., Gautier, E., and Dolvio, M., 1979, Biochemical characterization of a myelin fraction isolated from rat brain aggregating cell cultures, *J. Neurochem.* **32**:869–881.

Matthieu, J.-M., Honegger, P., Favrod, P., Poduslo, J. F., Costantino-Ceccarini, E., and Krstic, R., 1980, Myelination and demyelination in aggregating cultures of rat brain cells, in: *Tissue Culture in Neurobiology* (E. Giacobini, A. Vernadakis, and A. Shahar, eds.), pp. 441–459, Raven Press, New York.

Maturana, H. R., 1960, The fine anatomy of the optic nerve of *Anurans*—an electron microscopic study, *J. Biophys. Biochem. Cytol.* **7**:107–120.

McCarthy, K. D., and de Vellis, J., 1978, Alpha-adrenergic receptor modulation of beta-adrenergic, adenosine and prostaglandin E_1 increased adenosine 3'-5'-cyclic monophosphate levels in primary cultures of glia, *J. Cyclic Nucleotide Res.* **4**:15–26.

McCarthy, K. D., and de Vellis, J., 1980, Preparation of separate astroglial and oligodendroglial cell cultures from rat cerebral tissue, *J. Cell Biol.* **85**:890–892.

McDermott, J. R., and Smith, A. R., 1978, Absence of myelin basic protein from glial cell lines and cultures, *J. Neurochem.* **30**:1637–1639.

McKhann, G. M., and Ho, W., 1967, The *in vivo* and *in vitro* synthesis of sulphatides during development, *J. Neurochem.* **14**:717–724.

McMorris, F. A., 1977, Norepinephrine induces glial-specific enzyme activity in cultured glioma cells, *Proc. Natl. Acad. Sci. U.S.A.* **74**:4501–4504.

McMorris, F. A., Miller, S. L., Pleasure, D., and Abramsky, O., 1981, Expression of biochemical properties of oligodendrocytes in oligodendrocyte glioma cell hybrids proliferating *in vitro, Exp. Cell Res.* **133**:395–404.

Meier, H., and MacPike, A. D., 1970, A neurological mutation (msd) of the mouse causing a deficiency of myelin synthesis, *Exp. Brain Res.* **10**:512–525.

Mikoshiba, K., Nagaike, K., Aoki, E., and Tsukada, Y., 1979, Biochemical and immunohistochemical studies on dysmyelination of quaking mutant mice *in vivo* and *in vitro, Brain Res.* **177**:287–299.

Mikoshiba, K., Nagaike, K., Takamatsu, K., and Tsukada, Y., 1980, Developmental change of 2',3'-cyclic nucleotide 3'-phosphohydrolase activity in the nervous system of the Shiverer mutant mice *in vivo* and *in vitro,* in: *Neurological Mutations Affecting Myelination* (N. Baumann, ed.), INSERM Symposium No. 14, pp. 349–354, Elsevier/North, Holland, Amsterdam.

Mirsky, R., and Thompson, E. J., 1975, Thy-1 (theta) antigen on the surface of morphologically distinct brain cell types, *Cell* **4**:95–101.

Mirsky, R., Wendon, L. M. B., Black, P., Stolkin, C., and Bray, D., 1978, Tetanus toxin: A cell surface marker for neurones in culture, *Brain Res.* **148**:251–259.

Mirsky, R., Winter, J., Abney, E. R., Pruss, R. M., Gavrilovic, J., and Raff, M. C., 1980, Myelin-specific proteins and glycolipids in rat Schwann cells and oligodendrocytes in culture, *J. Cell Biol.* **84**:483–494.

Mitrova, E., 1967, Karyometric investigation of glia cells in the cerebellum in the course of myelination, *Z. Mikrosk. Anat. Forsch.* **77**:304–312.

Moore, B. W., 1965, A soluble protein characteristic of the nervous system, *Biochem. Biophys. Res. Commun.* **19**:739–744.

Morell, P., and Norton, W. T., 1980, Myelin, *Sci. Am.* **242**(5):88–118.

Mori, S., and Leblond, C. P., 1970, Electron microscopic identification of three classes of oligodendrocytes and a preliminary study of their proliferative activity in the corpus callosum of young rats, *J. Comp. Neurol.* **139**:1–30.

Morris, R. J., 1982, The surface antigens of nerve cells, in: *Neuroscience Approached through Cell Culture,* Vol I (S. E. Pfeiffer, ed.), pp. 1–80, CRC Press, Boca Raton, Florida.

Moscona, A. A., 1965*a*, Rotation-mediated histogenetic aggregation of dissociated cells, *Exp. Cell Res.* **22**:455–475.

Moscona, A. A., 1965*b*, Recombination of dissociated cells and the development of cell aggregates, in: *Cells and Tissues in Culture,* Vol. 1 (E. N. Willmer, ed.) pp. 489–529, Academic Press, New York.

Moscona, A. A., 1968, Cell aggregation: Properties of specific cell-ligands and their role in the formation of multicellular systems, *Dev. Biol.* **18**:250–277.

Murray, M. R., 1959, Factors bearing on myelin formation *in vitro,* in: *Progress in Neurobiology,* Vol. IV, *The Biology of Myelin* (S. R. Korey and J. I. Nurnberger, eds.), pp. 201–221, Hoeber, New York.

Murray, M. R., 1964, Myelin formation and neuron histogenesis in tissue culture, in: *Comparative Neurochemistry* (D. Richter, ed.), pp. 49–61, Pergamon Press, London.

Murray, M. R., 1965, Nervous tissue *in vitro,* in: *Cells and Tissues in Culture,* Vol. 2 (E. N. Willmer, ed.), pp. 373–455, Academic Press, New York.

Murray, M. R., 1971, Nervous tissues isolated in culture, in: *Handbook of Neurochemistry,* Vol. 5A (A. Lajtha, ed.), pp. 373–438, Plenum Press, New York.

Murray, M. R., 1977, Introduction, in: *Cell, Tissue, and Organ Cultures in Neurobiology* (S. Fedoroff and L. Hertz, eds.), pp. 1–8, Academic Press, New York.

Murray, M. R., Peterson, E. R., and Bunge, R. P., 1962, Some nutritional aspects of myelin sheath formation in cultures of central and peripheral nervous system, in: *Proceedings of the Fourth International Congress on Neuropathology,* Vol. II (H. Jacob, ed.), pp. 267–272, Georg Thieme, Stuttgart.

Nadler, N. J., 1978, Kinetics of oligodendrocytes in growing rats, *J. Comp. Neurol.* **180**:129–131.

Nagata, Y., and Tsukada, Y., 1978, Bulk separation of neuronal cell bodies and glial cells from mammalian brain and some of their biochemical properties, *Rev. Neurosci.* **3**:195–221.

Nixon, R. A., Suva, M., and Wolf, M. K., 1976, Neurotoxicity of a non-metabolizable amino acid, 1-aminocyclopentane-1-carboxylic acid: Antagonism by amino acids in cultures of cerebellum, *J. Neurochem.* **27**:245–251.

Noël-Courtney, B., and Heinen, E., 1977, Observations en microscope électronique à balayage de cellules nerveuses de moelle spinal d'embryons de poulet cultivées *in vitro* sur la polyly-sine-L, *C. R. Acad. Sci. Paris* **285**:385–387.

Norenberg, M. D., and Martinez-Hernandez, A., 1979, Fine structural localization of glutamine synthetase in astrocytes of rat brain, *Brain Res.* **161**:303–310.

Norton, W. T., 1983, Recent advances in the neurobiology of oligodendroglia, in: *Advances in Cellular Neurobiology,* Vol. 4 (S. Fedoroff and L. Hertz, eds.), pp. 3–55, Academic Press, New York.

Nussbaum, J. L., Delaunoy, J. P., and Mandel, P., 1977, Some immunochemical characteristics of W1 and W2 Wolfgram proteins isolated from rat brain myelin, *J. Neurochem.* **28**:183–191.

Orr, M. F., 1968, Histogenesis of sensory epithelium in reaggregates of dissociated embryonic chick otocysts, *Dev. Biol.* **17**:39–54.

Parkhouse, R. M. E., and Cooper, M. D., 1977, A model for the differentiation of B lymphocytes with implications for the biological role of IgD, *Immunol. Rev.* **37**:105–126.

Paterson, J. A., Privat, A., Ling, E. A., and Leblond, C. P., 1973, Investigation of glial cells in semithin sections. III. Transformation of subependymal cells into glial cells, as shown by radioautography after ^{3}H-thymidine injection into the lateral ventricle of the brain of young rats, *J. Comp. Neurol.* **149**:83–102.

Perier, O., 1959, Formation de la myelin *in vitro* en rapport avec les maladies demyelinisantes, *Acta Neurol. Belg.* **6**:747–755.

Peters, A., 1960, The formation and structure of myelin sheaths in the central nervous system, *J. Biophys. Biochem. Cytol.* **8**:431–446.

Peters, A., 1964, Observations on the connections between myelin sheaths and glial cells in the optic nerves of young rats, *J. Anat. (London)* **98**:125–134.

Peters, A., Palay, S. L., and Webster, H. de F., 1976, *The Fine Structure of the Nervous System: The Cells and Their Processes,* W. B. Saunders, Philadelphia.

Peterson, E. R., 1950, Production of myelin sheaths *in vitro* by embryonic spinal ganglion cells, *Anat. Rec.* **106**:232.

Peterson, E. R., and Murray, M. R., 1955*a*, Myelin sheath formation in cultures of avian spinal ganglia, *Am. J. Anat.* **96**:319–356.

Peterson, E. R., and Murray, M. R., 1955*b*, Patterns of peripheral demyelination *in vitro, Ann. N. Y. Acad. Sci.* **122**:39–50.

Peterson, E. R., and Murray, M. R., 1960, Modification of development in isolated dorsal root ganglia by nutritional and physical factors, *Dev. Biol.* **2**:461–476.

Peterson, E. R., Crain, S. M., and Murray, M. R., 1965, Differentiation and prolonged maintenance of bioelectrically active spinal cord cultures (rat, chick, and human), *Z. Zellforsch.* **66**:130–154.

Pettman, B., Delanoy, J. P., Couraget, J., Devilliers, G., and Sensenbrenner, M., 1980, Rat brain glial cells in culture: Effect of brain extracts on the development of oligodendroglia-like cells, *Dev. Biol.* **75**:278–287.

Pfeiffer, S. E., Betchart, B., Cook, J., Mancini, P., and Morris, R., 1977, Glial cell lines, in: *Cell, Tissue, and Organ Cultures in Neurobiology* (S. Fedoroff and L. Hertz, eds.), pp. 287–346, Academic Press, New York.

Pfeiffer, S. E., Barbarese, E., and Bhat, S., 1981*a*, Glial cell lines, in: *Functionally Differentiated Cell Lines* (G. Sato, ed.), pp. 141–154, Alan R. Liss, New York.

Pfeiffer, S. E., Barbarese, E., and Bhat, S., 1981*b*, Non-coordinate regulation of myelinogenic parameters in primary cultures of dissociated fetal rat brain, *J. Neurosci. Res.* **6**:369–380.

Phillips, R. J. S., 1954, Jimpy, a new totally sex-linked gene in the house mouse, *Z. Vererbungsl.* **86**:322–326.

Pieringer, R. A., Campbell, G. Le M., Bhat, N. R., Subba Rao, G., and Sarlieve, L. L., 1980, Biochemical, morphological, and regulatory aspects of myelination in cultures of dissociated brain cells from embryonic mice, in: *Cell Surface Glycolipids* (C. S. Sweeley, ed.), pp. 303–319, American Chemical Society Symposium Series 128, Washington, D.C.

Piper, R., 1962, Microtomy techniques and the problem of relation of cell outgrowth to events within explants *in vitro, J. Med. Lab. Technol.* **19**:1–18.

Pleasure, D. E., and Kim, S. U., 1976*a*, Sterol synthesis by myelinating cultures of mouse spinal cord, *Brain Res.* **103**:117–126.

Pleasure, D. E., and Kim, S. U., 1976*b*, Enzyme markers for myelination of mouse cerebellum *in vivo* and in tissue culture, *Brain Res.* **104**:193–196.

Pleasure, D. E., Towfighi, J., Silberberg, D., and Parris, J., 1974, The pathogenesis of hexachlorophene neuropathy: *In vivo* and *in vitro* studies, *Neurology* **21**:1068–1075.

Pomerat, C. M., 1951, Pulsatile activity of cells from the human brain in tissue culture, *J. Nerv. Ment. Dis.* **114**:430–449.

Pomerat, C. M., 1958, Functional concepts based on tissue culture studies of neuroglia cells, in: *Biology of Neuroglia* (W. F. Windle, ed.), pp. 162–175, Charles C. Thomas, Springfield, Illinois.

Pomerat, C. M., and Costero, I., 1956, Tissue culture of cat cerebellum, *Am. J. Anat.* **99**:211–247.

Pomerat, C. M., Ewalt, J. R., Snodgrass, S. R., and Orr, M. F., 1950, Tissue cultures of adult human cerebral cortex, *Tex. Rep. Biol. Med.* **8**:108–110.

Privat, A., 1975, Postnatal gliogenesis in the mammalian brain, *Int. Rev. Cytol.* **40:**281–323.

Privat, A., and Leblond, C. P., 1972, The subependymal layer and neighboring region in the brain of the young rat, *J. Comp. Neurol.* **146:**277–301.

Pruss, R. M., Bartlett, P. F., Gavrilovic, J., Lisak, R. P., and Rattray, S., 1982, Mitogens for glial cells: A comparison of the response of cultured astrocytes, oligodendrocytes and Schwann cells, *Dev. Brain Res.* **2:**19–35.

Raff, M. C., Abney, E., Brockes, J. P., and Hornby-Smith, A., 1978*a*, Schwann cell growth factors, *Cell* **15:**813–822.

Raff, M. C., Hornby-Smith, A., and Brockes, J. P., 1978*b*, Cyclic AMP as a mitogenic signal for cultured rat Schwann cells, *Nature (London)* **273:**672–673.

Raff, M. C., Mirsky, R., Fields, K. L., Lisak, R. P., Dorfman, S. H., Silberberg, D. H., Gregson, N. A., Leibowitz, S., and Kennedy, M. C., 1978*c*, Galactocerebroside is a specific cell-surface antigenic marker for oligodendrocytes in culture, *Nature (London)* **274:**813–816.

Raff, M. C., Brockes, J. P., Fields, K. L., and Mirsky, R., 1979*a*, Neural cell markers: The end of the beginning, *Prog. Brain Res.* **51:**17–22.

Raff, M. C., Fields, K. L., Hakomori, S., Mirsky, R., Pruss, R. M., and Winter, J., 1979*b*, Cell-type specific markers for distinguishing and studying neurons and the major classes of glial cells in culture, *Brain Res.* **174:**283–308.

Raff, M. C., Miller, R. H., and Noble, M., 1983, A glial progenitor cell that develops *in vitro* into an astrocyte or an oligodendrocyte depending on culture medium, *Nature (London)* **303:**390–396.

Raine, C. S., and Bornstein, M. B., 1974, Unusual profiles in organotypic cultures of central nervous tissue, *J. Neurocytol.* **3:**313–325.

Raine, C. S., and Bornstein, M. B., 1979, Experimental allergic neuritis: Ultrastructure of serum-induced myelin aberrations in peripheral nervous system culture, *Lab. Invest.* **40:**423–432.

Raine, C. S., Diaz, M., Pakingan, M., and Bornstein, M. B., 1978, Antiserum-induced dissociation of myelinogenesis *in vitro:* An ultrastructural study, *Lab. Invest.* **38:**397–403.

Raine, C. S., Johnson, A. B., Marcus, D. M., Suzuki, A., and Bornstein, M. B., 1981, Demyelination *in vitro:* Absorption studies demonstrate that galactocerebroside is a major target, *J. Neurol. Sci.* **52:**117–131.

Ranscht, B., Clapshaw, P. A., Price, J., Noble, M., and Siefert, W., 1982, The development of oligodendrocytes and Schwann cells studied with a monoclonal antibody against galactocerebroside, *Proc. Natl. Acad. Sci. U.S.A.* **79:**2709–2713.

Richter-Landsberg, C., and Yavin, E., 1979, Protein profiles of rat embryo cerebral cells during differentiation in culture, *J. Neurochem.* **32:**133–143.

Rioux, F., Derbin, C., Margules, S., Joubert, R., and Bisconte, J.-C., 1980, Kinetics of oligodendrocyte-like cells in primary culture of mouse embryonic brain, *Dev. Biol.* **76:**87–99.

Ross, L. L., and Bornstein, M. B., 1962, The application of tissue cultures to the study of experimental "allergic" encephalomyelitis. Part 3. Electron microscopic observations of demyelinization, in: *Proceedings of the 4th International Congress on Neuropathology,* Vol. 2, pp. 285–287, Georg Thieme, Stuttgart.

Roussel, G., Labourdette, G., Nussbaum, J. L., 1981, Characterization of oligodendrocytes in primary cultures from brain hemispheres of newborn rats, *Dev. Biol.* **81:**372–378.

Salzer, J. L., and Bunge, R. P., 1980, Studies of Schwann cell proliferation. I. An analysis in tissue culture of proliferation during development, *J. Cell Biol.* **84:**739–752.

Salzer, J. L., William, A. K., Glaser, L., and Bunge, R. P., 1980*a*, Studies of Schwann cell proliferation. II. Characterization of the stimulation and specificity of the response to a neurite membrane fraction, *J. Cell Biol.* **84:**767–778.

Salzer, J. L., Williams, A. K., Glaser, L., and Bunge, R. P., 1980*b*, Studies of Schwann cell proliferation. III. Characterization of the stimulation and specificity of the response to a neurite fraction, *J. Cell Biol.* **84:**753–766.

Sandru, L., Siegrist, H. P., Wiesmann, U. N., and Herschkowitz, N., 1980, Development of oligodendrocytes in jimpy brain cultures, in: *Neurological Mutations Affecting Myelination* (N. Baumann, ed.), INSERM Symposium No. 14, pp. 469–474, Elsevier/North-Holland, Amsterdam.

Sarlieve, L. L., Subba Rao, G., Campbell, G., and Pieringer, R. A., 1980*a*, Investigations on myelination *in vitro:* Biochemical and morphological changes in cultures of dissociated brain cells from embryonic mice, *Brain Res.* **189:**79–80.

Sarlieve, L. L., Fabre, M., Delaunoy, J. P., Pieringer, R. A., and Rebel, G., 1980*b*, Surface adhering primary cultures of dissociated brain cells from embryonic mice as a tool to study myelination *in vitro,* in: *Neurological Mutations Affecting Myelination* (N. Baumann, ed.), INSERM Symposium No. 14, pp. 489–499, Elsevier/North-Holland, Amsterdam.

Sarlieve, L. L., Delaunoy, J. P., Dierich, A., Ebel, A., Fabre, M., Mandel, P., Rebel, G., Vincendon, G., Wintzerith, M., and Yusufi, A. N. K., 1981, Investigations on myelination *in vitro.* III. Ultrastructural, biochemical, and immunohistochemical studies in cultures of dissociated brain cells from embryonic mice, *J. Neurosci. Res.* **6:**659–683.

Sato, G., 1975, The role of serum in cell culture, in: *Biochemical Actions of Hormones,* Vol. III (G. Litwack, ed.), pp. 391–396, Academic Press, New York.

Schachner, M., and Willinger, M., 1979, Cell type specific cell surface antigens in the cerebellum, *Prog. Brain Res.* **51:**23–44.

Schachner, M., Kim, S. K., and Zehnle, R., 1981, Developmental expression in central and peripheral nervous system of oligodendrocyte cell surface antigens (O antigens) recognized by monoclonal antibodies, *Dev. Biol.* **83:**328–338.

Schaper, A., 1897, The earliest differentiation in the central nervous system of vertebrates, *Science* **5:**430–431.

Schmechel, D., Marango, P. J., Brightman, M., and Goodwin, F., 1978, Brain enolases as specific markers of neuronal and glial cells, *Science* **199:**313–315.

Schmidt, G. L., 1975, Development of biochemical activities associated with myelination in chick brain aggregate cultures, *Brain Res.* **87:**110–113.

Schnitzer, J., and Schachner, M., 1982, Cell type specificity of a neural cell antigen recognized by the monoclonal antibody A2B5, *Cell Tissue Res.* **224:**625–636.

Schousboe, A., 1982, Metabolism and function of neurotransmitters, in: *Neuroscience Approached through Cell Culture,* Vol. I (S. E. Pfeiffer, ed.), pp. 107–141, CRC Press, Boca Raton, Florida (in press).

Seeds, N. W., 1971, Biochemical differentiation in reaggregating brain cell culture, *Proc. Natl. Acad. Sci. U.S.A.* **68:**1858–1861.

Seeds, N., 1973, Differentiation of aggregating brain cell cultures, in: *Tissue Culture of the Nervous System* (G. Sato, ed.), pp. 35–53, Plenum Press, New York.

Seeds, N. W., 1975, Expression of differentiated actvities in reaggregated brain cell cultures, *J. Biol. Chem.* **250:**5455–5458.

Seeds, N. W., and Gilman, A. G., 1971, Norepinephrine stimulated increase of cyclic AMP levels in developing mouse brain cell cultures, *Science* **174:**292.

Seeds, N. W., and Haffke, S. C., 1978, Cell junction and ultrastructural development of reaggregated mouse brain cultures, *Dev. Neurosci.* **1:**69–79.

Seeds, N. W., and Vatter, A. E., 1971, Synaptogenesis in reaggregating brain cell culture, *Proc. Natl. Acad. Sci. U.S.A.* **68:**3219–3222.

Seil, F. J., 1979, Cerebellum in tissue culture, in: *Reviews of Neuroscience,* Vol. 4 (D. M. Schnei-
    der, ed.), pp. 105–177, Raven Press, New York.
Seil, F., 1982, Demyelination, *Adv. Cell. Neurobiol.* **3:**235–274.
Seil, F. J., and Agrawal, H. C., 1980, Myelin-proteolipid protein does not induce demyelinating
    or myelination-inhibiting antibodies, *Brain Res.* **194:**273–277.
Seil, F. J., and Blank, N. K., 1981, Myelination of central nervous system axons in tissue culture
    by transplanted oligodendrocytes, *Science* **212:**1407–1408.
Seil, F., and Herndon, R. M., 1970, Cerebellar granule cells *in vitro:* A light and electron micro-
    scope study, *J. Cell Biol.* **45:**212–220.
Seil, F. J., Falk, G. A., Kies, M. W., and Alvord, E. C., Jr., 1968, The *in vitro* demyelinating
    activity of sera from guinea pigs sensitized with whole CNS and with purified encephalito-
    gen, *Exp. Neurol.* **22:**545–555.
Seil, F. J., Rauch, H. C., Einstein, E. R., and Hamilton, A. E., 1973, Myelination inhibition
    factor: Its absence in sera from subhuman primates sensitized with myelin basic protein, *J.
    Immunol.* **111:**96–100.
Seil, F. J., Smith, M. E., Leiman, A. L., and Kelly, J. M., 1975a, Myelination inhibiting and
    neuroelectric blocking factors in experimental allergic encephalomyelitis, *Science* **187:**951–
    953.
Seil, F. J., Kies, M. W., and Bacon, M., 1975b, Neural antigens and induction of myelination
    inhibition factor, *J. Immunol.* **114:**630–634.
Seil, F. J., Blank, N. K., and Leiman, A. L. 1979, Toxic effects of kainic acid on mouse cere-
    bellum *in vitro, Brain Res.* **161:**253–265.
Seil, F. J., Kies, M. W., Agrawal, H. C., Quarles, R. H., and Brady, R. O., 1980a, Myelin
    proteins dissociated from induction of antimyelin antibodies, in: *Tissue Culture in Neuro-
    biology* (E. Giacobini, A. Vernadakis, and A. Shahar, eds.), pp. 477–488, Raven Press, New
    York.
Seil, F. J., Leiman, A. L., and Woodward, W. R., 1980b, Cytosine arabinoside effects on devel-
    oping cerebellum in tissue culture, *Brain Res.* **186:**393–408.
Seil, F. J., Quarles, R. H., Johnson, D., and Brady, R. O., 1981, Immunization with purified
    myelin-associated glycoprotein does not evoke myelination-inhibiting or demyelinating anti-
    bodies, *Brain Res.* **209:**470–475.
Sensenbrenner, M., 1977, Dissociated brain cells in primary cultures, in: *Cell, Tissue, and Organ
    Cultures in Neurobiology* (S. Fedoroff and L. Hertz, eds.), pp. 191–213, Academic Press,
    New York.
Sensenbrenner, M., Booher, J., and Mandel, P., 1971, Cultivation and growth of dissociated
    neurons from chick embryo cerebral cortex in the presence of different substrates, *Z. Zell-
    forsch.* **117:**559–569.
Sensenbrenner, M., Springer, N., Booher, J., and Mandel, P., 1972, Histochemical studies during
    the differentiation of dissociated nerve cells cultivated in the presence of brain extracts, *Neu-
    robiology* **2:**49–60.
Sensenbrenner, M., Wittendorp, E., Barakat, I., and Rechenmann, R. V., 1980a, Autoradio-
    graphic study of proliferating brain cells in culture, *Dev. Biol.* **75:**268–277.
Sensenbrenner, M., Labourdette, G., Delaunoy, J. P., Pettman, B., Devilliers, G., Mooneu, G.,
    and Bock, E., 1980b, Morphological and biochemical differentiation of glial cells in primary
    cultures, in: *Tissue Culture in Neurobiology* (E. Giacobini, A. Vernadakis, and A. Shahar,
    eds.), pp. 385–395, Raven Press, New York.
Sensenbrenner, M., Barakat, I., Delaunoy, J. P., Labourdette, G., and Pettman, B., 1982, Influ-
    ence of brain extracts on nerve cell development, in: *Neuroscience Approached through Cell
    Culture,* Vol. I (S. E. Pfeiffer, ed.), pp. 85–105, CRC Press, Boca Raton, Florida.

Sheffield, W. D., and Kim, S. U., 1977, Basic protein radioimmunoassay as a monitor of myelin in tissue culture, *Brain Res.* **120**:193–196.

Sheppard, J. R., Brus, D., and Wehner, J. M., 1978, Brain reaggregate cultures: Biochemical evidence for myelin membrane synthesis, *J. Neurobiol.* **9**:309–315.

Sidman, R. L., 1970, Proliferation, migration and interaction in the developing mammalian central nervous system, in: *The Neurosciences Second Study Program* (F. O. Schmitt, ed.), pp. 100–107, Rockefeller University Press, New York.

Sidman, R. L., Dickie, M. M., and Appel, S. H., 1964, Mutant mice (quaking and jimpy) with deficient myelination in the central nervous system, *Science* **144**:309–311.

Sidman, R. L., Green, M. G., and Appel, S. H., 1965, *Catalog of the Neurological Mutants of the Mouse,* Harvard University Press, Cambridge.

Siegrist, H. P., Burkart, T., Hofmann, K., Wiesmann, U., and Herschkowitz, N. N., 1980, Theophylline reduces the activity of cerebroside-sulfotransferase, a key enzyme in myelination, in cell cultures from newborn mouse brain, *Pediatr. Res.* **14**:1226–1229.

Siegrist, H. P., Bologa-Sandru, L., Burkart, T., Wiesmann, U., Hofmann, K., and Herschkowitz, N., 1981, Synthesis of lipids in mouse brain cell cultures during development, *J. Neurosci. Res.* **6**:293–301.

Silberberg, D. H., 1975, Scanning electron microscopy of organotypic rat cerebellum cultures, *J. Neuropathol. Exp. Neurol.* **34**:189–199.

Silberberg, D. H., Benjamins, J., Herschkowitz, N., and McKhann, G. M., 1972, Incorporation of radioactive sulphate into sulphatide during myelination on cultures of rat cerebellum, *J. Neurochem.* **19**:11–18.

Silberberg, D. H., Dorfman, S. H., Latovitzki, N., and Younkin, L. H., 1980, Oligodendrocyte differentiation in myelinating cultures, in: *Tissue Culture in Neurobiology* (E. Giacobini, A. Vernadakis, and A. Shahar, eds.), pp. 489–500, Raven Press, New York.

Singh, H., and Pfeiffer, S. E., 1983, Expression of galactolipids by mixed primary cultures from rat brain, *Trans. Am. Soc. Neurochem.* **14**:218.

Skoff, R. P., Price, D. L., and Stocks, A., 1976a, Electron microscopic autoradiographic studies of gliogenesis in rat optic nerve. I. Cell proliferation, *J. Comp. Neurol.* **169**:291–312.

Skoff, R. P., Price, D. L., and Stocks, A., 1976b, Electron microscopic autoradiographic studies of gliogenesis in rat optic nerve. II. Time of origin, *J. Comp. Neurol.* **169**:313–333.

Snyder, D. S., Raine, C. S., Farooq, M., and Norton, W. T., 1980, The bulk isolation of oligodendroglia from whole rat forebrain: A new procedure using physiologic media, *J. Neurochem.* **34**:1614–1621.

Sommer, I., and Schachner, M., 1981, Monoclonal antibodies (O1 to O4) to oligodendrocyte cell surfaces: An immunocytological study in the central nervous system, *Dev. Biol.* **83**:311–327.

Sprinkle, T. J., Wells, M. R., Garver, F. A., and Smith, D. B., 1980, Studies on the Wolfgram high molecular weight CNS myelin proteins: Relationship to 2′,3′-cyclic nucleotide 3′-phosphohydrolase, *J. Neurochem.* **35**:1200–1208.

Steck, A., and Perruisseau, G., 1980, Characterization of membranes of isolated oligodendrocytes and clonal lines of the nervous system, *J. Neurol. Sci.* **47**:135–144.

Stefanelli, A., Cataldi, E., and Ieradi, L. A., 1977, Specific synaptic systems in reaggregated spherules from dissociated chick cerebellum cultivated *in vitro, Cell Tissue Res.* **182**:311–325.

Steinberg, M. S., 1963, Reconstruction of tissues by dissociated cells, *Science* **141**:401–408.

Sternberger, N. H., Itoyama, Y., Kies, M. W., and Webster, H. de F., 1978a, Immunocytochemical method to identify basic protein in myelin-forming oligodendrocytes of newborn rat C.N.S., *J. Neurocytol.* **7**:251–263.

Sternberger, N. H., Itoyama, Y., Kies, M., and Webster, H. de F., 1978*b*, Myelin basic protein demonstrated immunocytochemically in oligodendroglia prior to myelin sheath formation, *Proc. Natl. Acad. Sci. U.S.A.* **75:**2521–2524.

Storts, R. W., and A. Koestner, 1969, Development and characterization of myelin in tissue culture of canine cerebellum, *Z. Zellforsch.* **95:**9–18.

Sturrock, R. R., 1981, Electron microscopic evidence for mitotic division of oligodendrocytes, *J. Anat.* **132:**429–432.

Sturrock, R. R., 1982, Cell division in the normal central nervous system, *Adv. Cell. Neurobiol.* **3:**3–33.

Sturrock, R. R., and McRae, D. A.,1980, Mitotic division of oligodendrocytes which have begun myelination, *J. Anat.* **131:**579–584.

Sundarraj, N., Schachner, M., and Pfeiffer, S. E., 1975, Biochemically differentiated mouse glial lines carrying a nervous system specific cell surface antigen (NS-1), *Proc. Natl. Acad. Sci. U.S.A.* **72:**1927–1931.

Szuchet, S., and Stefansson, K., 1980, *In vitro* behavior of isolated oligodendrocytes, in: *Advances in Cellular Neurobiology* (S. Fedoroff and L. Hertz, eds.), pp. 313–346, Academic Press, New York.

Szuchet, S., Stefansson, K., Wollman, R. L., Dawson, G., and Arnason, B. G., 1980, Maintenance of isolated oligodendrocytes in long-term culture, *Brain Res.* **200:**151–164.

Towbin, H., Staehelin, T., and Gordon, J., 1979, Electrophoretic transfer of proteins from polyacrylamide gels to nitrocellulose sheets: Procedure and some applications, *Proc. Natl. Acad. Sci. U.S.A.* **76:**4350–4354.

Trapp, B. D., Honegger, P., Richelson, E., and Webster, H. de F., 1978, Effects of vitamin E on the fine structure of aggregating cell cultures, *Anat. Rec.* **190:**564.

Trapp, B. D., Honegger, P., Richelson, E., and Webster, H. de F., 1979, Morphological differentiation of mechanically dissociated fetal rat brain in aggregating cell cultures, *Brain Res.* **160:**117–130.

Traugott, U., Snyder, S., and Raine, C. S., 1979, Oligodendrocyte staining by multiple sclerosis serum is nonspecific, *Ann. Neurol.* **6:**13–20.

Van Heyningen, W. E., 1963, The fixation of tetanus toxin, strychnine, serotonin and other substances by ganglioside, *J. Gen. Microbiol.* **31:**375–387.

Varon, S., 1970, *In vitro* study of developing neural tissue and cells: Past and prospective contributions, in: *The Neurosciences* (F. O. Schmidt, ed.), pp. 83–99, Rockefeller University Press, New York.

Varon, S., and Bunge, R. P., 1978, Tropic mechanisms in the peripheral nervous system, *Annu. Rev. Neurosci.* **1:**327–361.

Varon, S., and Manthorpe, M., 1982, Schwann cells: An *in vitro* perspective, *Adv. Cell. Neurobiol.* **3:**35–95.

Varon, S., and Raiborn, C. W., Jr., 1969, Dissociation, fractionation, and culture of embryonic brain cells, *Brain Res.* **12:**180–199.

Vaughn, J. E., 1969, An electron microscopic analysis of gliogenesis in rat optic nerves, *Z. Zellforsch.* **94:**293–324.

Waehneldt, T. V., and Malotka, J., 1980, Comparative electrophoretic study of the Wolfgram proteins in myelin from several Mammalia, *Brain Res.* **189:**582–587.

Webster, H. de F., 1975, Development of peripheral myelinated and unmyelinated nerve fibers, in: *Peripheral Neuropathy* (P. J. Dyck, P. K. Thomas, and E. H. Lambert, eds.), pp. 37–61, W. B. Saunders, Philadelphia.

Weinberg, H. J., and Spencer, P. S., 1975, Studies on the control of myelinogenesis. I. Myelination of regenerating axons after entry into a foreign unmyelinated nerve, *J. Neurocytol.* **4:**395–418.

Weinberg, H. J., and Spencer, P. S., 1976, Studies on the control of myelinogenesis. II. Evidence for neuronal regulation of myelin production, *Brain Res.* 113:363–378.

Weinberg, E. L. [*sic*], and Spencer, P. S., 1979, Studies on the control of myelinogenesis. 3. Signalling of oligodendrocyte myelination by regenerating peripheral axons, *Brain Res.* 162:273–279.

Werner, I., Peterson, G. R., and Shuster, L., 1971, Choline acetyltransferase and acetylcholinesterase in cultured brain cells from chick embryos, *J. Neurochem.* 18:141–151.

Weston, J. A., 1963, A radioautographic analysis of the migration and localization of trunk neural crest cells in the chick, *Dev. Biol.* 6:279–310.

Wiesmann, U. N., Hofmann, K., Burkart, T., and Herschkowitz, N., 1975, Dissociated cultures of newborn mouse brain. I. Metabolism of sulfated lipids and mucopolysaccharides, *Neurobiology* 5:305–315.

Wiesmann, U. N., Burkart, T., Hofmann, K., Siegrist, H.-P., and Herschkowitz, N., 1979, Biochemical alterations of sulfatide metabolism in jimpy brain cell culture, in: *Models for the Study of Inborn Errors of Metabolism* (F. A. Hommes, ed.), pp. 279–280, Elsevier/North-Holland, Amsterdam.

Wiesmann, U. N., Hofmann, K., Burkart, T., Siegrist, H.-P., Sandru, L., Omlin, F. X., and Herschkowitz, N., 1980, Tissue culture models for the study of the jimpy mutant, in: *Neurological Mutants Affecting Myelination: Research Tools in Neurobiology,* INSERM Symposium, No. 14, pp. 461–468, Elsevier, Amsterdam.

Wiggins, R. C., Joffe, S., Davidson, D., and Del Valle, U., 1974, Characterization of Wolfgram proteolipid protein of bovine white matter and fractionation of molecular weight heterogeneity, *J. Neurochem.* 22:171–175.

Windle, W. F., 1958, *Biology of Neuroglia,* Charles C. Thomas, Springfield, Illinois.

Wolf, M. K., 1964, Differentiation of neuronal types and synapses in myelinating cultures of mouse cerebellum, *J. Cell Biol.* 22:259–279.

Wolf, M., 1970, Anatomy of mouse cerebellum. II. Organotypic migration of granule cells demonstrated by silver impregnation of normal and mutant cultures, *J. Comp. Neurol.* 140:281–297.

Wolf, M. K., 1974, Problems in culture analysis of neurological mutant disorders, in: *Methodological Approaches to the Study of Brain Maturation and Its Abnormalities* (D. P. Purpura and G. P. Reaser, eds.), pp. 29–32, University Park Press, Baltimore.

Wolf, M. K., 1977, Cell and organotypic culture studies of neurological mutations affecting structural development, in: *Cell, Tissue, and Organ Cultures in Neurobiology* (S. Fedoroff and L. Hertz, eds.), pp. 555–572, Academic Press, New York.

Wolf, M. K., and Billings-Gagliardi, S., 1983, A tissue culture strategy for studying mutant mice with CNS hypomyelination, in: *Neuroscience Approached through Cell Culture,* Vol. II (S. E. Pfeiffer, ed.), pp. 141–154, CRC Press, Boca Raton, Florida.

Wolf, M. K., and Holden, A. B., 1969, Tissue culture analysis of the inherited defect of central nervous system myelination in jimpy mice, *J. Neuropathol. Exp. Neurol.* 28:195–204.

Wolf, M. K., Schwing, G. B., Adcock, L. H., and Billings-Gagliardi, S., 1981, Hypomyelinated mutant mice. III. Increased myelination in mutant cerebellum co-cultured with normal optic nerve, *Brain Res.* 206:193–197.

Wolfgram, F., 1966, A new proteolipid fraction of the nervous system. I. Isolation and amino acid analyses, *J. Neurochem.* 13:461–470.

Wolfgram, F., and Rose, A. S., 1957, The morphology of neuroglia in tissue culture with comparison to histological preparations, *J. Neuropathol. Exp. Neurol.* 16:514–531.

Wollman, R. L., Szuchet, S., Barlow, J., and Jerkovic, M., 1981, Ultrastructural changes accompanying the growth of isolated oligodendrocytes, *J. Neurosci. Res.* 6:757–769.

Wood, P. M., 1976, Separation of functional Schwann cells and neurons from normal peripheral nerve tissue, *Brain Res.* **115**:361–375.

Wood, P. M., and Bunge, R. P., 1975, Evidence that sensory axons are mitogenic for Schwann cells, *Nature (London)* **256**:662–664.

Wood, P. M., Okada, E., and Bunge, R., 1980, The use of networks of disassociated rat dorsal root ganglion neurons to induce myelination by oligodendrocytes in culture, *Brain Res.* **196**:247–252.

Wood, P., Szuchet, S., Williams, A. K., Bunge, R. P., and Arnason, B. G. W., 1983, CNS myelin formation in cocultures of rat neurons and lamb oligodendrocytes, *Trans. Am. Soc. Neurochem.* **14**:212.

Yavin, E., and Menkes, J. H., 1973, The culture of dissociated cells from rat cerebral cortex, *J. Cell Biol.* **57**:232–237.

Yavin, E., and Yavin, Z., 1974, Attachment and culture of dissociated cells from rat embryo cerebral hemispheres on polylysine-coated surface, *J. Cell Biol.* **62**:540–546.

Yavin, E., and Yavin, E., 1977, Synaptogenesis and myelinogenesis in dissociated cerebral cells from rat embryo on polylysine coated surfaces, *Exp. Brain Res.* **29**:137–147.

Yonezawa, T., and Iwanami, H., 1966, An experimental study of thiamine deficiency in nervous tissue using culture techniques, *J. Neuropathol. Exp. Neurol.* **25**:362–372.

Yonezawa, T., Bornstein, M., Peterson, E., and Murray, M., 1962a, A histochemical study of oxidative enzymes in myelinating cultures of central and peripheral nervous tissue, *J. Neuropathol. Exp. Neurol.* **21**:479–487.

Yonezawa, T., Bornstein, M. B., Peterson, E. R., and Murray, M. R., 1962b, Temporal and spatial distribution of oxidative enzymes during myelin formation and maintenance, in: *Proceedings of the 4th International Congress on Neuropathology,* Vol. II, pp. 273–274, Georg Thieme, Stuttgart.

Yonezawa, T., Saida, T., and Hasagawa, M., 1976, Myelination inhibiting factor in experimental allergic encephalomyelitis and demyelinating diseases, in: *The Aetiology and Pathogenesis of the Demyelinating Diseases* (H. Shikari, T. Yonezawa, and Y. Kuriowa, eds.), pp. 255–263, Japan Science Press, Tokyo.

Younkin, L., and Silberberg, D. H., 1973, Myelination in developing cultured newborn rat cerebellum inhibited by 5-bromodeoxyuridine, *Exp. Cell Res.* **76**:455–458.

Younkin, L. H., and Silberberg, D. H., 1976, Delay of oligodendrocyte differentiation by 5-bromodeoxyuridine (BudR), *Brain Res.* **101**:600–605.

REGULATION OF DIFFERENTIATED PROPERTIES OF OLIGODENDROCYTES

DANIEL P. WEINGARTEN,
SHALINI KUMAR, JOSEPH BRESSLER, and
JEAN DE VELLIS

1. INTRODUCTION

How a given eukaryotic cell achieves its ultimate differentiated state from primitive embryonic origins and how the expression of specific gene products is regulated are two of the fundamental and, as yet, unresolved issues in biology. Despite extraordinary advances in our knowledge of primary nucleotide

DANIEL P. WEINGARTEN • Life Technologies Incorporated, Chagrin Falls, Ohio 44022   SHALINI KUMAR and JEAN DE VELLIS • Laboratory of Biomedical and Environmental Sciences, Mental Retardation Research Center, and the Departments of Anatomy and Psychiatry, University of California, Los Angeles, School of Medicine, Los Angeles, California 90024   JOSEPH BRESSLER • Surgical Neurology Branch, National Institutes of Health, Bethesda, Maryland 20205 sequences and genomic organization, we cannot at present predict or explain the various patterns of gene expression from one cell type to another. Most research in this area has been confined to the study of highly specialized systems in which large amounts of a particular protein are made (Shapiro, 1982). In brain, the search for specific, identifiable proteins has largely concentrated on neuronal elements. However, in the past decade, glial physiology has gained a more prominent role in neurobiology. An appreciation of how certain genes are regulated in the oligodendrocyte has become increasingly important to our understanding of the role these proteins play in a number of normal and pathological processes in the CNS. Of particular interest is the myelin-forming function of the oligodendrocyte in health and disease. The genotypic and phenotypic alterations that occur during glial neoplasia can be interpreted with respect to changes in these differentiated oligodendrocyte properties. That oligodendrocytes are now recognized as capable of secreting soluble protein factors that influence the morphology and physiology of neuronal elements underscores an even greater need to know whether and how these factors are themselves subject to regulatory signals (Arenander and de Vellis, 1982). Finally, the temporal patterns of the expression of these proteins from embryonic development onward will aid in the tracing of oligodendrocyte-cell lineages.

A detailed, unambiguous analysis of these regulated processes in the oligodendrocyte is now emerging, thanks to several recent developments. First, a method has been devised that permits the preparation from the same brain tissue of separate cultures of oligodendrocytes and astrocytes (McCarthy and de Vellis, 1980). Second, the successful identification of markers specific to the oligodendrocyte has helped to direct neurobiologists' research interests (see Chapter 4). Third, the use of model glial tumor cell lines, such as C6, has made a great contribution to our understanding of the detailed molecular mechanisms that underlie the regulation of differentiated oligodendrocyte marker proteins. It is noteworthy that C6 glial cells exhibit a number of features of myelin-producing glia such as 2′,3′-cyclic nucleotide 3′-phosphohydrolase, a proteolipid protein, and two basic proteins that are identical in their electrophoretic mobilities with the respective proteins found in myelin (Volpe *et al.,* 1975).

The great majority of regulatory agents of oligodendrocyte markers fall in the category of the classic hormones such as steroids and cyclic AMP (cAMP), the second messenger of many hormones. However, it is now apparent that oligodendrocytes and their neuronal neighbors additionally influence each other's morphological and biochemical differentiation via cell–cell interactions mediated through actual contact or by the release of bioactive soluble molecules. This review will attempt to summarize the most significant findings with respect to factors that control oligodendrocyte proteins, both those that are unique to oligodendrocytes and those that they share with other CNS cell types.

2. REGULATORY AGENTS

2.1. Steroid Hormones

Steroid hormones, particularly the glucocorticoids and sex hormones, are known to have profound influences on the development and differentiation of the brain (Gorski, 1971; McEwen *et al.,* 1971). Many of these hormones, after being radiolabeled, can be recovered in brain following injection into blood and show a specific, regional pattern of uptake with both nuclear and cytoplasmic binding sites (McEwen *et al.,* 1971). In a number of tissues, these hormones influence the rate of production of a variety of proteins; one manner by which this is accomplished is succinctly summarized as follows: All steroid hormones appear to diffuse passively into cells and bind to a limited number of high-affinity cytoplasmic receptors; such binding initiates an apparent conformational change in the receptor that permits it to translocate into the nucleus, where it interacts with certain (as yet unspecified) chromatin acceptor sites and in this manner stimulates the increased production of specific messenger RNAs (mRNAs) (Yamamoto and Alberts, 1976). The specific proteins subsequently produced vary from tissue to tissue.

2.1.1. α-Glycerol Phosphate Dehydrogenase

In brain, in primary oligodendrocyte cultures, and in C6 glioma cells, the activity of the cytoplasmic enzyme α-glycerol phosphate dehydrogenase (GPDH) is regulated by physiological concentrations of hydrocortisone (HC) (McCarthy and de Vellis, 1980; de Vellis and Inglish, 1968, 1969). GPDH was the first protein to be identified as steroid-inducible in brain. Like most inducible enzymes in mammalian cells, GPDH has a basal level of activity (de Vellis, 1973). Although it is high in C6 cells, it varies considerably in C6 subclones and hybrids; however, its activity is low in primary culture (de Vellis *et al.,* 1977) because of the heterogeneity of cell types in these cultures. However, pure oligodendrocyte cultures possess high basal and induced levels (McCarthy and de Vellis, 1980). The basal and induced levels appear to be regulated independently, since inducibility does not relate to basal levels of the enzyme. This enzyme in adult rat brain has been localized to rat oligodendrocytes as shown by immunoperoxidase staining at the light-microscopic (LM) and electron-microscopic (EM) levels (Meyer *et al.,* 1982; Leveille *et al.,* 1980); its regulation by HC marks these cells as targets for glucocorticoid hormones both *in vitro* and *in vivo.* Inhibitor studies have demonstrated that this induction requires RNA and protein synthesis in C6 cells (de Vellis, 1973; de Vellis and Brooker, 1973; de Vellis *et al.,* 1971) as well as in explant and dissociated cultures (Breen and de Vellis, 1974, 1975). By virtue of the characteristics of their GPDH induction, C6 clonal cells, explant, dissociated, and reaggregated cultures are all appropriate models to study induction mechanisms that occur *in vivo* (de Vellis *et al.,* 1977). Use of monospecific rabbit antisera to GPDH has shown that the HC induction of GPDH activity in C6 cells is due to an increase in the number of GPDH molecules that results from an increase in the rate of synthesis of new enzyme molecules (McGinnis and de Vellis, 1978). This HC induction of GPDH appears to be mediated by the classic steroid-receptor complex interacting with chromatin acceptor sites (O'Malley *et al.,* 1972; Baxter *et al.,* 1972), since cytochalasin B inhibits the HC-mediated increases in GPDH activity and synthesis by interfering with a critical step in the induction process, namely, nuclear binding of HC (Bennett *et al.,* 1977). Furthermore, C6 cytosol receptor concentration and binding of the hormone–receptor complex in the cell nucleus correlate well with GPDH inducibility (de Vellis *et al.,* 1974).

While catecholamines (or dibutyryl AMP) do not by themselves induce GPDH, in combination with HC, the rate of synthesis of GPDH is enhanced 2-fold (Breen *et al.,* 1978). This increase begins after a lag of approximately 5 hr and appears to be mediated by cAMP at the transcriptional level. The exact mechanism by which this interaction occurs has yet to be elucidated.

In the developing rat brain, the GPDH level coincides with myelination, rising rapidly between 10 and 30 days (de Vellis *et al.,* 1967); injection of HC in rat pups in the 2nd postnatal week (when the pituitary–adrenal axis has not yet matured) results in the precocious appearance of GPDH (de Vellis and Inglish, 1973). A similar developmental increase in GPDH inducibility with age of cultures from 20-day rat fetuses has been shown in both dissociated cells and explants (Breen and de Vellis, 1975), thus further validating their use as models for developmental studies. GPDH inducibility in C6 likewise increases with age in culture until confluency (Davidson and Benda, 1970; de Vellis and Inglish, 1973), but declines thereafter. These effects appear to be the result of changes in receptor concentration and nuclear binding of the hormone with time in culture (de Vellis *et al.,* 1974). The starting age of primary cultures from rat cerebral cortex also shows a developmental profile for GPDH inducibility (McCarthy and de Vellis, 1977); cultures from prenatal pups show less inducibility than cultures from postnatal pups. C6 is not the only glial cell line that exhibits GPDH inducibility; it has been discovered in others as well (West *et al.,* 1977; Claisse and Roscoe, 1976). Recent studies from our laboratory (Kumar, Weingarten, and de Vellis, unpublished observations) demonstrate that the HC-mediated induction of new GPDH molecules in C6 cells is the result of an increase in the functional GPDH mRNA as determined in a reticulocyte lysate cell-free translation assay. Whether the same is true for this induction in oligodendrocytes awaits corroboration. Nevertheless, it appears that glial cells, in particular oligodendrocytes, respond to glucocorticoid hormones at the transcriptional level in a manner reminiscent of other hormone-induction systems. The induction by HC of GPDH has also recently been observed in rat optic nerve (Meyer *et al.,* 1982) in morphologically identified oligodendrocytes. As before, this induction can be accounted for by the presence of an increased number of enzyme molecules.

In the classic model of steroid hormone action, the precise nature of the nuclear chromatin "acceptor" sites for the cytoplasmic steroid–receptor complex is inadequately known (Yamamoto and Alberts, 1976). With respect to this interaction in glial target cells, our understanding has been deepened by the use of sodium butyrate (NaB). This naturally occurring short-chain fatty acid blocks the HC-mediated induction of GPDH in C6 cells and primary glial cultures (Weingarten and de Vellis, 1980). This inhibition is not the result of nonspecific cellular toxicity or enzyme inactivation, is not due to an effect on cytoplasmic receptors or nuclear steroid accumulation, and is not the result of changes in the sedimentation properties of either form of the receptor on sucrose gradients. This effect is specific, since the norepinephrine induction of lactate dehydrogenase (LDH) was unaffected by the presence of NaB. Furthermore, this inhibition is completely and rapidly reversed with the removal of NaB from the culture medium. Additional studies (Weingarten *et al.,* 1981) demonstrated that the absence of an increase in GPDH specific activity is the result of a complete blockade in the induced rate of synthesis of GPDH molecules, suggesting an inhibition in the production of functional GPDH mRNA. To test this possibility, we have extracted total mRNA from C6 cells under various experimental treatments, and utilizing this RNA in a cell-free translation system, we have seen that NaB does indeed inhibit the production of functional GPDH mRNA (Weingarten and co-workers, unpublished observations). Currently, experiments are under way to obtain a complementary DNA (cDNA) to GPDH mRNA in order to quantitate directly the amount and locus of this inhibitory action. A plausible explanation of this inhibition arises from an understanding of how NaB might interfere with the access of the steroid–receptor complex to those critical chromatin-binding sites necessary to the GPDH induction process. In a wide variety of vertebrate cell lines, NaB, as well as other short-chain fatty acids, produces a hyperacetylation of histone proteins by a rapid, reversible inhibition of nuclear deacetylase enzymes (Sealy and Chalkley, 1978). This chromatin structural change may conceivably underlie the ineffectiveness of HC in the presence of NaB. That this is a plausible hypothesis is suggested by the fact that these other short-chain fatty acids also inhibit GPDH induction and, further, that the extent of histone hyperacetylation produced by any given fatty acid correlates closely with the extent of its particular inhibition of HC-mediated GPDH induction (Weingarten, unpublished observations).

2.1.2. Glutamine Synthetase

Glutamine synthetase (GS) catalyzes the synthesis of L-glutamine from L-glutamate, ATP, and ammonia and is widely distributed in mammalian tissues (Lund, 1970; Wu, 1963). Its product, glutamine, not only is a necessary amino acid in protein synthesis but also serves as the principal nitrogen source in numerous biosynthetic pathways (Stadtman, 1973). Other more specific CNS functions postulated for GS include ammonia detoxification (Sadasividu *et al.,* 1977) and metabolism of the putative neurotransmitters γ-aminobutyric acid and glutamate (Kemel *et al.,* 1979; Reubi *et al.,* 1978; Tapia and Gonzales, 1978). To date, the most thoroughly studied system of GS hormonal regulation is the induction by HC of GS in the chick neural retina (A. A. Moscona, 1975). This induction is considered a convenient biochemical marker of differentiation and specialization of retinal glial cells (Linser and Moscona, 1981) and is the result of an increase in newly synthesized GS mRNA (Soh and Sarkar, 1978) with a concomitant increase in the rate of enzyme synthesis (M. Moscona *et al.,* 1972).

In brain, LM examination of immunocytochemical GS staining suggests a predominantly glial localization (Martinez-Hernandez *et al.,* 1977). Immunocytochemical studies at the EM level suggest that GS is localized in astrocytes (Norenberg and Martinez-Hernandez, 1979), while in primary astrocyte cultures, HC induces GS (Juurlinck *et al.,* 1981). Nevertheless, the discovery that in C6 cells GS is also inducible by HC (Pishak and Phillips, 1980) prompts us to include GS regulation in this chapter, since C6 cells appear to have both oligodendrocytelike and astrocytelike differentiated properties (Parker *et al.,* 1980; Volpe *et al.,* 1975; Bissell *et al.,* 1974; Zanetta *et al.,* 1972; Benda *et al.,* 1971). Furthermore, using our purified oligodendrocyte- and astrocyte-cell culture systems, this laboratory has discovered significant basal and HC-inducible GS specific activity in both oligodendrocytes and astrocytes (de Vellis, unpublished observations). However, caution must be exercised here, since we have yet to rule out astrocyte contamination or the possibility that a small subpopulation of oligodendrocytes possessing GS are merely selected for by our culture conditions. Because of this potential discrepancy with previously published material on GS localization in the CNS (Norenberg and Martinez-Hernandez, 1979), we are currently pursuing additional immunocytochemical evidence *in vivo* and *in vitro* to resolve this issue.

In C6 cells, another inducer of GS specific activity has been recently documented, namely, NaB in millimolar concentrations (Weingarten *et al.,* 1981).

Like HC, this induction requires RNA and protein synthesis. Unlike HC, NaB operates through at least a partially separate mechanism, since the antigluco-corticoid progesterone is ineffective in blocking this induction. Further, in combination with HC, NaB yields an additive response. In addition, histone hyper-acetylation once again appears to be a promising candidate as the underlying mechanism of this induction. The increase in the amount of histone hypera-cetylation in C6 cells correlates well with the increase in C6 GS specific activity (Weingarten, unpublished observations). This work on NaB has now been extended to primary glial cultures as well. Preliminary observations show that NaB strongly decreases basal GS level in both oligodendrocytes and astrocytes, a result strikingly different from the case with C6 cells. Whether GS induci-bility by NaB is a consequence of the transformation process awaits further study. The existence of multiple inducers for the same enzyme (GS in this case) makes the C6 cell system an attractive one to molecular neurobiologists seeking to dissect out in greater detail the mechanisms of enzyme induction in mammalian cells, in general, and in glial cells, in particular.

2.1.3. Sulfotransferase

This enzyme catalyzes the production of sulfogalactosylceramide (sulfa-tide), a compound that may be an important functional component of the mye-lin sheath (Dawson and Kearns, 1978); therefore, hormonal regulation in this case could have a potentially significant role in the initiation of myelination. In the mouse glioblastoma cell lines G26-20 and G26-24, which Dawson and Kearns (1978) claim are of presumptive oligodendroglial origin, physiological doses of HC cause a 3- to 6-fold increase in the activity of 3'-phosphoadeno-sine 5'-phosphosulfate:galactosylceramide sulfotransferase (sulfotransferase), apparently by a translational mechanism. This sulfotransferase induction is specific to glucocorticoids among the steroid hormones. The potential impor-tance of this enzyme is suggested by the elegant work of Tennekoon *et al.* (1977) on developing rat optic nerve in which its maximal activity correlates with oligodendrocyte differentiation and the period of most active myelination. The enzyme can also be found in bulk-prepared oligodendrocytes (Pleasure *et al.*, 1977). In dissociated mouse brain-cell cultures, the developmental pattern of this sulfotransferase is correlated with the number of galactocerebroside (GalCer)-positive oligodendrocytes (Herschkowitz *et al.*, 1982). GalCer, the major glycolipid in myelin, has been established as a cell-surface marker for cultured oligodendrocytes (Raff *et al.*, 1978). In these same cultures (Hersch-kowitz *et al.*, 1982), the developmental pattern of 2',3'-cyclic nucleotide 3'-phosphohydrolase (CNP) activity and the number of myelin-basic-protein-pos-itive oligodendrocytes were also positively correlated. A pertinent recent result with HC in dissociated embryonic mouse cerebral cultures, grown in surface-adhering, reaggregating primary cultures using a completely defined medium, reveals a dose-dependent increase in sulfolipid synthesis and CNP activity (Stephens and Pieringer, 1981). Taken together, these results indicate that the detailed molecular mechanisms that regulate this enzyme should now be further studied in clonal and primary (nontransformed) cultures to determine the role of the enzyme in the initiation and maintenance of myelination. Combined with techniques in which myelination can be studied *in vitro* (Sarlieve *et al.,* 1980; Matthieu *et al.,* 1978, 1979; Sheppard *et al.,* 1978), future studies can be directed to the hormonal regulation of myelination vis-à-vis specific biochemical markers.

See Chapters 2, 5, and 7 for further discussion of the sulfotransferase.

2.1.4. Nerve Growth Factor

Nerve growth factor (NGF) is a peptide hormone that is recognized as necessary for the development and survival of sympathetic neurons (Levi-Montalcini, 1976). The discovery that 17β-estradiol causes both increased *de novo* NGF synthesis (requiring RNA synthesis) and release of NGF in C6 glioma cells (Perez-Polo *et al.,* 1977) is exciting in light of the fact that this clonal cell line possesses a number of differentiated glial properties. These authors suggest that this steroid induction of a peptide hormone important to neural development could provide neurobiologists with a formidable model system for the study of the hormonal regulation of neuronal development and, further, that this clonal model system can provide clues to the *in vivo* regulatory mechanisms.

2.2. Cyclic Nucleotides

Cyclic 3',5'-adenosine monophosphate (cAMP) is the classic example of this group of hormones. Cyclic AMP, its analogues such as dibutyryl cAMP, and agents that alter its intracellular levels have long been known to exert profound influences on the biochemistry and morphology of nerve tissue (for reviews, see Prasad, 1977; J. P. Schwartz *et al.,* 1973). It acts as a second messenger after the primary hormone has interacted with cell-surface receptors. The intracellular level of cAMP is increased by agents that stimulate membrane adenylate cyclase. This intracellular cAMP then stimulates protein kinase(s) that subsequently phosphorylate certain cell proteins. It is these phosphorylated products that presumably alter cellular functions, among them various aspects of gene expression. There is strong evidence that this basic scheme is, on the whole, consistent with research findings on cAMP effects in oligodendrocytes. Since a wide variety of agents can influence cyclic nucleotide levels, research in this area has the added significance of providing the information needed to understand how these levels could eventually be manipulated pharmacologically for clinical purposes.

C6 cells contain all the known components of the cAMP-generating system (Jard *et al.*, 1972; Terasaki *et al.*, 1978), in which the initial event occurs with agonist binding to a β-adrenergic receptor (Gilman and Nirenberg, 1971). These cells respond to norepinephrine, a β-adrenergic agonist, with the activation of adenylate cyclase and the concomitant elevation of intracellular cAMP (Gilman and Nirenberg, 1971). Removal of the norepinephrine results in cAMP levels decreasing rapidly, reaching basal levels within minutes (Schultz *et al.*, 1972). Continued application of the β-adrenergic agonist causes a peak of cAMP within 20 min followed by a 90% decline over the next 2 hr (de Vellis and Brooker, 1974). At this point, the cells are refractory and unable to mount a second response to a subsequent agonist challenge. This "refractoriness" phenomenon is common to many cell types and was first described by Kakiuchi and Rall (1968). In the C6-2B subclone, this refractoriness appears to depend on RNA and protein synthesis (de Vellis and Brooker, 1974). Primary glial-cell cultures respond with increased cAMP accumulation to a variety of agents such as β-adrenergic agonists, adenosine, and prostaglandin E_1 (McCarthy and de Vellis, 1979).

α-Receptor activation simultaneous with β-receptor activation substantially lowers the β-activation of cAMP in both C6 and primary glial cultures (McCarthy and de Vellis, 1978). The mechanism that underlies this α-adrenergic modulation of β-responsiveness is unknown. Utilizing pure, separate oligodendrocyte and astrocyte populations, McCarthy and de Vellis (1980) were able to show that both cell types can accumulate cAMP via membrane receptors, but that the nature and magnitude of response varied with a given pharmacological agent. Developmentally, the magnitude of the cAMP increase to either norepinephrine, adenosine, or prostaglandin E_1 increases as a function of the age of the donor tissue for primary glial cultures (McCarthy and de Vellis, 1977); this may, as these authors suggest, reflect a maturation of the glial receptor-linked adenylate cyclase system. In summary, glial-cell cultures (normal or transformed) can accumulate cAMP in response to a number of chemical agents.

2.2.1. *Lactate Dehydrogenase*

LDH is a constitutive cytoplasmic enzyme of all cells that catalyzes the reversible dehydrogenation of lactate to pyruvate in an NAD^+-dependent reaction. LDH is composed of five isoenzymes, each of which is formed by the tetrameric association of two subunits referred to as M and H, their relative distribution being tissue-specific (Venkov *et al.*, 1976). LDH permits cells to maintain anaerobic glycolysis, thus ensuring production of metabolic energy under anoxic conditions; hence, this may explain how the brain endures anoxia and, in particular, how the brains of newborns show greater tolerance to anoxia than do those of adults (Nissen and Schousboe, 1979). Newborn brains have less of the H subunit type, which, in contrast to the M type, is markedly dependent on normal oxygen tension (Cahn et al., 1962).

Catecholamines, acting through cAMP, cause a rise in the activity of LDH in the C6-2B subclone (de Vellis and Brooker, 1973). Cyclic AMP and RNA synthesis are required only for the first 2.5 hr following addition of norepinephrine to the cell cultures. After a lag of 4 hr, LDH activity begins to rise and reaches a plateau in approximately 20 hr. This second phase shows a requirement for protein synthesis. Cytochalasin B reversibly inhibits this induction (Bennett and de Vellis, 1977) and is effective when added during the transcription-dependent phase (first 3 hr), but not during the translation-dependent phase (after 3 hr) of LDH induction. Cytochalasin B accomplishes this inhibition without affecting the transient (intracellular and extracellular) rise in cAMP generated in response to norepinephrine. Careful experiments using RNA- and protein-synthesis inhibitors led the authors to conclude that the mode of action of cytochalasin B is localized between the rise in cAMP and the triggering of nuclear events associated with this rise. Furthermore, it was postulated that cytochalasin B interferes with the translocation of cytoplasmic protein kinase to the nucleus (Salem and de Vellis, 1976). This translocation may indeed be physiologically significant, since these authors also discovered that the nucleus displayed increased phosphorylation of specific protein bands. Protein kinase translocation to the nucleus and subsequent nuclear protein phosphorylation have been observed in other cell systems as well (Rosenfeld and Barrieux, 1979) and have been hypothesized to represent a general mechanism by which cAMP potentially regulates transcription. Dibutyryl cAMP treatment has been shown to increase the functional levels of mRNA for tyrosine aminotransferase (Ernest and Feigelson, 1978), phosphoenolpyruvate carboxykinase (Iynedjian and Hanson, 1977), and albumin (Brown and Papaconstantinou, 1979). A second hypothesis is that this transcriptional activation by cAMP in eukaryotes involves activation of cAMP-dependent nuclear protein kinases that, in turn, phosphorylate and thus modify nuclear regulatory proteins that participate in the control of genetic expression (Jungmann and Kranias, 1977; Kleinsmith, 1975). Tentative support for this concept can be found in the altered pattern of histone phosphorylation in isoproterenol-induced C6 glioma cells due to a cAMP-mediated activation of nuclear protein kinase (Harrison et al., 1980). Nor only nuclear proteins but also plasma-membrane proteins are phosphorylated in C6 cells by cAMP-dependent protein kinase(s) (Salem and de Vellis, 1980). These latter events may mediate cAMP action in regulating membrane functions, such as amino acid transport in C6 cells (Borg et al., 1979; Schousboe et al., 1977).

In preparations of pure oligodendrocyte cultures, 48-hr treatment with dibutryl cAMP increases LDH specific activity by 153% (McCarthy and de Vellis, 1980). This is the result of a 2-fold increase in the rates of synthesis as well as a near doubling in the percentage relative rates of synthesis of LDH-1, LDH-5, and total LDH (Kumar and de Vellis, 1981). This increase in the enzyme's rate of synthesis is exclusively localized to oligodendrocytes and is not shared by astrocytes or neurons and thus has been proposed as an oligodendroglial marker along with CNP and GalCer (Kumar and de Vellis, 1981).

The mechanism of catecholamine induction of LDH in C6 cells has been examined by quantitative immunoprecipitation (Kumar et al., 1980), which revealed that an increase in the specific rate of synthesis of total LDH, rather than a decreased rate of degradation, has occurred. LDH is coded for by two structural genes (coding for the M and H subunits, respectively) that are independently regulated (Everse and Kaplan, 1973); investigations in our laboratory showed that norepinephrine increases the rate of synthesis of both subunits (Kumar et al., 1980). These studies have been extended by other investigators who demonstrated that isoproterenol and dibutyryl cAMP increase the level of functionally active mRNA coding for the M subunit in glioma cells, which in turn determines the extent of synthesis of the LDH M subunit (Derda et al., 1980). Using a cloned DNA complementary to the mRNA coding for rat C6 glioma LDH M subunit, Jungmann's group (Miles et al., 1981) presented evidence that this cAMP-mediated increase in functional mRNA is indeed a transcriptional phenomenon and not the result of changes in posttranscriptional processing.

See Chapter 6 for other aspects of LDH activity in oligodendroglia.

2.2.2. 2′,3′-Cyclic Nucleotide 3′-Phosphohydrolase

CNP, bound to both plasma and intracellular membranes (Pfeiffer, 1973), has traditionally been viewed as a myelin marker (Matthieu et al., 1979; Kim and Pleasure, 1978a,b; D. M. Moore and Kirksey, 1977; Olafson et al., 1969; Kurihara and Tsukada, 1968). Yet CNP appears in pure oligodendrocyte cultures apparently free of visible myelin (McCarthy and de Vellis, 1980), thereby supporting an earlier suggestion (Zanetta et al., 1972) that CNP is present in glial plasma membranes in the myelin-free C6 glial cell line. In C6 cells, CNP can be induced by norepinephrine in a cAMP-mediated process (McMorris, 1977) that requires RNA and protein synthesis and the increased production of newly synthesized CNP molecules (McMorris and Sprinkle, 1982). The physiological significance of this enzyme has yet to be determined, although it is known to develop along a time–course that parallels that of myelin protein (Everly et al., 1977; Sarlieve et al., 1976) and is reduced in myelin-deficient mutants (Sarlieve et al., 1976; Kurihara et al., 1970). Furthermore, CNP is significantly reduced in normal-appearing white matter from multiple sclerosis patients (Gopfert *et al.,* 1980; Chou *et al.,* 1981). A recent study (Sprinkle *et al.,* 1980) undertaken to establish the apparent relationship between CNP and the Wolfgram protein doublet designated W1 and W2 (nomenclature of Waehneldt and Malotka, 1980) showed CNP to be a major component of this protein doublet.* These observations on the potential structural and functional role of CNP in myelin, its oligodendrocyte localization, and its induction in C6 by a major neurotransmitter make the study of the regulation of this enzyme both *in vivo* and *in vitro* of paramount importance in neurobiology (see also Chapters 4, 6, and 7).

2.2.3. Ornithine Decarboxylase

The biological importance of the naturally occurring polyamines spermidine and spermine is now well established. A large body of research literature points to their role in the control of transcription and translation (Bachrach, 1973), in the regulation of cellular proliferation in mammalian cells (Tabor and Tabor, 1976), and in differentiation (Stoscheck *et al.,* 1980; Takigawa *et al.,* 1980). In mammalian cells, the precursor of these polyamines, putrescine, is formed by the enzymatic decarboxylation of L-ornithine by ornithine decarboxylase (ODC). This enzyme has been shown to be the rate-limiting step in polyamine biosynthesis (Pegg and Williams-Ashman, 1969).

In the nervous system, there is evidence to indicate that brain maturation is reflected by ODC activity and that periods of greatest cell proliferation are accompanied by the highest ODC activity levels (for a review, see Shaw, 1979). Polyamines appear to be associated with glia, since brain spermidine concentration peaks during gliogenesis (Sobue and Nakajima, 1978), while large increases in brain polyamine content occur in astrocytoma (Kremzner *et al.,* 1970). In addition, brain protein synthesis is influenced by the polyamines (Goertz, 1979). In brain, a number of inducers of ODC have been uncovered, among them NGF (Lewis *et al.,* 1978; Ikeno *et al.,* 1978), vasopressin (Ikeno and Guroff, 1979), and the glucocorticoids (Cousin *et al.,* 1982). However, the localization of these effects is unclear. Treatment of C6-BU1 glioma cells, derived from the original C6 line (Benda *et al.,* 1968), with dibutyryl cAMP, norepinephrine, or isoproterenol results in increased ODC activity (Bachrach, 1975). This stimulation is cAMP-dependent and is blocked by drugs that inhibit protein or RNA synthesis. This fact and the prolonged lag between stimulation and the onset of enzyme induction led these authors to argue against "an activation of the decarboxylase by a direct phosphorylation of the enzyme or its precursor through a cAMP-dependent protein kinase." In the

---

*For a fuller discussion of this relationship, see Chapter 7 (Section 2.3.2c).

C6-2B subclone, dibutyryl cAMP, isoproterenol, and epinephrine are all ODC inducers (Gibbs *et al.,* 1980). In this system, the microtubule-disrupting agents vinblastine and colchicine and the microfilament-disrupting agent cytochalasin B block this cAMP-mediated induction. These authors conclude that ODC induction requires an intact cytoskeleton. This inhibition by cytoskeletal-disrupting agents is not unique, but is reminiscent of cytochalasin B's inhibition of the cAMP-mediated induction of LDH in C6 cells cited in Section 2.2.1 (Bennett and de Vellis, 1977). One potential explanation of these phenomena comes from the observation that in C6 cells, vinblastine and colchicine appear to inhibit nuclear kinase activity by interfering with the translocation of catalytic subunits of protein kinase to the nucleus (J. P. Schwartz and Costa, 1979). This translocation of the cytoplasmic protein kinase thus appears dependent on a normal microtubule system. The following considerations are relevant to future studies of the cytoskeleton in glia: (1) Are the sites of inhibition the same for these various effects, such as blockade of cAMP-mediated induction of LDH and ODC? (2) What general role do intact microtubules play in enzyme regulation in glial cells? (3) Will similar kinds of regulation be uncovered in brain *in situ* and in primary oligodendrocyte cultures as well? The presence of multiple cAMP-mediated inductions and their apparent universal requirement for cytoskeletal integrity makes the C6 glial-cell line an excellent model system to pursue this inquiry.

2.2.4. Nerve Growth Factor

The synthesis and release of NGF by C6 cells in monolayer culture increase in the presence of isoproterenol by a cyclic-nucleotide-dependent mechanism (J. P. Schwartz *et al.,* 1977). That a glial cell line can not only synthesize NGF but also release it to the external milieu as well (Murphy *et al.,* 1977) supports the earlier notion of Varon and co-workers (Varon *et al.,*1974; Burnham *et al.,* 1972) that NGF is released by ganglionic glial cells to provide NGF to ganglionic neurons, where it promotes the survival of these neurons. To date, this is still a provocative, though unproved, hypothesis.

2.2.5. Glutamine Synthetase

Dibutryl cAMP and isoproterenol (via a β-adrenergic receptor) induce GS in C6 cells by a mechanism that requires protein synthesis (Browning and Nicklas, 1982). This effect is also mimicked by increasing passage number. These results make understanding the regulation of GS even more interesting, since it now appears that GS is controlled by at least two classes of hormones, cyclic nucleotides and the glucocorticoids (Pishak and Phillips, 1980).

2.3. Thyroid Hormones

The thyroid hormones, L-thyroxine (T_4) and L-triiodothyronine (T_3), affect a wide range of physiological and biochemical processes, most notably those functions involved with growth and development (for a review, see H. L. Schwartz and Oppenheimer, 1978). Thyroid deficiency in early life produces irreversible cerebral damage and poor myelination (Rosman *et al.*, 1972; Flynn *et al.*, 1977). A variety of biochemical components in brain are reduced in neonatal hypothyroidism, such as cholesterol, cerebrosides, sulfatides, gangliosides, phospholipids, lipoproteins, and myelin-associated glycoprotein (Balazs *et al.*, 1969; Dalal *et al.*, 1971; Walters and Morrell, 1981).

Thyroid hormones most likely alter the level and pattern of gene expression through their interaction with low-capacity, high-affinity nuclear binding sites (H. L. Schwartz and Oppenheimer, 1978) followed by increased RNA synthesis *in vivo* (Tata *et al.*, 1963), probably as a consequence of increased activity of DNA-dependent RNA polymerase (Viarengo *et al.*, 1975).

In dissociated embryonic mouse brain cells, the synthesis of myelin-associated glycolipids was shown to be dependent on the availability of T_3 in the culture medium (N. R. Bhat *et al.*, 1979, 1981a). By contrast, precocious myelination is observed in intact rats (Schapiro, 1968) and in cultured cerebellar explants obtained from newborn rats (Hamburgh, 1966) following the administration of thyroid hormones. Since CNS myelin is produced by oligodendrocytes, these myelin disturbances indicate that a lack of thyroid hormones may interfere with the normal maturation and differentiation of these cells. Thus, the effect of thyroid hormones on oligodendrocyte differentiated macromolecules is a logical next step of inquiry.

2.3.1. 2′,3′-Cyclic Nucleotide 3′-Phosphohydrolase

This myelin and oligodendroglial plasma-membrane marker has been shown to be markedly reduced in dissociated embryonic mouse brain cultures in which serum in the culture medium comes from a thyroidectomized calf (N. R. Bhat *et al.*, 1981b). These low enzyme levels were restored to normal when the medium was supplemented with T_3. Therefore, oligodendrocytes themselves may be target cells for thyroid hormone; however, the presence of other cell types in this culture system allows for the possibility that this effect is an indirect one. The use of pure, primary cultures of oligodendrocytes will help to resolve this issue.

2.3.2. α-Glycerol Phosphate Dehydrogenase

The normal developmental increase in rat brain GPDH in cerebral cortex and cerebellum was markedly impaired in hypothyroid rats (Schwark *et al.*,

1971). T$_3$ treatment of these animals increased GPDH activity in both brain regions, but this reversal is time-dependent; i.e., if T$_3$ treatment is delayed until adulthood, the hormone fails to produce any appreciable change in enzyme activity. Since GPDH is believed to play an important role in the synthesis of brain phospholipid and myelin (Laatsch, 1962; Casper *et al.,* 1967; de Vellis and Inglish, 1968) (also see Chapter 6), this effect of hypothyroidism raises the interesting possibility that defective myelination may be associated with a decrease in the activity of this enzyme.

2.3.3. 5'-Nucleotidase

This enzyme, which catalyzes the hydrolysis of adenosine-5-monophosphate to adenosine, is apparently exclusively localized to the plasma membrane of CNS neuroglia as demonstrated by histochemistry (Kreutzberg *et al.,* 1978). It has been suggested (Schubert *et al.,* 1979) that glial-membrane adenosine is then released into the extracellular space, where it functions in the stimulation of cAMP synthesis in neighboring cells (Sattin and Rall, 1970). Its association with myelin has also been well established; 5'-nucleotidase increases with increasing myelin deposition, and myelin is a major locus in the brain (Cammer *et al.,* 1980; Cammer and Zimmerman, 1981). However, in dysmyelinating mouse mutant brains, 5'-nucleotidase is only minimally reduced (S. Bhat and Pfeiffer, 1982; Bourre *et al.,* 1981). In primary reaggregating cultures from embryonic mouse brain, cells maintained in serum with low T$_3$ concentrations have low enzyme activity and achieve only partial reversal when T$_3$ is added to cells previously exposed to hypothyroid serum (Shanker *et al.,* 1982). Though the extent of thyroid-hormone action on 5'-nucleotidase has not been as great as on other markers, these smaller effects may still be physiologically significant and thus merit the continued attention of neurobiologists.

3. CELL–CELL INTERACTIONS

3.1. Lectins and Cell Contact

The cell surface and its properties, components, and organization are acknowledged to have special significance in a number of cellular phenomena such as cancer metastasis, cell recognition, contact inhibition, escape from immune destruction, differentiation, movement, and growth regulation (for reviews, see Nicholson, 1976*a,b;* Pardee, 1975). It is the role of the cell surface in the differentiation of oligodendrocytes or their clonal model cells, C6, on which we have narrowed our focus.

It was originally postulated that surface-acting lectins such as concanavalin A (Con A) and its succinylated derivative (succinyl Con A) might prove to be useful probes in simulating external stimuli acting on the cell surface, i.e., cell–cell contact (Edelman *et al.,* 1973). Extending this hypothesis, these authors proposed that these stimuli are transduced to the metabolic machinery of the cytoplasm and the nucleus via cell–surface receptor interactions with cytoskeletal structures. As we shall see, this approach has generated a number of useful observations in glial biology. We have already cited how cytoskeletal poisons inhibit cAMP-mediated ornithine decarboxylase and lactate dehydrogenase induction in C6 cells. This section summarizes work on other glial proteins affected by cell-surface events, lectins, and cytoskeletal-disrupting agents.

3.1.1. S-100 Protein

Although the function of this acidic, soluble protein is unknown, its localization in glial cells in the nervous system (Cicero *et al.,* 1970), its developmental expression during neural maturation, and its widespread occurrence in vertebrate brain mark it as an important object of study. Though the use of C6 cells as a model for normal glia or, for that matter, normal oligodendrocytes arouses controversy (Labourdette and Mandel, 1978), we shall see momentarily that the C6 cell shows at least one interesting similarity in culture with whole brain in terms of S-100 accumulation.

C6 cells accumulate S-100 protein (B. W. Moore, 1965) as the cells progress from low density to confluency in monolayer cultures (Benda *et al.,* 1968; B. W. Moore, 1965). The cells accumulate S-100 protein at the end of the logarithmic phase when the cultures enter a phase of density-dependent inhibition of cell proliferation (Pfeiffer *et al.,* 1970). Other results confirm that the onset of S-100 protein synthesis coincides with a transition from low density to confluent growth in monolayer cultures (Labourdette and Marks, 1975). However, unlike earlier reports, these authors were able to unequivocally demonstrate S-100 synthesis in the logarithmic phase of growth and thus concluded that confluency modulates the level of cellular differentiation, not the "quantal" all-or-none expression of this specific protein. More refined analysis using an immunoprecipitation assay showed that regulation is occurring at the level of S-100 synthesis with no apparent change in the rate of degradation (Labourdette and Marks, 1975). Furthermore, these authors conclude that since S-100 protein in stationary C6 cells attains a value equal to that reported for brain (Zomzely-Neurath *et al.,* 1972), the study of S-100 regulation *in vitro* in C6 cells may be relevant to the mechanisms operating in the postnatal development of the rodent brain (Stewart and Urban, 1972). Other evidence, albeit indirect, suggests that homologous cell–cell contact at confluency mediates the induction of S-100 synthesis (Pfeiffer *et al.,* 1971).

Testing the transmembrane hypothesis of Edelman *et al.* (1973) in C6 cells, Marks and Labourdette (1977) have shown that succinyl Con A induces the synthesis of S-100 protein in logarithmic but not stationary cultures, while its relative synthesis in stationary cultures is inhibited by drugs that disrupt microtubules, such as colchicine and vinblastine. Apparently, the lectin is effective only in logarithmic cultures in which S-100 protein is low and not fully induced. The effects of the antimicrotubular agents are specific, because incorporation of [^{3}H]leucine into total soluble protein was not markedly affected. Presumably, the lectin, via interactions with cell-surface receptors, mimics the effects of cell–cell contact on S-100 levels. This process may be analogous to the ability of succinyl Con A to inhibit cellular growth in a manner resembling density-dependent inhibition in monolayer cultures (Mannino and Burger, 1975). The complexities of the intimate associations between nerve and glia are poorly understood, yet our attention must now be drawn to the possibility that cell–cell contact itself can transmit signals that regulate biochemical differentiation.

3.1.2. Adenylate Cyclase

The activity of this enzyme in C6 increases when the cells reach confluency (S. Morris and Mackman, 1976). With the use of hybrids with fibroblast cells, adenylate cyclase can be activated in the logarithmic phase of growth, but as soon as cell contacts become close, the hybrids behave as the fibroblast parent (Benda, 1978). Studies using hybrids to dissect out the genetic apparatus at each point of the cAMP-generating system could prove valuable in this regard.

3.1.3. 2′,3′-Cyclic Nucleotide 3′-Phosphohydrolase

In C6 cells grown to high density, there is a 4-fold increase in CNP specific activity (Maltese and Volpe, 1979). However, these authors caution that cell–cell contact may not necessarily be the critical determinant to this induction, since removal of serum also induces the enzyme in the absence of a high degree of cell contact. In addition, extremely high levels of cell density (well into stationary phase) are required to induce CNP, in contrast to S-100, induction of which starts at the very beginning of confluency (Labourdette *et al.*, 1977). This serum effect in sparse cultures of C6 cells has also been observed for S-100 (Gysin *et al.*, 1980). These multiple serum effects seem to be due to the presence of inhibitors in the serum operating, at least in the case of S-100, independently of cell-contact effects. Nevertheless, in terms of CNP production, C6 cells possess the ability to express a high degree of oligodendroglial biochemical differentiation.

Comparing CNP activity between fetal-rat-brain primary cultures and cultures of isolated oligodendrocytes of comparable age has generated some exciting results. The CNP activity in isolated oligodendrocytes is lower than in oligodendrocytes from mixed cultures (S. Bhat *et al.,* 1981). The presence of other brain cells thus enhances the capacity of oligodendrocytes to express a myelin-related differentiation function. Myelin basic protein (MBP) and sulfatide synthesis were similarly lower in the isolated oligodendrocytes (N. R. Bhat *et al.,* 1981*a*). Since MBP is a well-established specific marker of myelin and sulfatides are a major myelin component (Fry *et al.,* 1972), these results taken together indicate that nonoligodendrocyte signals may influence a whole spectrum of myelin-related differentiated functions and thus play a key role in myelination in the developing CNS. The exact nature of the mixed-culture factor is still unknown; nevertheless, a number of researchers have emphasized neuronal input in the initiation and maintenance of myelination (Saltzer *et al.,* 1980; Poser, 1978; Aguayo *et al.,* 1976). The long-term culture of myelinogenic oligodendrocytes offers a promising system to pinpoint critical regulatory factors by utilizing coculture with other CNS cell types or with components such as purified neuronal membranes or other subcellular fractions (also see Chapter 7).

3.1.4. Hydroxymethylglutaryl-CoA Reductase

Cholesterol is a critical component of cellular membranes; its levels are very high in neural tissue (Suzuki, 1976). Cholesterol synthesis is important in glial-cell differentiation, because it is a major component of all cellular membranes, including myelin (Volpe and Hennessy, 1977; Volpe *et al.,* 1978). Thus, the study of the regulation of hydroxymethylglutaryl (HMG)-CoA reductase, the rate-limiting enzyme of cholesterol biosynthesis in C6 glia and other mammalian cells (Volpe, 1978), is warranted. The antimicrotubular agent colcemid produces a concomitant fall in both cholesterol and HMG-CoA reductase activity in C6 cells (Volpe, 1979*a,b*). This drug effect did not appear to be the consequence of nonspecific toxicity. How the microtubules accomplish this change and whether it is the synthesis, degradation, or catalytic efficiency of the reductase that is altered are unknown at present. Likewise unknown are the consequences of disturbances in microtubular structure or function during development or disease to the synthesis of this critical membrane lipid. Further studies on the importance of cytoskeletal structures to glial differentiation and cholesterol biosynthesis revealed that disruption of microfilaments in C6 cells with cytochalasin D also dramatically inhibits the activity of HMG-CoA reductase (Volpe and Obert, 1981). Since cycloheximide blocked recovery of activity after removal of cytochalasin D, the observed decrease may be related to a decrease in the content of the enzyme. No change was seen in five other glial enzymes; hence, this effect is apparently specific.

See Chapters 2 and 5 for further discussion of the regulation of cholesterol metabolism.

3.1.5. α-Glycerol Phosphate Dehydrogenase

Recently, our laboratory discovered that the hydrocortisone (HC)-mediated induction of α-glycerol phosphate dehydrogenase (GPDH) can be completely and reversibly inhibited by lectins in both C6 cells and pure oligodendrocyte cultures (McGinnis and de Vellis, 1981). This inhibition by Con A of GPDH induction can be accounted for by a 90% reduction in cytoplasmic glucocorticoid receptors. Primary astrocyte cultures reveal a similar depression in quantifiable glucocorticoid receptors. That this "down-regulation" occurs *in vivo* as well suggests that one consequence of cell–cell contact may be the modulation of the role of glucocorticoids in the development and maintenance of specific cellular functions in the brain.

In mouse brain, GPDH exists as two isozymes the relative amounts of which depend on the developmental age of the tissue (Kozak and Erdelsky, 1975; Kozak, 1972). When mouse cerebellar cells are coaggregated with three types of tumor cells, synthesis of the major adult isozyme of GPDH is blocked, whereas coaggregation of cerebellar cells with telencephalon cells has little or no effect (Kozak, 1979). The ineffectiveness of conditioned media in these experiments suggested to Kozak that a diffusible factor is not involved and that tumor cell-surface components are the responsible elements in repressing the biochemical differentiation of the undifferentiated cerebellar cells.

Coculturing of live C6 cells with live or fixed B104 neuroblastoma results in the inability of the C6 cells to induce GPDH with HC treatment, presumably the result of surface determinants on the B104 cells (Ciment and de Vellis, 1982). Heterotypic associations appear necessary, since C6 cells as a live or fixed bedlayer had no effect.

3.1.6. Glutamine Synthetase

Probably the best-known example of the role of cell interactions in the hormonal control of gene expression comes from work on the induction of GS in embryonic neural retina by glucocorticoids. In dissociated retinal cells dispersed in monolayers, GS was not inducible (J. E. Morris and Moscona, 1971); however, if the cells were reaggregated, induction occurred as usual, suggesting that histiotypic cell contacts are necessary (Linser and Moscona, 1979). The molecular organization of the cell surface of the

Mueller cells in juxtaposition with the cell surface of retinal neurons appears to be a prerequisite for Mueller-cell responsiveness to the hormonal inducer.

3.1.7. Cyclic-AMP-Generating System

Coculturing C6 glioma cells with B104 neuroblastoma cells results in the uncoupling of β-adrenergic receptors from adenylate cyclase in C6 cells (Ciment and de Vellis, 1978). As a consequence, C6 cells show a marked impairment in their ability to accumulate cAMP. A careful series of conditioned media controls have ruled out a B104 diffusible, soluble factor. These authors suggest that this uncoupling is due to the intimate cellular interactions between C6 glioma and B104 neuroblastoma. To better understand the nature of this interaction, Ciment and de Vellis (1982) used a p-formaldehyde-fixed bedlayer of B104 cells prior to the addition of live C6 glioma cells. This procedure eliminated the possibility that the bedlayer B104 releases trophic factors over a short distance (Grobstein, 1968) or passes electrical currents or small molecules through gap junctions (Lawrence *et al.,* 1978; Revel and Brown, 1976). When B104 cells are pretreated with dibutyryl cAMP for 24–28 hr prior to fixation, the β-responsiveness of C6 cells is once again diminished. Careful controls ruled out nonspecific cytotoxicity by fixed or live B104 cells on C6 cells. The ability of trypsin to reverse these effects of dibutyryl-cAMP treatment suggests that the cell-surface determinant may be one or more proteins.

3.2. Soluble Factors

The notion that glial cells themselves can act to release soluble materials that affect the growth and differentiation of neighboring cells has received considerable attention (for a review, see Arenander and de Vellis, 1982). A number of peptides and proteins can modulate neural activity (Iverson *et al.,* 1978). We have previously discussed the regulation in C6 of nerve growth factor (NGF) by HC and β-adrenergic agonists; it is also accepted that C6 and other glial cell lines *in vitro* can secrete NGF (Norrgren *et al.,* 1980; Murphy *et al.,* 1977; Reynolds and Perez-Polo, 1975), where it is likely to have potent effects on neuronal survival, growth, and differentiation (Varon, 1975). Conditioned medium has been a favorite choice as a source of neuroactive, soluble macromolecules from a variety of neural and nonneural cell types (for reviews, see Patterson, 1978; Varon and Adler, 1981).

3.2.1. Glial-Released Protein and Conditioned Media

C6 cells have been used as a model system to investigate the nature of macromolecules released by glial cells into the culture medium (Arenander and de Vellis, 1980, 1981*a,b*). These macromolecules were first analyzed by one-dimensional gel electrophoresis, and a reproducible pattern of proteins was observed and collectively termed glial-released protein (GRP) (Arenander and de Vellis, 1980). Since these cells are known to be glucocorticoid target cells, the GRP was examined with respect to its responsiveness to hormonal manipulations. It was previously established that the GRP is sensitive to the position of the cells in the cell cycle and to differences in monolayer density, or to both. HC in physiological doses has a significant effect on C6-GRP patterns; a number of peaks increase, while others decrease. This effect is specific, since 17β-estradiol, isoproterenol, dibutyryl cAMP, and melatonin had either no effect or a distinctly different one, depending, in some cases, on the subclone examined. Using the higher resolution of two-dimensional sodium dodecyl sulfate–polyacrylamide gel electrophoresis (SDS-PAGE) (Arenander and de Vellis, 1981*a*), the specific members of the GRP that are modulated by HC were identified. About 50% of the GRP domain is affected by HC, unusually high when compared to the intracellular HC domain in other cells (Ivarie and O'Farrell, 1978). It remains to be seen whether this large intracellular HC domain is characteristic of normal glial cells and, in particular, oligodendrocytes.

A number of studies indicate that conditioned medium (CM) has biological activity in neurons. C6 cells release into the culture medium a protease-sensitive non-NGF substance that supports the survival and process formation of dissociated neurons from chick embryo sensory ganglia (Barde *et al.,* 1978). There is also an age-dependent change in sensitivity of dissociated dorsal-root-ganglion neurons to NGF compared to glial CM or brain extracts (Barde *et al.,* 1980); an increasing effect of glial CM or brain extract is seen on older sensory neurons, while NGF becomes less effective. This permits a clear distinction in functional terms between NGF and non-NGF growth factors. The evidence that the active factor or factors from brain extract are glial in origin is indirect; i.e., older brain extracts that contain more glia than newborns are more effective in this bioassay. The morphological differentiation of neuroblastoma cells by C6-CM factor(s) has long been appreciated (Reynolds and Perez-Polo, 1975; Monard *et al.,* 1973). The factor or factors that cause this effect on process formation are linearly dependent on the amount of factor used and are not correlated with an increase in intracellular cAMP (Monard *et al.,* 1973). This latter observation is significant, because dibutyryl cAMP induces morphological differentiation in neuroblastoma (Prasad and Hsie, 1971). Whether these effects are the result of unidentified components of glial CM or the consequence of glial NGF was not determined in these latter reports. In a recent paper, CM from primary glial rat brain culture was shown to be essential for the development of nearly pure neuronal cultures from embryonic rat-brain hippocampus (Muller and Siefert, 1982); in this work, the soluble factor or factors support both survival and neurite outgrowth in a serum-free medium. In the pheochromocytoma-derived PC12 cell line, C6-CM induced neurite outgrowth and choline acetyltransferase in a non-NGF-mediated process (Arenander and de Vellis, 1981*b;* Edgar *et al.,* 1979). Prenatal spinal-cord explants from chick and rat extend processes when treated with C6-CM (Arnason *et al.,* 1981); various other peripheral neuronal preparations are also similarly affected by C6-CM (Varon and Adler, 1981). Thus, glial-cell CM can alter the morphological and biochemical differentiation and the growth and survival of neural tissues by the action of trophic agents (Varon and Adler, 1980).

In the developing autonomic nervous system, the nature of the neurotransmitter substances that neurons synthesize is altered by changes in their environmental milieu (Landis and Keefe, 1980; LeDourain, 1980; LeDourain *et al.,* 1978; Patterson, 1978; LeDourain and Teillet, 1974). A similar plasticity has been observed in long-term primary cultures from newborn rat superior cervical ganglia. In culture conditions that prevent the growth of nonneuronal ganglion cells, the adrenergic phenotype predominates (Patterson *et al.,* 1975; Burton and Bunge, 1975; Reese and Bunge, 1974; Mains and Patterson, 1973). In contrast, the cholinergic phenotype is selected for by the presence of nonneuronal cells or CM from such cells (Patterson and Chun, 1974, 1977*a,b*). Weber (1981) has partially purified the active cholinergic factor from C6-CM utilizing conventional biochemical techniques. In future studies, the greater utilization of long-term primary cultures of sympathetic neurons will become an important part of an overall strategy dedicated to understand how glial CM can aid in neuronal differentiation.

3.2.2. Glial Maturation Factor(s)

The existence of glial maturation factor(s) (GMF) was discovered as a consequence of the search for active growth and differentiation factors in the nervous system (Lim and Mitsunobu, 1974, 1975; Lim *et al.,* 1973). This acidic protein from adult brain promotes the phenotypic expression of cultured glioblasts and aids in the expression of a number of glial differentiation products.

Morphological differentiation of glial cells by brain extracts has been reported from a number of laboratories in the last ten years (Lim *et al.,* 1973; Sensenbrenner *et al.,* 1972). Treatment of primary rat-brain cultures with either rat- or chick-brain extract causes an increase in the number of oligodendrocytes (Pettman *et al.,* 1980*a*). This effect is even stronger when brain extracts are taken from older animals. Extracts recently prepared from prenatal, postnatal, and adult tissues were separated on the basis of molecular weight, and fractions were assayed for mitogenic activity on pure astrocyte cultures (Morrison *et al.,* 1982). It is worth noting here that the observed fractions differed greatly in mitogenic activity among the three groups. This suggests that the CNS possesses a wide spectrum of growth-stimulatory activities that vary with developmental stage of donor tissue and thus offers the neurobiologist a more dynamic view of the complexities of growth control. Similar experiments are currently under way to identify and purify those factors that stimulate oligodendrocyte growth and development.

Characterization of the GMF suggests that substances of molecular weight greater than 15,000 have a stimulatory effect on glial-cell differentiation (Cam *et al.*, 1977). These dialyzable active factors are heat-labile and trypsin-sensitive, suggestive of proteins. Similar results have been obtained (Lim and Mitsunobu, 1974, 1975) in which a high-molecular-weight protein in adult rat and pig brain was found to be biologically active on newborn rat glial cultures. Pettman *et al.* (1980*b*) have partially purified from beef-brain extract an active thermolabile GMF that appeared as two molecular-weight species of 16,000 and 20,000 in SDS-PAGE. Cell cultures in their experiments were tentatively identified as astroglial by virtue of their increased levels of S-100 protein. From pig brain, other workers (Kato *et al.*, 1979) report purified active factors in two molecular-weight forms of 40,000 and 200,000, respectively. These fractions have both morphological and mitogenic effects.

Though the exact nature of the GMF is not yet fully characterized, the biological effects are potent and merit an intensive research program by virtue of their probable role in oligodendrocyte differentiation and growth.

4. NEOPLASTIC TRANSFORMATION

Since the mechanisms of cell differentiation are obscure, the study of neoplasia as an abnormality in this process (Mintz and Illmensee, 1975) has of necessity been rather slow. Viewing cancer as a disease of differentiation is only one of many conceptualizations of the etiology and pathology of cancer (Pitot, 1981). This section will not attempt even a modest review. We will only briefly discuss some aspects of oligodendroglial differentiated properties that appear to be altered by malignant transformation.

4.1. Modes of Investigation

4.1.1. In Vivo–in Vitro Model System

To dissect out mechanisms of transformation in glia, our laboratory combined certain features of two published methods: (1) the growth in culture of pure, separate populations of oligodendrocytes and astrocytes (McCarthy and de Vellis, 1980) and (2) the *in vivo–in vitro* system of Laerum and Rajewsky

(1975) in which *N*-ethyl-*N*-nitrosourea (ENU) is injected into pregnant rats, after which mixed, primary cultures from prenatal pups are made. In our laboratory, Bressler *et al.* (1980) injected pregnant rats with ENU and then cultured oligodendrocytes separately from astrocytes in 1- to 2-day-old pups. Between 100 and 150 days in culture, oligodendroglial-derived cells from pups of ENU-treated mothers transformed. Transformation was measured by a variety of standard criteria, for example, proliferation rate in culture and tumor formation in animals. Cell lines produced in this manner all retain normal 2′,3′-cyclic nucleotide 3′-phosphohydrolase levels and dibutyryl cAMP induction of lactate dehydrogenase. However, α-glycerol phosphate dehydrogenase inducibility by hydrocortisone was lost in all lines. All lines were S-100-positive; none was glial fibrillary acidic protein (GFAP)- or myelin basic protein (MBP)-positive. These authors believe that the carcinogen has "hit" a glial stem cell already expressing some glial functions, after which the cell is inhibited from differentiating further and eventually transforms. As-yet-unexplained spontaneous transformation could be observed in oligodendrocytes derived from saline-injected control mothers if horse serum was added to the culture medium. These cell lines were also positive for S-100 protein and negative for GFAP and MBP. Additional results (Bressler, Cole, and de Vellis, personal communication) show that these various transformed oligodendrocytes are morphologically similar to primary cultures of oligodendrocytes despite possessing anchorage-independent growth conventionally believed to be an *in vitro* characteristic of malignancy.

4.1.2. Monoclonal Antibody against Tumor-Associated Antigen

A monoclonal antibody has been developed in our laboratory that specifically binds to the surface of transformed glial cells and to tumor tissue of transformed oligodendrocytes, but not to the surface of normal glial cells (Peng *et al.*, 1982). C6 cells were used as the antigen source here. This antibody also recognizes ENU-induced transformed oligodendrocytes as well as spontaneously transformed astrocytes. That the specific C6 antigen that binds this antibody is absent in normal glia is likely to stimulate further research on the importance of this tumor-specific cell-surface antigen in the transformation process.

4.2. Specific Changes

4.2.1. Glial Maturation Factor(s)

A recent report (Lim *et al.*, 1981) indicates that glial maturation factor(s) (GMF) can prevent or minimize the disturbed growth properties of glial cancer cells. Work on the glioma cell line 354A revealed that addition of GMF to the culture medium prevents overgrowth once the cells reach confluency, thus restoring contact inhibition representative of a more normal phenotype.

4.2.2. Hydroxymethylglutaryl-CoA Reductase

In metastatic human brain glioblastoma, the activity of this enzyme is markedly elevated and can be compared with the finding that dividing C6 glioma cells, cultured without lipoprotein, exhibit a much higher rate of *de novo* sterol synthesis than nondividing glial cells (Maltese, 1982). The significance of these findings is at present unknown.

4.2.3. Glutamine Synthetase

Glutamine and GS may be involved in the events of neoplastic trans-formation. In a variety of tumor tissues, GS basal levels are consistently shown to be lower than in their nontransformed counterparts (Wu *et al.*, 1965). In rapidly growing malignant cells *in vivo,* glutamine is one of the most important substrates in their oxidative and energy metabolism (Kovacevic and Morris, 1972). Furthermore, in a variety of hepatomas, GS is inducible by hydrocortisone, whereas normal liver or primary hepatocyte cultures show no such regulatory response (Wu, 1976). Because of the unique position of GS in anabolic nitrogen metabolism with glutamine as the key nitrogen source in a great variety of biosynthetic pathways (Stadtman, 1973), this enzyme is a logical site of inquiry into normal cellular regulation and possible aberrations thereof.

Millimolar concentrations of sodium butyrate, which induce GS (Weingarten and de Vellis *et al.*, 1981), dramatically decrease GS specific activity in both pure oligodendrocyte and pure astrocyte cultures as mentioned previously. The mechanism by which this decrease occurs is currently under investigation. As shown in other cell types as well, GS specific activity is considerably lower in tumor tissue (C6 glioma cell) than in either normal glia in culture or whole brain. Hence, a number of intriguing differences are already apparent in these initial comparisons of GS between normal and transformed glial cells.

5. FUTURE PERSPECTIVES

As is evident from this review, a variety of agents regulate oligodendrocyte functions, both those that are unique to this cell type and those that oligodendrocytes share with other cell types, particularly the astrocytes. A number of differentiated functions are regulated by multiple effectors, and it will be interesting to discover whether these agents operate through common or independent mechanisms.

With respect to hormonal regulation of enzyme levels, a more detailed analysis of molecular mechanisms will undoubtedly require the application of recombinant DNA technology. In conjunction with the aforementioned use of pure, primary oligodendrocyte cultures and the model C6 cell line, cDNAs to such important oligodendrocyte mRNAs as those that code for α-glycerol phosphate dehydrogenase and $2',3'$-cyclic nucleotide phosphohydrolase will enable neurobiologists to delineate the molecular machinery of hormonal regulation, make comparisons between C6 cells and normal oligodendrocytes, and compare the mode of action of multiple effectors. The development of a serum-free medium for cultured oligodendrocytes, as has been successfully accomplished for astrocytes (Morrison and de Vellis, 1981), is a priority here in order to experimentally isolate the action(s) of individual hormones. *In situ,* the sequential developmental appearance of the mRNAs that code for oligodendrocyte-specific markers can be followed pre- and postnatally to ascertain oligodendrocyte cell lineages. Furthermore, the application of molecular biology techniques is needed in neurobiology if we are to understand the process of myelination in its embryological development and its maintenance in adulthood. These tools will be required to comprehend the pattern of production and coordinate expression of the mRNAs that code for myelin protein components and for biosynthetic and degradative enzymes regulating nonprotein components. Cell-culture systems that exhibit *in vitro* myelination provide the opportunity to begin these kinds of investigation.

The phenomenon of cell contact with respect to biochemical differentiation of glia in general and of certain myelin-associated components in particular is in our judgment potentially very significant to our understanding of nervous system development. In the near future, immediate aims should center on identifying active subcellular fractions and further purifying specific biochemical components from these fractions. These latter molecules may, for example, be specific membrane gangliosides or glycoproteins on neurons and astrocytes that ultimately modulate oligodendrocyte development and differentiation. Identifying such components allows us the possibility of manipulating their biological effects, for example, by producing antisera or monoclonal antibodies against them. Quite recently, our laboratory, in collaboration with Dr. Harvey Herschman, has discovered that both oligodendrocytes and astrocytes, but not neurons, possess cell-surface receptors for epidermal growth factor (EGF) (Simpson *et al.,* 1982*a*). This surprising result means that EGF could modulate glial effects on neurons and, in addition, offers us the opportunity of using EGF–toxin conjugates (Simpson *et al.,* 1982*b*; Cawley *et al.,* 1980) to grow pure neuronal cultures by selectively killing glial cells while leaving neurons intact.

The production and use of monoclonal antibodies (Kohler and Milstein, 1975, 1976) represent a technological breakthrough for all of bioscience, including neurobiology. Clearly, the goal of much of this work is to generate highly specific probes characteristic of a particular cell type (either normal or tumorigenic) and use these probes to (1) monitor the developmental expression of a differentiation antigen, (2) isolate functional subclasses of a given cell type, (3) develop diagnostic and therapeutic antibody molecules, and (4) utilize antibody-mediated cell separation to produce homogeneous primary cell cultures. As we have shown in our laboratory, a glial-tumor-specific antibody is now a reality (Peng *et al.*, 1982). In addition, a series of monoclonal antibodies have been generated to bovine CNS white matter that react with oligodendrocyte cell surfaces but not with surfaces of astrocytes, neurons, or fibroblasts (Sommer and Schachner, 1981). A monoclonal antibody has also recently been generated against galactocerebroside (Ranscht *et al.*, 1982), an oligodendrocyte marker (Raff *et al.*, 1978) and major glycolipid component of myelin (Norton and Autilio, 1966). These monoclonal antibodies will permit developmental studies of oligodendrocytes and myelin with respect to the sequential appearance of their antigens both *in vivo* and *in vitro*. Future development of other monoclonal antibodies will permit us to identify novel antigens on oligodendrocyte cell surfaces. With regard to tumor immunobiology, the potential now exists for chemically conjugating diphtheria toxin A chain or ricin A chain to antibody molecules, thus permitting the action of the toxic A chain to be directed to the antibody's specific target cell (Gilliland *et al.*, 1980). Such a cell-type-specific toxin is now being developed for our glial-tumor-specific monoclonal antibody.

It is hoped that the continued endeavor to identify regulated proteins in oligodendrocytes and to elucidate the underlying molecular mechanisms of these processes will serve to focus the attention of neurobiologists on the importance of these gene products to the differentiated state and physiological functioning of oligodendrocytes.

Acknowledgments

This work was supported by Department of Energy Contract DE-AM03-76-SF00012, U.S. Public Health Service Training Grant NS 6238, and U.S. Public Health Service Grants HD-05615 and AG-01754. We gratefully acknowledge Joyce Adler for her preparation of this manuscript and her stoic calm throughout its numerous revisions.

6. REFERENCES

Aguayo, A. J., Epps, J., Charron, L., and Bray, G. M., 1976, Multipotentiality of Schwann cells in cross-anastomosed and grafted myelinated and unmyelinated nerves: Quantitative microscopy and radioautography, *Brain Res.* **104**:1–20.

Arenander, A. T., and de Vellis, J., 1980, Glial-released proteins in clonal cultures and their modulation by hydrocortisone, *Brain Res.* **200**:401–419.

Arenander, A. T., and de Vellis, J., 1981*a,* Glial-released proteins. II. Two-dimensional electrophoretic identification of proteins regulated by hydrocortisone, *Brain Res.* **224**:105–116.

Arenander, A. T., and de Vellis, J., 1981*b,* Glial-released proteins. III. Influence on neuronal morphological differentiation, *Brain Res.* **224**:117–127.

Arenander, A. T., and de Vellis, J., 1982, Glial-released proteins in neural intercellular communication: Molecular mapping, modulation and influence on neuronal differentiation, in: *Proteins in the Nervous System: Structure and Function* (B. Haber, J. R. Perez-Polo, and J. D. Coulter, eds.), pp. 243–269, Alan R. Liss, New York.

Arnason, B. G. W., Yu, R. C., Amico, L., Arenander, A., and de Vellis, J., 1981, The effect of a glial cell released factor on spinal cord neuron growth and its modulation by steroids, *Soc. Neurosci. Symp.* **11** (abstr. 179.10).

Bachrach, U., 1973, *Function of Naturally Occurring Polyamines,* Academic Press, New York, 211 pp.

Bachrach, U., 1975, Cyclic AMP-mediated induction of ornithine decarboxylase of glioma and neuroblastoma cells, *Proc. Natl. Acad. Sci. U.S.A.* **72**:3087–3091.

Balazs, R., Brookshank, B. W. L., Davison, A. L., Eayrs, J. T., and Wilson, D. A., 1969, The effect of neonatal thyroidectomy on myelination in the rat brain, *Brain Res.* **15**:219–232.

Barde, Y. A., Lindsay, R. M., Monard, D., and Thoenen, H., 1978, New factor released by cultured glioma cells supporting survival and growth of sensory neurons, *Nature (London)* **274**:818.

Barde, Y. A., Edgar, D., and Thoenen, H., 1980, Sensory neurons in culture: Changing requirements for survival factors during embryonic development, *Proc. Natl. Acad. Sci. U.S.A.* **77**:1199–1203.

Baxter, J., Rousseau, G., Benson, H., Garcia, R., Ito, J., and Tomkins, G., 1972, Role of DNA and specific cytoplasmic receptors in glucocorticoid action, *Proc. Natl. Acad. Sci. U.S.A.* **69**:1892–1896.

Benda, P., 1978, Rodent glial cell lines, in: *Dynamic Properties of Glial Cells* (E. Schoffeniels, G. Franck, D. B. Tower, and L. Hertz, eds.), pp. 67–81, Pergamon Press, New York.

Benda, P., Lightbody, J., Sato, G., Levine, L., and Sweet, W., 1968, Differentiated rat glial cell strain in tissue culture, *Science* **161**:350–371.

Benda, P., Someda, K., Messer, J., and Sweet, W. H., 1971, Morphological and immunochemical studies of rat glial tumors and conal strains propagated in culture, *J. Neurosurg.* **34**:310–323.

Bennett, K., and de Vellis, J., 1977, Reversible inhibition of the norepinephrine induction of lactate dehydrogenase by cytochalasin B in rat glial C6 cells, *J. Cell. Physiol.* **93**:261–268.

Bennett, K., McGinnis, J. F., and de Vellis, J., 1977, Reversible inhibition of the hydrocortisone induction of glycerol phosphate dehydrogenase by cytochalasin B in rat glial C6 cells, *J. Cell. Physiol.* **93**:247–260.

Bhat, N. R., Sarlieve, L. L., Rao, G. S., and Pieringer, R., 1979, Investigations on myelination *in vitro:* Regulation by thyroid hormone in cultures of dissociated brain cells from embryonic mice, *J. Biol. Chem.* **254**:9342–9346.

Bhat, N. R., Rao, G. S., and Pieringer, R. A., 1981*a,* Investigations on myelination *in vitro:* Regulation of sulfolipid synthesis by thyroid hormone in cultures of dissociated brain cells from embryonic mice, *J. Biol. Chem.* **256:**1167–1171.

Bhat, N. R., Shankar, G., and Pieringer, R. A., 1981*b,* Investigations of myelination *in vitro:* Regulation of 2′,3′-cyclic nucleotide 3′-phosphohydrolase by thyroid hormone in cultures of dissociated brain cells from embryonic mice, *J. Neurochem.* **37:**695–701.

Bhat, S., and Pfeiffer, S. E., 1982, Myelinogenic gene expression intrinsic to cultured oligodendrocytes, *Trans. Am. Soc. Neurochem.* **13:**154.

Bhat, S., Barbarese, E., and Pfeiffer, S. E., 1981, Requirement for nonoligodendrocyte cell signals for enhanced myelinogenic gene expression in long-term cultures of purified rat oligodendrocytes, *Proc. Natl. Acad. Sci. U.S.A.* **78:**1283–1287.

Bissell, M. G., Rubinstein, L. J., Bignami, A., and Herman, M. M., 1974, Characteristics of the rat C-6 glioma maintained in organ culture systems: Production of glial fibrillary acidic protein in the absence of gliofibrillogenesis, *Brain Res.* **82:**77–89.

Borg, J., Bakar, V. J., and Mandel, P., 1979, Effect of cyclic nucleotides on the high affinity uptake of L-glutamate and taurine in glial and neuroblastoma cells, *Brain Res.* **166:**113–120.

Bourre, J. M., Chanez, C., Dumont, O., and Flexor, M. A., 1981, 5-Nucleotidase Na^+, K^+-ATPase in nervous tissue from demyelinating mouse, *Trans. Am. Soc. Neurochem.* **12:**80.

Breen, G. A. M., and de Vellis, J., 1974, Regulation of glycerol phosphate dehydrogenase by hydrocortisone in dissociated rat cerebral cell cultures, *Dev. Biol.* **41:**255–266.

Breen, G. A. M., and de Vellis, J., 1975, Regulation of glycerol phosphate dehydrogenase by hydrocortisone in rat brain explants, *Exp. Cell Res.* **91:**159–169.

Breen, G. A. M., McGinnis, J. F., and de Vellis, J., 1978, Modulation of the hydrocortisone induction of glycerol phosphate dehydrogenase by N^6,O^2-dibutyryl cyclic AMP, norepinephrine and isobutylmethylxanthine in rat brain cell cultures, *J. Biol. Chem.* **253:**2554–2562.

Bressler, J. P., Cole, R., and de Vellis, J., 1980, Cell culture systems to study glial transformation, in: *Mechanisms of Toxicity and Hazard Evaluation* (B. Holmstedt, R. Lavwerys, M. Mercier, and M. Roberfroid, eds.), pp. 187–197, Elsevier/North-Holland, Amsterdam.

Brown, P. C., and Papaconstantinou, J., 1979, Coordinated modulation of albumin synthesis and mRNA levels in cultured hepatoma cells by hydrocortisone and cyclic AMP analogs, *J. Biol. Chem.* **254:**9379–9384.

Browning, E. T., and Nicklas, W. J., 1982, Induction of glutamine synthetase by dibutyryl cyclic AMP in C-6 glioma cells, *J. Neurochem.* **39:**336–341.

Burnham, P., Raiborn, C., and Varon, S., 1972, Replacement of nerve growth factor by ganglionic non-neuronal cells for the survival *in vitro* of dissociated ganglionic neurons, *Proc. Natl. Acad. Sci. U.S.A.* **69:**3556–3560.

Burton, H., and Bunge, R. P., 1975, A comparison of the uptake and release of [^{3}H]-norepinephrine in rat autonomic and sensory ganglia in tissue culture, *Brain Res.* **97:**157–162.

Cahn, R. D., Kaplan, N. O., Levine, L., and Zwilling, E., 1962, Nature and development of lactic dehydrogenases, *Science* **136:**962–969.

Cam, Y., Sensenbrenner, M., Ledig, M., and Mandel, P., 1977, Partial characterization of a brain extract that stimulates nerve cell differentiation in culture, *Neuroscience* **2:**801–805.

Cammer, W., and Zimmerman, T. R., 1981, Rat brain 5′-nucleotidase: Developmental changes in myelin and activities in subcellular fractions and myelin subfractions, *Brain Res.* **227:**381–389.

Cammer, W., Sirota, S. R., Zimmerman, T. R., and Norton, W. T., 1980, 5′-Nucleotidase in rat brain myelin, *J. Neurochem.* **35:**367–373.

Casper, R., Vernadakis, A., and Timiras, P. S., 1967, Influence of estradiol and cortisol on lipids and cerebrosides in the developing brain and spinal cord of the rat, *Brain Res.* **5**:524–526.

Cawley, D. B., Herschman, H. R., Gilliland, D. G., and Collier, R. J., 1980, EGF-ricin A is a potent toxin while EGF-diphtheria fragment A is nontoxic, *Cell* **22**:563–570.

Chou, C. H. J., Chou, F., Peacocke, N., Eltzroth, D., Tourtellotte, W., and Kibler, R. F., 1981, CNPase activity of multiple sclerosis brains, *Trans. Am. Soc. Neurochem.* **12**:91.

Cicero, T. J., Cowan, W. M., Moore, B. W., and Suntzeff, V., 1970, The cellular localization of two brain specific proteins, S-100 and 14-3-2, *Brain Res.* **18**:25–34.

Ciment, G., and de Vellis, J., 1978, Cellular interactions uncouple β-adrenergic receptors from adenylate cyclase, *Science* **202**:765–768.

Ciment, G., and de Vellis, J., 1982, Cell surface-mediated cellular interactions: Effects of B104 neuroblastoma surface determinants on C6 glioma cellular properties, *J. Neurosci. Res.* **7**: 371–386.

Claisse, P. J., and Roscoe, J. P., 1976, The inducibility of glycerol phosphate dehydrogenase in two rat-glial tumors, *Brain Res.* **109**:423–425.

Cousin, M. A., Lando, D., and Moguilewsky, M., 1982, Ornithine decarboxylase induction by glucocorticoids in brain and liver of adrenalectomized rats, *J. Neurochem.* **38**:1296–1304.

Dalal, K. B., Vulcana, T., Timiras, P. S., and Einstein, E. R., 1971, Regulatory role of thyroxine on myelogenesis in the developing rat, *Neurobiology* **1**:211–224.

Davidson, R. L., and Benda, P., 1970, Regulation of specific functions of glial cells in somatic hybrids. II. Control of inducibility of glycerolphosphate dehydrogenase, *Proc. Natl. Acad. Sci. U.S.A.* **67**:1870–1877.

Dawson, G., and Kearns, S. M., 1978, Mechanism of action of hydrocortisone potentiation of sulfogalactosylceramide synthesis in mouse oligodendroglioma cell lines, *J. Biol. Chem.* **254**:163–167.

Derda, D. F., Miles, M. F., Schweppe, J. S., and Jungmann, R. A., 1980, Cyclic AMP regulation of lactate dehydrogenase, *J. Biol. Chem.* **255**:11,112–11,121.

De Vellis, J., 1973, Mechanisms of enzymic differentiation in the brain and in cultured cells, in: *Developing and Aging in the Nervous System* (M. Rockstein, ed.), pp. 171–198, Academic Press, New York.

De Vellis, J., and Brooker, G., 1973, Induction of enzymes by glucocorticoids in a rat glial cell line, in: *Tissue Culture of the Nervous System* (G. Sato, ed.), pp. 231–245, Plenum Press, New York.

De Vellis, J., and Brooker, G., 1974, Reversal of catecholamine refractoriness by inhibitors of RNA and protein synthesis, *Science* **186**:1221–1223.

De Vellis, J., and Inglish, D., 1968, Hormonal control of glycerolphosphate dehydrogenase in the rat brain, *J. Neurochem.* **15**:1061–1070.

De Vellis, J., and Inglish, D., 1969, Effect of cortisol and epinephrine on the biochemical differentiation of cloned glial cells in culture and of the developing rat brain, in: *Transactions of the 2nd International Meeting Society of Neurochemistry*, pp. 151–152, Tamburini, Milan.

De Vellis, J., and Inglish, D., 1973, Age-dependent changes in the regulation of glycerolphosphate dehydrogenase in the rat brain and in a glial cell line, *Prog. Brain Res.* **40**:321–330.

De Vellis, J., Schjeide, O. A., and Clemente, C. D., 1967, Protein synthesis and enzymic patterns in the developing brain following head X-irradiation of newborn rats, *J. Neurochem.* **14**:499–511.

De Vellis, J., Inglish, D., Cole, R., and Molson, J., 1971, Effects of hormones on the differentiation of cloned lines of neurons and glial cells, in: *Influence of Hormones on the Central Nervous System* (D. Ford, ed.), pp. 25–39, S. Karger, Basel.

De Vellis, J., McEwen, B. S., Cole, R., and Inglish, D., 1974, Relations between glucocorticoid nuclear binding, cytosol receptor and enzyme induction in a rat glial cell line, *J. Steroid Biochem.* **5**:392–393.

De Vellis, J., McGinnis, J. F., Breen, G. A. M., Leveille, P., Bennett, K., and McCarthy, K. D., 1977, Hormonal effects on differentiation in neural cultures, in: *Cell, Tissue, and Organ Cultures in Neurobiology* (S. Fedoroff and L. Hertz, eds.), pp. 485–511, Academic Press, New York.

Edelman, G. M., Yahara, I., and Wang, J. L., 1973, Receptor mobility and receptor–cytoplasmic interactions in lymphocytes, *Proc. Natl. Acad. Sci. U.S.A.* **70**:1442–1446.

Edgar, D., Barde, Y. A., and Thoenen, H., 1979, Induction of fiber outgrowth and choline acetyltransferase in PC12 pheochromocytoma cells by conditioned media from glial cells and organ extracts, *Exp. Cell Res.* **121**:353–361.

Ernest, M. J., and Feigelson, P., 1978, Increase in hepatic tyrosine aminotransferase in RNA during enzyme induction by N^6,O^2 2'-dibutryl cyclic AMP, *J. Biol. Chem.* **253**:319–322.

Everly, J. L., Quarles, R. H., and Brady, R. O., 1977, Proteins and glycoproteins in myelin purified from the developing bovine and human central nervous systems, *J. Neurochem.* **28**:95–101.

Everse, J., and Kaplan, N. O., 1973, Lactate dehydrogenases: Structure and function, *Adv. Enzymol. Relat. Areas Mol. Biol.* **37**:61–133.

Flynn, T. J., Deshmukh, D. S., and Pieringer, R. A., 1977, Effects of altered thyroid function on galactosyl diacylglycerol metabolism in myelinating rat brain, *J. Biol. Chem.* **252**:5864–5870.

Fry, J. M., Lehrer, G. M., and Bernstein, M. B., 1972, Sulfatide synthesis: Inhibition by experimental allergic encephomyelitis serum, *Science* **175**:192–194.

Gibbs, J. B., Shu, C.-Y., Terasaki, W. L., and Brooker, G., 1980, Calcium and microtubule dependence for increased ornithine decarboxylase EC-4.1.1.17 activity stimulated by beta adrenergic agonists dibutyryl cyclic AMP or serum in a rat astrocytoma cell line, *Proc. Natl. Acad. Sci. U.S.A.* **77**:995–999.

Gilliland, D. G., Steplewski, R. J., Collier, R. J., Mitchell, K. F., Chang, T. H., and Koprowski, H., 1980, Antibody-directed cytotoxic agents: Use of monoclonal antibody to direct the action of toxin A chains to colorectal carcinoma cells, *Proc. Natl. Acad. Sci. U.S.A.* **77**:4539–4543.

Gilman, A. G., and Nirenberg, M., 1971, Effect of catecholamines on the cAMP concentrations of clonal satellite cells of neurons, *Proc. Natl. Acad. Sci. U.S.A.* **68**:2165–2168.

Goertz, B., 1979, Effect of polyamines on cell-free protein synthesizing systems from rat cerebral cortex, cerebellum, and liver, *Brain Res.* **173**:125–135.

Gopfert, E., Pytlik, S., and Debuch, H., 1980, 2',3'-Cyclic nucleotide 3'-phosphohydrolase and lipids of myelin from multiple sclerosis and normal brains, *J. Neurochem.* **34**:732–739.

Gorski, R. A., 1971, Steroid hormones and brain function: Progress, principles and problems, in: *Steroid Hormones and Brain Function* (C. H. Sawyer and R. A. Gorski, eds.), pp. 1–26, University of California Press, Los Angeles.

Grobstein, C., 1968, Developmental significance of interface materials in epithelio–mesenchymal interactions, in: *Epithelial–Mesenchymal Interactions* (R. Fleischmajer and R. E. Billingham, eds.), pp. 173–176, Williams and Wilkins, Baltimore.

Gysin, R., Moore, B. W., Proffitt, R. T., Devel, T. F., Caldwell, K., and Glaser, L., 1980, Regulation of the synthesis of S-100 protein in rat glial cells, *J. Biol. Chem.* **255**:1515–1520.

Hamburgh, M., 1966, Evidence for a direct effect of temperature and thyroid hormone on myelinogenesis *in vitro*, *Dev. Biol.* **13**:15–30.

Harrison, J. J., Suter, P., Suter, S., and Jungmann, R. A., 1980, Isoproterenol induced selective phosphorylative modification *in vivo* of rat C6 glioma cell histones, *Biochem. Biophys. Res. Commun.* **96**:1253–1260.

Herschkowitz, N., Bologa, L., and Siegrist, H. P., 1982, Characterization of mouse oligodendrocytes during development, *Trans. Am. Soc. Neurochem.* **13**:173.

Ikeno, T., and Guroff, G., 1979, The effect of vasopressin on the activity of ornithine decarboxylase in rat brain and liver, *J. Neurochem.* **33**:973–975.

Ikeno, T., MacDonnell, P. C., Nagaiah, K., and Guroff, G., 1978, The permissive effect of cortical steroids on the induction of brain ornithine decarboxylase by nerve growth factor, *Biochem. Biophys. Res. Commun.* **82**:957–963.

Ivarie, R. D., and O'Farrell, P. H., 1978, The glucocorticoid domain: Steroid-mediated changes in the rate of synthesis of rat hepatoma proteins, *Cell* **13**:41–55.

Iverson, L. L., Nicoll, R. A., and Vale, W. W., 1978, Neurobiology of peptides, *Neurosci. Res. Program Bull.* **16**:214–370.

Iynedjian, P. B., and Hanson, R. W., 1977, Increase in level of functional mRNA coding for phosphoenolpyruvate carboxykinase (GTP) during induction by cyclic adenosine 3:5'-monophosphate, *J. Biol. Chem.* **252**:655–662.

Jard, S., Premont, J., and Benda, J., 1972, Adenylate cyclase, phosphodiesterase and protein kinase of rat glial cells in culture, *FEBS Lett.* **26**:344–348.

Jungmann, R. A., and Kranias, E. G., 1977, Minireview: Nuclear phosphoprotein kinases and the regulation of gene expression, *Int. J. Biochem.* **8**:819–830.

Juurlinck, B. H. J., Schousboe, A., Jorgensen, O. D., and Hertz, L., 1981, Induction by hydrocortisone of glutamine synthetase in mouse primary astrocyte cultures, *J. Neurochem.* **36**:136–142.

Kakiuchi, S., and Rall, T. W., 1968, The influence of chemical agents on the accumulation of adenosine 3',5'-phosphate in slices of rabbit cerebellum, *Mol. Pharmacol.* **4**:367–378.

Kato, T., Chiu, T. C., Lim, R., Troy, S. S., and Turiff, D. E., 1979, Multiple molecular forms of glial maturation factor, *Biochim. Biophys. Acta* **579**:216–227.

Kemel, M. L., Gauchy, C., Glowinski, J., and Besson, M. J., 1979, Spontaneous and potassium evoked release of ³H-GABA newly synthesized from ³H-glutamine in slices of the rat substantia nigra, *Life Sci.* **24**:2139–2150.

Kim, S. U., and Pleasure, D. E., 1978a, Tissue culture analysis of neurogenesis: Myelination and synapse formation are retarded by serum deprivation, *Brain Res.* **145**:15–25.

Kim, S. U., and Pleasure, D. E., 1978b, Tissue culture analysis of neurogenesis: Lipid-free medium retards myelination in mouse spinal cord cultures, *Brain Res.* **157**:206–211.

Kleinsmith, L. J., 1975, Phosphorylation of non-histone proteins in the regulation of chromosome structure and function, *J. Cell. Physiol.* **85**:459–476.

Kohler, G., and Milstein, C., 1975, Continuous culture of fused cells secreting antibody of predefined specificity, *Nature (London)* **256**:495–497.

Kohler, G., and Milstein, C., 1976, Derivation of specific antibody-producing tissue culture and tumor lines by cell fusion, *Eur. J. Immunol.* **6**:511–519.

Kovacevic, Z., and Morris, H. P., 1972, The role of glutamine in the oxidative metabolism of malignant cells, *Cancer Res.* **32**:326–333.

Kozak, L. P., 1972, Genetic control of α-glycerolphosphate dehydrogenase in mouse brain, *Proc. Natl. Acad. Sci. U.S.A.* **69**:3170–3174.

Kozak, L. P., 1979, Coaggregation with tumor cells inhibits expression by cerebellar cells of the adult isozyme locus, *Gdc-1, Dev. Biol.* **68**:407–421.

Kozak, L. P., and Erdelsky, K. J., 1975, The genetics and developmental regulation of L-glycerol-3-phosphate dehydrogenase, *J. Cell. Physiol.* **85**:437–448.

Kremzner, L. T., Barrett, R. E., and Terano, M. J., 1970, Polyamine metabolism in the central and peripheral nervous system, *Ann. N.Y. Acad. Sci.* **171:**735–748.

Kreutzberg, G. W., Barron, K. D., and Schubert, P., 1978, Cytochemical localization of 5′-nucleotide in glial plasma membranes, *Brain Res.* **158:**247–257.

Kumar, S., and de Vellis, J., 1981, Induction of lactate dehydrogenase by dibutyryl cAMP in primary cultures of central nervous tissue is an oligodendroglial marker, *Dev. Brain Res.* **1:**303–307.

Kumar, S., McGinnis, J. F., and de Vellis, J., 1980, Catecholamine regulation of lactate dehydrogenase in rat brain cell culture: Norepinephrine differentially increases the rate of synthesis of the individual subunits in the C6 glial tumor cell line, *J. Biol. Chem.* **255:**2315–2321.

Kurihara, T., and Tsukada, Y., 1968, 2′,3′-Cyclic nucleotide 3′-phosphohydrolase in the developing chick brain and spinal cord, *J. Neurochem.* **15:**827–832.

Kurihara, T., Nussbaum, J. L., and Mandel, P., 1970, 2′,3′-Cyclic nucleotide 3′-phosphohydrolase in brains of mutant mice with deficient myelination, *J. Neurochem.* **17:**993–997.

Laatsch, R. H., 1962, Glycerol phosphate dehydrogenase activity of developing rat in the central nervous system, *J. Neurochem.* **9:**487–492.

Labourdette, G., and Mandel, P., 1978, S-100 protein in monolayer cultures of glial cells: Basal level in primary and secondary cultures, *Biochem. Biophys. Res. Commun.* **85:**1307–1313.

Labourdette, G., and Marks, A., 1975, Synthesis of S-100 protein in monolayer cultures of rat glial cells, *Eur. J. Biochem.* **58:**73–79.

Labourdette, G., Mahony, J. B., Brown, I. R., and Marks, A., 1977, Regulation of synthesis of a brain-specific protein in monolayer cultures of clonal rat glial cells, *Eur. J. Biochem.* **81:**591–597.

Laerum, O. D., and Rajewsky, M. F., 1975, Neoplastic transformation of fetal rat brain cells in culture after exposure to ethylnitrosourea *in vivo*, *J. Natl. Cancer Inst.* **55:**1177–1188.

Landis, S. C., and Keefe, D., 1980, Development of cholinergic sympathetic innervation of eccrine sweat glands in rat footpad, *Soc. Neurosci. Symp.* **10** (abstr. 131.20).

Lawrence, T. S., Beers, W. H., and Gilula, N. B., 1978, Transmission of hormonal stimulation by cell-to-cell communication, *Nature (London)* **272:**501–506.

LeDourain, N. M., 1980, The ontogeny of the neural crest in avian embryo chimaeras, *Nature (London)* **286:**663–669.

LeDourain, N. M., and Teillet, M. A. M., 1974, Experimental analysis of the migration and differentiation of neuroblasts of the autonomic nervous system and of neuroectodermal mesenchymal derivatives using a biological cell marking technique, *Dev. Biol.* **41:**162–184.

LeDourain, N. M., Teillet, M. A., Ziller, C., and Smith, J., 1978, Adrenergic differentiation of cells of the cholinergic ciliary and Remak ganglia in avian embryo after *in vivo* transplantation, *Proc. Natl. Acad. Sci. U.S.A.* **75:**2030–2034.

Leveille, P. J., McGinnis, J. F., Maxwell, D. S., and de Vellis, J., 1980, Immunocytochemical localization of glycerol-3-phosphate dehydrogenase in rat oligodendrocytes, *Brain Res.* **196:**287–305.

Levi-Montalcini, R., 1976, The nerve growth factor: Its role in growth, differentiation, and function of the sympathetic adrenergic neuron, *Prog. Brain Res.* **45:**235–258.

Lewis, M. E., Lakshmanan, J., Nagiah, K., MacDonnel, P. C., and Guroff, G., 1978, Nerve growth factor increases activity of ornithine decarboxylase in rat brain, *Proc. Natl. Acad. Sci. U.S.A.* **75:**1021–1023.

Lim, R., and Mitsunobu, K., 1974, Brain cells in culture: Morphological transformation by a protein, *Science* **185:**63–66.

Lim, R., and Mitsonobu, K., 1975, Partial purification of a morphological transforming factor from pig brain, *Biochem. Biophys. Acta* **400:**200–207.

Lim, R., Mitsonobu, K., and Li, W. K. P., 1973, Maturation stimulating effect of brain extract and dibutyryl cyclic AMP on dissociated embryonic brain cells in culture, *Exp. Cell Res.* **79**:243–246.

Lim, R., Nagawara, S., Anason, B., Barry, G. W., and Turtiff, D. E., 1981, Effect of glial maturation factor on glioma cells, *Trans. Am. Soc. Neurochem.* **12**:225.

Linser, P., and Moscona, A. A., 1979, Induction of glutamine synthetase in embryonic neural retina: Localization in Muller fibers and dependence on cell interactions, *Proc. Natl. Acad. Sci. U.S.A.* **76**:6476–6480.

Linser, P. J., and Moscona, A. A., 1981, Induction of glutamine synthetase in embryonic neural retina: Its suppression by the gliatoxic agent α-aminoadipic acid, *Dev. Brain Res.* **1**:103–120.

Lund, P., 1970, A radiochemical assay for glutamine synthetase, and activity of the enzyme in rat tissues, *Biochem. J.* **118**:35–39.

Mains, R. E., and Patterson, P. H., 1973, Primary cultures of dissociated sympathetic ganglia. I. Establishment of long-term growth in culture and studies of differentiated properties, *J. Cell Biol.* **59**:329–345, 346–360, 361–366.

Maltese, W. A., 1982, 3-Hydroxy-3-methylglutaryl-CoA reductase in human intracranial tumors, *Trans. Am. Soc. Neurochem.* **13**:158.

Maltese, W. A., and Volpe, J. J., 1979, Induction of an oligodendroglial enzyme in C6 glioma cells maintained at high density or in serum-free medium, *J. Cell. Physiol.* **101**:459–470.

Mannino, R. J., and Burger, M. M., 1975, Growth inhibition of normal cells by succinylated concanavalin A, *Nature (London)* **256**:19–22.

Marks, A., and Labourdette, G., 1977, Succinyl concanavalin A stimulates and antimicrotubular drugs inhibit the synthesis of a brain-specific protein in rat glial cells, *Proc. Natl. Acad. Sci. U.S.A.* **74**:3855–3856.

Martinez-Hernandez, A., Bell, K. P., and Norenberg, M. D., 1977, Glutamine synthetase: Glial localization in brain, *Science* **195**:1356–1358.

Matthieu, J. M., Honegger, P., Trapp, B. D., Cohen, S. R., and Webster, H. de F., 1978, Myelination in rat brain aggregating cell cultures, *Neuroscience* **3**:565–572.

Matthieu, J. M., Honegger, P., Farrod, P., Gautier, E., and Dolivo, M., 1979, Biochemical characterization of a myelin fraction isolated from rat brain aggregating cell cultures, *J. Neurochem.* **32**:869–881.

McCarthy, K. D., and de Vellis, J., 1977, Age dependent changes in neuronal and glial cell markers in cultures from rat cerebral cortex, *Trans. Am. Soc. Neurochem.* **8**:88.

McCarthy, K. D., and de Vellis, J., 1978, Alpha-adrenergic modulation of beta-adrenergic, adenosine and prostaglandin E_1 increased adenosine $3':5'$ cyclic monophosphate levels in primary cultures of glia, *J. Cyclic Nucleotide Res.* **4**:15–26.

McCarthy, K. D., and de Vellis, J., 1979, The regulation of adenosine $3':5'$-cyclic monophosphate accumulation in glia by alpha-adrenergic agonists, *Life Sci.* **24**:639–650.

McCarthy, K. D., and de Vellis, J., 1980, Preparation of separate astroglial and oligodendroglial cell cultures from rat cerebral tissue, *J. Cell Biol.* **85**:890–902.

McEwen, B. S., Magnus, C., and Wallack, C., 1971, Biochemical studies of corticosterone binding to cell nuclei and cytoplasmic macromolecules in specific regions of the rat brain, in: *Steroid Hormones and Brain Function* (C. H. Sawyer and R. A. Gorski, eds.), pp. 247–258, University of California Press, Los Angeles.

McGinnis, J. F., and de Vellis, J., 1978, Glucocorticoid regulation in rat brain cell cultures: Hydrocortisone increases the rate of synthesis of glycerol phosphate dehydrogenase in C6 glioma cells, *J. Biol. Chem.* **253**:8483–8492.

McGinnis, J. F., and de Vellis, J., 1981, Cell surface modulation of gene expression in brain cells by down regulation of glucocorticoid receptors, *Proc. Natl. Acad. Sci. U.S.A.* **78:**1288–1292.

McMorris, F. A., 1977, Norepinephrine induces glial specific enzyme activity in cultured glioma cells, *Proc. Natl. Acad. Sci. U.S.A.* **74:**4501–4504.

McMorris, F. A., and Sprinkle, T. J., 1982, Mechanism of CNP induction in C6 glioma cells, *Trans. Am. Soc. Neurochem.* **13:**114.

Meyer, J. S., Leveille, P. J., de Vellis, J., Gerlach, J. L., and McEwen, B. S., 1982, Evidence for glucocorticoid target cells in the rat optic nerve: Hormone binding and glycerolphosphate dehydrogenase induction, *J. Neurochem.* **39:**423–434.

Miles, M. F., Hung, P., and Jungmann, R. A., 1981, Cyclic AMP regulation of lactate dehydrogenase, *J. Biol. Chem.* **256:**12,545–12,552.

Mintz, B., and Ilmensee K., 1975, Normal genetically mosaic mice produced from malignant teratocarcinoma cells, *Proc. Natl. Acad. Sci. U.S.A.* **72:**3585–3589.

Monard, D., Solomon, F., Rentsch, M., and Gysin, R., 1973, Glial-induced morphological differentiation in neuroblastoma cells, *Proc. Natl. Acad. Sci. U.S.A.* **70:**1894–1897.

Moore, B. W., 1965, A soluble protein characteristic of the nervous system, *Biochem. Biophys. Res. Commun.* **19:**729–744.

Moore, D. M., and Kirksey, A., 1977, The effect of a deficiency of vitamin B-6 on the specific activity of 2′,3′-cyclic nucleotide 3′-phosphohydrolase of neonatal rat brain, *Brain Res.* **146:**200–204.

Morris, J. E., and Moscona, A. A., 1971, The induction of glutamine synthetase in aggregates of embryonic neural retina cells: Correlations with differentiation and multicellular organization, *Dev. Biol.* **25:**420–444.

Morris, S., and Mackman, M., 1976, Cell density and receptor adenylate cyclase relationships in the C6 astrocytoma cell, *Mol. Pharmacol.* **12:**362–372.

Morrison, R., and de Vellis, J., 1981, Growth of purified astrocytes in chemically defined media, *Proc. Natl. Acad. Sci. U.S.A.* **78:**7205–7209.

Morrison, R. S., Saneto, R. P., and de Vellis, J., 1982, Developmental expression of rat brain mitogens for cultured astrocytes, *J. Neurosci. Res.* **8:**435–442.

Moscona, A. A., 1975, Comments on embryonic cell associations in enzyme induction and histogenesis: Experimental systems for studies on teratogenesis, in: *Tests of Teratogenicity in Vitro* (J. D. Ebert and M. Marois, eds.), pp. 67–72, North-Holland, Amsterdam.

Moscona, M., Frenkel, N., and Moscona, A. A., 1972, Regulatory mechanisms in the induction of glutamine synthetase in the embryonic retina: Immunochemical studies, *Dev. Biol.* **28:**229–241.

Muller, B. W., and Siefert, W., 1982, A neurotrophic factor (NTF) released from primary glial cultures supports survival and fiber outgrowth of cultured hippocampal neurons, *J. Neurosci. Res.* **8:**195–204.

Murphy, R. A., Oger, J., Saide, J. D., Blanchard, M. H., Arnason, B. G., Hogan, C., Pantazis, N. J., and Young, M., 1977, Secretion of nerve growth factor by central nervous system glioma cells in culture, *J. Cell Biol.* **72:**769–773.

Nicholson, G.,1976*a*, Transmembrane control of the receptors on normal and tumor cells. I. Cytoplasmic influence over cell surface components, *Biochim. Biophys. Acta* **457:**57–108.

Nicholson, G., 1976*b*, Transmembrane control of the receptors on normal and tumor cells. II. Surface changes associated with transformation and malignancy, *Biochim. Biophys. Acta* **458:**1–72.

Nissen, C., and Schousboe, A., 1979, Activity and isozyme pattern of lactate dehydrogenase in astroblasts cultured from brains of newborn mice, *J. Neurochem.* **32:**1787–1792.

Norenberg, M. D., and Martinez-Hernandez, A., 1979, Fine structural localization of glutamine synthetase in astrocytes of rat brain, *Brain Res.* **161**:303–310.

Norrgren, G., Ebendal, T., Belew, M., Jacobson, C. O., and Porath, J., 1980, Release of nerve growth factor by human glial cells in culture, *Exp. Cell Res.* **130**:31–39.

Norton, W. T., and Autilio, L. A., 1966, The lipid composition of purified bovine brain myelin, *J. Neurochem.* **13**:213–222.

Olafson, R. W., Drummond, G. I., and Lee, J. F., 1969, Studies on 2′,3′-cyclic nucleotide 3′-phosphohydrolase from brain, *Can. J. Biochem.* **47**:961–966.

O'Malley, B. T., Speisburg, W., Schrader, F., Chytil, F., and Stegglas, A., 1972, Mechanisms of interaction of a hormone receptor complex with the genome of a eukaryotic target cell, *Nature (London)* **235**:141–144.

Pardee, A. B., 1975, The cell surface and fibroblast proliferation—some current research trends, *Biochim. Biophys. Acta* **417**:153–172.

Parker, K. K., Norenberg, M. D., and Vernadakis, A., 1980, "Transdifferentiation" of C6 glial cells in culture, *Science* **208**:179–181.

Patterson, P. H., 1978, Environmental determination of autonomic neurotransmitter functions, *Annu. Rev. Neurosci.* **1**:1–17.

Patterson, P. H., and Chun, L. L. Y., 1974, The influence of non-neuronal cells on catecholamine and acetylcholine synthesis and accumulation in cultures of dissociated sympathetic neurons, *Proc. Natl. Acad. Sci. U.S.A.* **71**:3607–3610.

Patterson, P. H., and Chun, L. L. Y., 1977a, The induction of acetylcholine synthesis in primary cultures of dissociated rat sympathetic neurons, *Dev. Biol.* **56**:263–280.

Patterson, P. H., and Chun, L. L. Y., 1977b, The induction of acetylcholine synthesis in primary cultures of dissociated rat sympathetic neurons. II. Developmental aspects, *Dev. Biol.* **60**:473–481.

Patterson, P. H., Reichardt, L. F., and Chun, L. L. Y., 1975, Biochemical studies on the development of primary sympathetic neurons in cell culture, *Cold Spring Harbor Symp., Quant. Biol.* **40**:389–397.

Pegg, A. E., and Williams-Ashman, H. G., 1969, On the role of s-adenosylmethionine in the biosynthesis of spermidine in the rat prostate, *J. Biol. Chem.* **244**:682–693.

Peng, W. W., Bressler, J. P., Tiffany-Castiglioni, E., and de Vellis, J., 1982, Development of a monoclonal antibody against a tumor-associated antigen, *Science* **215**:1102–1104.

Perez-Polo, J. R., Hull, K., Livingston, K., and Westlund, K., 1977, Steroid induction of nerve growth factor in cell culture, *Life Sci.* **21**:1535–1544.

Pettman, B., Sensenbrenner, M., and Labourdette, G., 1980a, Isolation of a glial maturation factor from beef brain, *FEBS Lett.* **118**:195–199.

Pettman, B., Delaunoy, J. P., Courageot, J., Devilliers, G., and Sensenbrenner, M., 1980b, Rat brain glial cells in culture: Effects of brain extracts on the development of oligodendroglial-like cells, *Dev. Biol.* **75**:278–287.

Pfeiffer, S. E., 1973, Clonal lines of glial cells, in: *Tissue Culture of the Nervous System* (G. Sato, ed.), pp. 203–230, Plenum Press, New York.

Pfeiffer, S. E., Herschman, H. R., Lightbody, J., and Sato, G., 1970, Synthesis by clonal line of rat glial cells of a protein unique to the nervous system, *J. Cell. Physiol.* **75**:329–340.

Pfeiffer, S. E., Herschman, H. R., Lightbody, J. E., Sato, G., and Levine, L., 1971, Modification of cell surface ontogenicity as a function of culture conditions, *J. Cell Physiol.* **78**:145–151.

Pishak, M. R., and Phillips, A. T., 1980, Glucocorticoid stimulation of glutamine synthetase production in cultured rat glioma cells, *J. Neurochem.* **34**:866–872.

Pitot, H. C., 1981, The biochemistry of cancer, in: *Fundamentals of Oncology* (H. C. Pitot, ed.), pp. 159–193, Marcel Dekker, New York.

Pleasure, D., Abramsky, O., Silberberg, D., Quinn, B., and Parvis, J., 1977, Biochemical studies of oigodendrocytes from calf brain, *Trans. Am. Soc. Neurochem.* **8**:143.

Poser, C. M., 1978, Dysmyelination revisited, *Arch. Neurol.* **35**:401–408.

Prasad, K., 1977, Role of cyclic nucleotides in the differentiation of nerve cells, in: *Cell, Tissue, and Organ Cultures in Neurobiology* (S. Fedoroff and L. Hertz, eds.), pp. 447–484, Academic Press, New York.

Prasad, K. N., and Hsie, A. W., 1971, Morphological differentiation of mouse neuroblastoma cells induced *in vitro* by dibutyryl adenosine 3':5'-cyclic monophosphate, *Nature (London)* **233**:141–142.

Raff, M. C., Mirsky, R., Fields, K. L., Lisak, R. F., Dorfman, S. H., Silberberg, D. H., Gregson, N. A., Leibowitz, S., and Kennedy, M. S., 1978, Galactoce rebroside is a specific cell-surface antigenic marker for oligodendrocytes in culture, *Nature (London)* **274**:813–816.

Ranscht, B., Clapshaw, P. A., Price, J., Noble, M., and Seifert, W., 1982, Development of oligodendrocytes and Schwann cells studied with a monoclonal antibody against galactocerebroside, *Proc. Natl. Acad. Sci. U.S.A.* **79**:2709–2713.

Reese, R., and Bunge, R. P., 1974, Morphological and cytochemical studies of synapses formed in culture between isolated rat superior cervical ganglion neurons, *J. Comp. Neurol.* **157**:1–12.

Reubi, J. C., Van den Berg, C., and Cuenco, M., 1978, Glutamine as precursor for the GABA and glutamate transmitter pools, *Neurosci. Lett.* **10**:171–174.

Revel, J. P., and Brown, S. S., 1976, Cell junction in development with particular reference to the neural tube, *Cold Spring Harbor Symp. Quant. Biol.* **40**:443–455.

Reynolds, C. P., and Perez-Polo, J. R., 1975, Human neuroblastoma: Glial induced morphological differentiation, *Neurosci. Lett.* **1**:91–97.

Rosenfeld, M. G., and Barricux, A., 1979, Binding of proteins to mRNA, *Methods Enzymol.* **60**:392–440.

Rosman, N. P., Malone, M. J., Hepenstein, M., and Kraft, E., 1972, The effect of thyroid deficiency on myelination of brain, *Neurology* **22**:99–105.

Sadasivudu, B., Rao, T. I., and Murthy, C. R., 1977, Acute metabolic effects of ammonia in mouse brain, *Neurochem. Res.* **2**:639–645.

Salem, R., and de Vellis, J., 1976, Protein kinase activity and cAMP-dependent protein phosphorylation in subcellular fractions after norepinephrine treatment of glial cells, *Fed. Proc. Fed. Am. Soc. Exp. Biol.* **35**:296.

Salem, R., and de Vellis, J., 1980, Phosphorylation of plasma membrane proteins dependent on adenosine 3',5'-monophosphate in rat-glial C6 cells, *Eur. J. Biochem.* **107**:271–278.

Saltzer, J. L., Williams, A. K., Glaser, L., and Bunge, R. P., 1980, Studies of Schwann cell proliferation. II. Characterization of the stimulation and specificity of the response to a neurite membrane fraction, *J. Cell Biol.* **84**:753–766.

Sarlieve, L. L., Faroqui, A. A., Rebel, G., and Mandel, P., 1976, Arylsulfatase A and 2',3'-cyclic nucleotide 3'-phosphohydrolase activities in the brains of myelin deficient mutant mice, *Neuroscience* **1**:519–522.

Sarlieve, L. L., Rao, G. S., Campbell, G. L., and Pieringer, R. A., 1980, Investigations on myelination *in vitro:* Biochemical and morphological changes in cultures of dissociated brain cells from embryonic mice, *Brain Res.* **189**:79–90.

Sattin, A., and Rall, T. W., 1970, The influence of adenine nucleotides on the accumulation of adenosine-3',5'-phosphate in brain slices, *Mol. Pharmacol.* **6**:13–23.

Schapiro, S., 1968, Some physiological, biochemical, and behavioral consequences of neonatal hormone administration: Cortisol and thyroxine, *Gen. Comp. Endocrinol.* **10**:214–228.

Schousboe, A., Beck, E., and Hertz, C., 1977, Effect of Bt₂cAMP and serum withdrawal on morphological and biochemical differentiation of normal astrocytes in culture, *Proc. Int. Soc. Neurochem.* **6**:435.

Schubert, P., Komp, W., and Kreutzberg, G. W., 1979, Correlation of 5′-nucleotidase activity and selective transneuronal transfer of adenosine in the hippocampus, *Brain Res.* **168**:419–424.

Schultz, J., Hamprecht, B., and Daly, J. W., 1972, Accumulation of cAMP in clonal glial cells: Labelling of intracellular adenine nucleotides with radioactive adenine, *Proc. Natl. Acad. Sci. U.S.A.* **69**:1266–1270.

Schwark, W. S., Singhal, R. L., and Ling, G. M., 1971, Metabolic control mechanisms in mammalian systems: Thyroid hormone control of alpha-glycerolphosphate dehydrogenase activity in rat cerebral cortex and cerebellum, *Can. J. Physiol. Pharmacol.* **49**:598–607.

Schwartz, H. L., and Oppenheimer, J. H., 1978, Physiologic and biochemical actions of thyroid hormones, *Pharmacol. Ther. B* **3**:349–376.

Schwartz, J. P., and Costa, E., 1979, Activation of nuclear protein kinase and induction of cAMP phosphodiesterase in C6 glioma cells following stimulation of adrenergic beta receptors, *Fed. Proc. Fed. Am. Soc. Exp. Biol.* **38**:263.

Schwartz, J. P., Morris, N. R., and Breckenridge, B. McL., 1973, Adenosine 3′,5′-monophosphate in glial tumor cells, *J. Biol. Chem.* **248**:2699–2704.

Schwartz, J. P., Chuang, D., and Costa, E., 1977, Increase in nerve growth factor content in C6 glioma cells by the activation of a β-adrenergic receptor, *Brain Res.* **137**:369–375.

Sealy, L., and Chalkley, R., 1978, The effect of sodium butyrate on histone modification, *Cell* **14**:115–121.

Sensenbrenner, M., Springer, N., Booher, J., and Mandel, P., 1972, Histochemical studies during the differentiation of dissociated nerve cells cultivated in the presence of brain extracts, *Neurobiology* **2**:49–60.

Shanker, G., Subba Rao, G., and Pieringer, R. A., 1982, Regulation of 5′-nucleotidase in dissociated brain cells of embroynic mice, *Trans. Am. Soc. Neurochem.* **13**:134.

Shapiro, D., 1982, Steroid hormone regulation of vitellogenin gene expression, *CRC Crit. Rev. Biochem.* **12**:187–204.

Shaw, G. S., 1979, The polyamines in the central nervous system: Commentary, *Biochem. Pharmacol.* **28**:1–6.

Sheppard, J. R., Brus, D., and Wehner, J. M., 1978, Brain reaggregate cultures: Biochemical evidence for myelin membrane synthesis, *J. Neurobiol.* **9**:309–315.

Simpson, D. L., Morrison, R., de Vellis, J., and Herschman, H. R., 1982a, Epidermal growth factor binding and mitogenic activity on purified populations of cells from the central nervous system, *J. Neurosci. Res.* **8**:453–462.

Simpson, D. L., Cawley, E. B., and Herschman, H. R., 1982b, Killing of cultured hepatocytes by conjugates of asialofetuin and EGF linked to the A chains of ricin or diphtheria toxin, *Cell* **29**:469–473.

Sobue, K., and Nakajima, T., 1978, Changes in concentrations of polyamines and gamma-aminobutyric acid and their formation in chick embryo brain during development, *J. Neurochem.* **30**:277–279.

Soh, B. M., and Sarkar, P. K., 1978, Control of glutamine synthetase messenger RNA by hydrocortisone in the embryonic chick retina, *Dev. Biol.* **64**:316–328.

Sommer, I., and Schachner, M., 1981, Monoclonal antibodies (O1 to O4) to oligodendrocyte cell surfaces: An immunocytological study in the central nervous system, *Dev. Biol.* **83**:311–327.

Sprinkle, T. J., Wells, M. R., Garver, F. A., and Smith, D. B., 1980, Studies on the Wolfgram high molecular weight CNS myelin proteins: Relationship to 2′,3′-cyclic nucleotide 3′-phosphodiesterase, *J. Neurochem.* **35**:1200–1208.

Stadtman, E. R., 1973, Introduction: A note on the significance of glutamine in intermediary metabolism, in: *The Enzymes of Glutamine Metabolism* (S. Prusirer and E. R. Stadtman, eds.), pp. 1–6, Academic Press, New York.

Stephens, J. L., and Pieringer, R. A., 1981, Hydrocortisone stimulates myelination *in vitro* in defined media, *Trans. Am. Soc. Neurochem.* **12:**226.

Stewart, J. A., and Urban, M. I., 1972, The postnatal accumulation of S-100 protein in mouse central nervous system: Modulation of protein synthesis and degradation, *Dev. Biol.* **29:**372–384.

Stoscheck, C. M., Florini, J. R., and Richman, R. A., 1980, The relationship of ornithine decarboxylase activity to proliferation and differentiation of L6 muscle cells, *J. Cell. Physiol.* **102:**11–18.

Suzuki, K., 1976, Chemistry and metabolism of brain lipids, in: *Basic Neurochemistry* (G. J. Siegel, R. W. Albers, R. Katzman, and B. W. Agranoff, eds.), pp. 308–328, Little, Brown, Boston.

Tabor, C. W., and Tabor, H., 1976, 1,4-Diaminobutane (putrescine), spermidine, and spermine, *Annu. Rev. Biochem.* **45:**285–306.

Takigawa, M., Ishida, H., Takano, T., and Suzuki, F., 1980, Polyamines and differentiation: Induction of ornithine decarboxylase by parathyroid hormone is a good marker of differentiated chrondrocytes, *Proc. Natl. Acad. Sci. U.S.A.* **77:**1481–1485.

Tapia, R., and Gonzales, R. M., 1978, Glutamine and glutamate as precursors of the releasable pool of GABA in brain cortex slices, *Neurosci. Lett.* **10:**165–169.

Tata, J. R., Ernster, L., Lindberg, O., Arrhenius, E., Pedersen, S., and Hedman, R., 1963, The action of thyroid hormones at the cell level, *Biochem. J.* **86:**408–428.

Tennekoon, G. I., Cohen, S. R., Price, D. L., and McKhann, G. M., 1977, Myelinogenesis in optic nerve: A morphological, autoradiographic, and biochemical analysis, *J. Cell Biol.* **72:**604–616.

Terasaki, W. L., Brooker, G., de Vellis, J., Inglish, D., Hsu, C. Y., and Moylan, R. D., 1978, Involvement of cyclic AMP and protein synthesis in catecholamine refractoriness, in: *Advances in Cyclic Nucleotide Research* (W. J. George and L. J. Igharron, eds.), pp. 33–52, Raven Press, New York.

Varon, S., 1975, Nerve growth factor and its mode of action, *Exp. Neurol.* **48:**75–92.

Varon, S., and Adler, R., 1980, Nerve growth factors and control of nerve growth, *Curr. Top. Dev. Biol.* **16:**207–252.

Varon, S., and Adler, R., 1981, Trophic and specifying factors directed to neuronal cells, *Adv. Cell. Neurobiol.* **2:**115–163.

Varon, S., Raiborn, C., and Norr, S., 1974, Association of antibody to nerve growth factor with ganglionic non-neurons (glia) and consequent interference with their neuron-supportive action, *Exp. Cell. Res.* **88:**247–256.

Venkov, L., Rosental, L., and Manolova, M., 1976, Subcellular distribution of LDH isoenzymes in neuronal- and glial-enriched fractions, *Brain Res.* **109:**323–333.

Viarengo, A., Zoncheddu, A., Taningher, M., and Orunesu, M., 1975, Sequential stimulation of nuclear RNA polymerase activities in livers from thyroidectomized rats treated with triiodothyronine, *Endocrinology* **97:**955–961.

Volpe, J. J., 1978, Lipid metabolism: Fatty acid and cholesterol biosynthesis, in: *Diabetes, Obesity, and Vascular Disease* (H. M. Katzen and R. J. Mahler, eds.), pp. 37–125, Halstead Press, New York.

Volpe, J. J., 1979a, Microtubules and the regulation of 3-hydroxy-3-methylglutaryl coenzyme A reductase, *J. Biol. Chem.* **254:**2568–2571.

Volpe, J. J., 1979b, A role for microtubules in the regulation of 3-hydroxy-3-methylglutaryl coenzyme A reductase and cholesterol biosynthesis in cultured glial cells, *J. Neurochem.* **33**:97–106.

Volpe, J. J., and Hennessy, S. W., 1977, Cholesterol biosynthesis and 3-hydroxy-3-methylglutaryl coenzyme A reductase in cultured glial and neuronal cells: Regulation by lipoprotein and by certain free sterols, *Biochim. Biophys. Acta* **486**:408–420.

Volpe, J. J., and Obert, K. A., 1981, Relation of cholesterol biosynthesis to HMG-CoA reductase in glia, *Trans. Am. Soc. Neurochem.* **12**:215.

Volpe, J. J., Fujimoto, K., Marasa, J. C., and Agrawal, H. C., 1975, Relation of C6 glial cells in culture to myelin, *Biochem. J.* **152**:701–703.

Volpe, J. J., Hennessy, S. W., and Wong, T., 1978, Regulation of cholesterol ester synthesis in cultured glial and neuronal cells: Relation to control of cholesterol synthesis, *Biochim. Biophys. Acta* **528**:424–435.

Waehneldt, T. V., and Malotka, J., 1980, Comparative electrophoretic study of the Wolfgram proteins in myelin from several mammalia, *Brain Res.* **189**:582–587.

Walters, S. N., and Morrell, P., 1981, Effects of altered thyroid states on myelinogenesis, *J. Neurochem.* **36**:1792–1801.

Weber, W. J., 1981, A diffusible factor responsible for the determination of cholinergic functions in cultured sympathetic neurons, *J. Biol. Chem.* **256**:3447–3453.

Weingarten, D., and de Vellis, J., 1980, Selective inhibition by sodium butyrate of the glucocorticoid induction of glycerol phosphate dehydrogenase in glial cultures, *Biochem. Biophys. Res. Commun.* **93**(4):1297–1304.

Weingarten, D. P., Kumar, S., and de Vellis, J., 1981, Paradoxical effects of sodium butyrate on the glucocorticoid inductions of glutamine synthetase and glycerol phosphate dehydrogenase in C6 cells, *FEBS Lett.* **126**(2):289–291.

West, G. J., Uki, J., Stahn, R., and Herschman, H., 1977, Neurochemical properties of cell lines from *N*-ethyl-*N*-nitrosourea induced rat tumors, *Brain Res.* **130**:387–392.

Wu, C., 1963, Glutamine synthetase. I. A comparative study of its distribution in animals and its inhibition by DL-allo-8-hydroxylysine, *Comp. Biochem. Physiol.* **8**:335–351.

Wu, C., 1976, Hormonal regulation of glutamine synthetase and ornithine aminotransferase in normal and neoplastic rat tissues, in: *Control Mechanisms in Cancer* (W. F. Griss, T. Ono, and J. R. Sabine, eds.), pp. 125–138, Raven Press, New York.

Wu, C., Roberts, E. H., and Bauer, J. M., 1965, Enzymes related to glutamine metabolism and tumor-bearing rats, *Cancer Res.* **25**:677–684.

Yamamoto, K. R., and Alberts, B. M., 1976, Steroid receptor elements for modulation of eukaryotic transcription, *Annu. Rev. Biochem.* **45**:721–746.

Zanetta, J. P., Benda, P., Gombos, G., and Morgan, I. G., 1972, The presence of 2',3'-cyclic AMP 3'-phosphohydrolase in glial cells in tissue culture, *J. Neurochem.* **19**:881–883.

Zomzely-Neurath, C., York, C., and Moore, B. W., 1972, Synthesis of a brain-specific protein (S-100) in a homologous cell-free system programmed with cerebral polysomal messenger RNA, *Proc. Natl. Acad. Sci. U.S.A.* **69**:2326–2330.

INDEX

Acetoacetate
  as a cholesterol precursor, 59, 60
  as a lipid precursor, 186
Acetoacetyl-CoA-synthetase,
  in oligodendrocytes, 186, 218
Acetoacetyl-CoA-thiolase,
  activity in oligodendrocytes, 218
Acetylcholinesterase, 219–220
Acid lipase,
  activity of in oligodendrocytes, 219
"Active" oligodendrocytes,
  morphology of, 19, 20
Adenosine, action on glial cell cultures, 307
Adenylate cyclase,
  histochemistry of, 212
  regulation of by cell–cell contact, 315
Adrenalectomy
  effect of on myelination, 186
β-Adrenergic receptors
  on C6 cells, 307
  in primary cultures, 307
Aggregate cultures, *see* Reaggregated cell
  cultures
1-Alkyl-2-acylglycerol-3-phosphate, 54
Alkylacylglycerolphosphoethanolamine,
  in oligodendrocytes, 188
Alkyldihydroxyacetone phosphate, 54
1-Alkyl-*sn*-glycerophosphoethanolamine
  as a plasmalogen precursor, 180–181
1-Amino-cyclopentane-1-carboxylic acid
  effect of in explants, 270
Anticerebroside sera
  inhibit development of CNP, 270
  inhibit myelination in culture, 269, 270

Anticerebroside sera (*cont.*)
  inhibit sulfatide synthesis, 270
  and oligodendrocyte lysis, 183
  as an oligodendrocyte marker, 145
  reactions of in culture, 145, 147
Antimyelin-basic-protein serum,
  effect of on protein entry into myelin,
  109
Antimyelin serum,
  reaction of with oligodendrocytes, 145
Anti-oligodendrocyte sera, 92
  immunostaining patterns of, 126–128
  Schwann cell staining with, 117
Arylsulfatase
  activity of in oligodendrocytes, 218
  in cultures treated with EAE sera, 270
  during development, 72
Assembly of myelin lipids, 61–67
Astroblasts in gliogenesis, 12
Astrocytes,
  description of, 3
  glutamine synthetase in, 304
  origins of in optic nerve, 17
Astroglial lineage, 18
ATPase
  Mg-activated
    histochemistry of, 212
    in isolated cells, 212 *(table)*
  Na,K-activated
    immunocytochemical localization of 154,
    155, 156, 211, 212
    in isolated cells, 209, 211
    in myelin, 50, 211
Axolemma in myelin fractions, 91

339